1/18/83

To Bob Michels

For all the help over the years

John

PSYCHIATRIC ADMINISTRATION

A Comprehensive Text for the Clinician–Executive

PSYCHIATRIC ADMINISTRATION

A Comprehensive Text for the Clinician–Executive

Edited by

John A. Talbott, M.D.
Professor of Psychiatry
Cornell University Medical College
New York, New York

Seymour R. Kaplan, M.D.
Professor of Psychiatry
Albert Einstein College of Medicine
Bronx, New York

G&S

GRUNE & STRATTON
A Subsidiary of Harcourt Brace Jovanovich, Publishers
New York London
Paris San Diego San Francisco São Paulo
Sydney Tokyo Toronto

Library of Congress Cataloging in Publication Data
Main entry under title:

Psychiatric administration.

Bibliography: p.
Includes index.
1. Mental health services—Administration. 2. Mental health services—United States I. Talbott, John A. II. Kaplan, Seymour R. [DNLM: 1. Mental health services —Organization and administration. 2. Hospitals, Psychiatric—Organization and administration. WM 30 A239]
RA790.5.P757 1983 362.2′1′068 82-15410
ISBN 0-8089-1529-0

Grune & Stratton, Inc.
111 Fifth Avenue
New York, New York 10003

Distributed in the United Kingdom by
Academic Press Inc. (London) Ltd.
24/28 Oval Road, London NW 1

Library of Congress Catalog Number 82-15410
International Standard Book Number 0-8089-1529-0

Printed in the United States of America

Contents

Part IV: Leadership and Training

Part V: Facility Management, Budget, and Finance

Part VI: The Law and Psychiatry

Foreword

The editors and authors of *Psychiatric Administration* exemplify the deepest traditions and value-systems of psychiatry in the United States. This volume anticipates the evolution of the mental health field during the next decade, and provides current and potential clinician–executives with role analyses and management plans for psychiatric systems, roles, and boundaries.

At its very inception, American psychiatry became ineluctably tied to administration. Necessity forced the early pioneers to learn about maintenance of the physical plant, budgets, recordkeeping, and public attitudes about the mentally ill. Humanistic roots, institutional practice, and the vicissitudes of psychiatric illness also played a role in establishing the clinician–executive model for the superintendents who organized the forerunner of the American Psychiatric Association in 1844.

During the past century and a half, there have been many changes in the field of mental health as a whole and in psychiatry in particular. In the 1980s psychiatrists in the United States will be profoundly affected by a scientific explosion in the neurosciences, and there will be a strong re-emphasis on the medical identity of the psychiatrist. Integrating the new knowledge and the new alignments without biological reductionism will be one of psychiatry's major adaptive tasks. The psychological, behavioral, and social processes, in addition to biological systems, will remain a part of the psychiatrist's professional core; the integrative functions will continue to differentiate this field from other medical specialties. An increasingly strong and mature psychiatry can become much closer to medicine as a whole while simultaneously maintaining its distinctive qualities and special interests. Commitment to psychiatric administration is one of the major examples of these distinctions, and the editors have made a most significant contribution to the future shape of the profession in this comprehensive textbook.

The book's structure permits special areas of concentration for various interests; it is hoped that the majority of readers will take in its full sweep and deepen their understanding of what psychiatric administration has become and what it can be in the future. The historical span, from the nineteenth century innovations of Galt and Woodward to the newer automated systems, exemplifies, in part, psychiatry's dependence on current technology. The editors have emphasized, however, that administrative technology is always embedded in a larger matrix that continues to require forceful leadership, an understanding of organizational structure, and a blending of humanism, empathy, and perceptiveness.

Several of the chapters reflect the interplay of external accountability and internal responsibility which has come to the forefront during the past decade. Every clinician–executive must understand these forces and be able to deal with them on a continuous basis. Budgeting and fiscal management are also central to the core of administrative functions. Whatever the auspices and objectives of a psychiatric facility, a detailed and comprehensive financial plan is a *sine qua non*. Knowledge of current and potential resources tests the administrator's imagination, energy, and overall leadership.

Psychiatric administration is at a significant crossroad in its historical development. I join the editors and the authors in the hope of fortifying the knowledge and the self-esteem of our current cadre of clinician–executives and encouraging a newer generation to enter this challenging and important field. This text is well suited for such encouragement and should become a part of the broad educational activities that affect career choices. Practitioners and students will benefit from the detailed analyses of psychiatric services, the theoretical bases of administrative practice, the wealth of practical information, and the organizational perspectives. From my own personal standpoint, I am delighted with the broad-range description of the diversity of administrative roles. This text contains much for me to learn in order to improve my function as an administrator of a professional association. The inclusion of a section on the law and psychiatry exemplifies the editors' breadth of vision and their good judgment about this field of opportunity.

Psychiatry in the United States has passed adolescence and matured into a more self-reliant adulthood. In becoming more influential, psychiatrists must indeed press for active involvement with a host of power-brokers and decision-makers. To abandon the administrative aspects of this objective to other professionals, including generic managers, would be unsound at many levels. Psychiatry cannot achieve its next series of adaptive tasks without a strong cadre of administrative leaders who can deal with the full complexity of serving our patients, our profession, and our many allies. Psychiatry must put its identity crises of the past decade behind and unite in its efforts to achieve new resources, new alignments, and parity with other parts of medicine. Effective administrative leadership can and will make a difference in achieving these goals. The editors have put forward powerful arguments supporting the need for clinician–executives. I applaud them and the other authors for this forceful and lucid text, and I hope that their message will be effective.

Melvin Sabshin, M.D.
Medical Director
American Psychiatric Association

Preface

The publication of this text is the culmination of long years of practical experience on the part of the editors and reflects our attempt to give structure and meaning to this experience. During these years, we participated in, and reacted to, the accelerated growth of mental health services since World War II. The nature of our functions over the years also changed rapidly. Suddenly (or so it seemed) we were no longer working as individual clinicians with a small number of patients in a moderately controlled situation; we were making decisions about multimillion dollar budgets involving services for large numbers of patients. We became members of executive policy-making groups in large organizations, which are subject to unpredictable, and often uncontrollable, internal and external forces. We have become "clinician–executives," a term used by Levinson and Klerman[1] to describe the administrative position in which increasing numbers of clinicians find themselves.

In common with most of our professional colleagues we had had no formal administrative training. More importantly, the didactic teaching programs that we attended, conducted by schools of business administration, proved for the most part unsatisfactory; we were oriented to the clinical teaching methods of medical training, but the administrative course material was derived from the management of the industrial or commercial service organization. Discussions about administrative decision-making were predicated on the (unspoken) assumption that the procedures took place in an organizational structure in which the "chain of command" is clearly delineated, "job descriptions" are specifically defined, and the dollar value of the product or service is the bottom line.

Our informal contacts and meetings with other clinician–executives proved most rewarding. In particular, we benefited from our experiences as examiners for the American Psychiatric Association's Committee on Certification in Administrative Psychiatry. In the interim, we also initiated and conducted teaching programs in the administration and leadership of psychiatric services for residents and postgraduates. Throughout this time there has been a persistent need for teaching materials appropriate for the clinician–executive. This text is addressed to that need.

The book is designed not only for those who are or hope to become leaders in psychiatric settings but also for all those who work in psychiatric organizations who desire to understand their operation better. It is our belief that to understand the operation of psychiatric organizations one first should understand the background and characteristics of the setting. Therefore, the book begins with an examination of the history, structure, and organization of different psychiatric settings.

To enable the reader who desires a comprehensive look at the administrative practice in one type of setting to comprehend it fully, we have encouraged redundancies among the various chapters. The reader who intends to master the entire field should not find these redundancies overwhelming.

Finally, we would like to remind the reader that in a field so influenced by external events, today's truth concerning accreditation or civil law will become tomorrow's anachronism, and frequent updates of this volume will be forthcoming.

John A. Talbott, M.D.
Seymour R. Kaplan, M.D.

REFERENCE

1. Levinson DJ, Klerman GL: The clinician-executive: Some problematic issues for psychiatrists in mental health organizations. Psychiat 30:3–15, 1967

Contributors

BORIS M. ASTRACHAN, M.D.
Professor of Psychiatry, Yale University School of Medicine; Director, Connecticut Mental Health Center, New Haven, Connecticut

C. CLIFFORD ATTKISSON, PH.D.
Associate Dean, Graduate Division; Associate Professor, Health Psychology Graduate Program, University of California, San Francisco, California

HAROUTUN M. BABIGIAN, M.D.
Professor and Chairman, Department of Psychiatry, University of Rochester School of Medicine and Dentistry, Strong Memorial Hospital, Rochester, New York

GAIL M. BARTON, M.D., M.P.H.
Medical Director, Howard Mental Health Services, Burlington, Vermont

WALTER E. BARTON, M.D.
Professor of Psychiatry, Emeritus, Dartmouth Medical School, Hanover, New Hampshire

CESAR L. BENARROCHE, M.D.
Assistant Professor of Psychiatry, Yale University School of Medicine; Staff Psychiatrist, Connecticut Mental Health Center, New Haven, Connecticut

JUDITH R. BLAU, PH.D.
Associate Professor of Sociology, The State University of New York at Albany, Albany, New York

HARVEY BLUESTONE, M.D.
Director of Psychiatry, Bronx-Lebanon Hospital Center; Associate Professor of Psychiatry, Albert Einstein College of Medicine, Bronx, New York

ETHEL M. BONN, M.D.
Chief of Psychiatry, Albuquerque Veterans Administration Medical Center; Associate Professor of Psychiatry, University of New Mexico, Albuquerque, New Mexico

ROBERT C. BRICE, M.S.
Vice President, Crothall American, Inc.; Clinical Assistant Professor of Allied Health Professions, State University of New York at Stony Brook, Stony Brook, New York

THOMAS J. CONKLIN, M.D.
Medical Director, The Institute of Living; Assistant Professor of Psychiatry, University of Connecticut School of Medicine, Hartford, Connecticut

PETER M. CRAIN, M.D.
Clinical Assistant Professor of Psychiatry, Albert Einstein College of Medicine; Adjunct Associate Professor, Benjamin N. Cardozo School of Law, New York, New York

SAMUEL DAVIS, M.S.
President, Mount Sinai Hospital; Guggenheim Professor and Chairman, Department of Health Care Management, The Mount Sinai School of Medicine, New York, New York

ROBERT W. GIBSON, M.D.
President and Chief Executive Officer, The Sheppard and Enoch Pratt Hospital, Towson, Maryland

MILTON GREENBLATT, M.D.
Director, Neuropsychiatric Institute, Hospital and Clinics; Professor and Executive Vice Chairman, Department of Psychiatry and Behavioral Sciences, University of California, Los Angeles, California

WILLIAM A. HARGREAVES, PH.D.
Professor of Psychology, Director of Program Evaluation, Department of Psychiatry, University of California, San Francisco, California

SEYMOUR R. KAPLAN, M.D.
Professor of Psychiatry, Albert Einstein College of Medicine, Bronx, New York

STUART L. KEILL, M.D.
Clinical Professor of Psychiatry, School of Medicine, State University of New York at Buffalo; Chief, Psychiatry Service, Buffalo Veterans Administration Medical Center, Buffalo, New York

ALAN M. KRAFT, M.D.
Professor and Chairman, Department of Psychiatry, Albany Medical College; Psychiatrist-in-Chief, Albany Medical Center Hospital, Albany, New York

ALAN I. LEVENSON, M.D.
Professor and Head, Department of Psychiatry, University of Arizona College of Medicine, Tucson, Arizona

JOHN O. LIPKIN, M.D.
Associate Director for Psychiatry, Veterans Adminstration Central Office, Washington, D.C.

ERICA LOUTSCH, M.D.
Assistant Attending Psychiatrist, New York Hospital-Westchester Division; Assistant Professor of Psychiatry, Cornell University Medical College, New York, New York

JOHN T. MELELLA, M.S.W.
Chief, Forensic Psychiatry Clinic, Bronx-Lebanon Hospital Center, Bronx, New York

ARTHUR T. MEYERSON, M.D.
Associate Professor and Vice Chairman, Department of Psychiatry, Mount Sinai School of Medicine; Clinical Director, Department of Psychiatry, Mount Sinai Hospital, New York, New York

HERBERT C. MODLIN, M.D.
Senior Psychiatrist, The Menninger Foundation, Topeka, Kansas

DAVID F. MUSTO, M.A., M.D.
Professor of Psychiatry (Child Study Center) and Professor of the History of Medicine, Yale Medical School, New Haven, Connecticut

ROGER PEELE, M.D.
Chairman, Department of Psychiatry, St. Elizabeths Hospital; Clinical Professor of Psychiatry, George Washington University, Washington, D.C.

FREDERICK D. RAINE, M.B.A.
Administrator, The New York Hospital-Cornell Medical Center, Westchester Division, White Plains, New York

PEDRO RUIZ, M.D.
Professor of Psychiatry, Baylor College of Medicine; Chief, Psychiatry Service, Ben Taub General Hospital, Houston, Texas

HERZL R. SPIRO, M.D., PH.D.
Distinguished Professor of Psychiatry, Medical College of Wisconsin, Milwaukee, Wisconsin

ZEBULON C. TAINTOR, M.D.
Research Professor of Psychiatry, New York University, New York, New York; Assistant Director for Cost Consideration, Alcohol, Drug Abuse and Mental Health Administration, National Institute of Mental Health, Rockville, Maryland

JOHN A. TALBOTT, M.D.
Professor of Psychiatry, Cornell University Medical College; Associate Medical Director, The Payne Whitney Psychiatric Clinic, The New York Hospital, New York, New York

SUSAN W. TALBOTT, M.B.A., R.N.
Principal, Management Development Institutes, New York, New York

THOMAS T. TOURLENTES, M.D.
Clinical Associate Professor of Psychiatry, University of Illinois, College of Medicine; Executive Director, Community Mental Health Center, Rock Island, Illinois

RICHARD SCOTT WEBSTER, PH.D.
Principal, Management Development Institutes, New York, New York

PART I

Historical and Organizational Perspectives

John A. Talbott, M.D.

1

Trends in the Delivery of Psychiatric Services

Since this country's founding, the shape of the delivery of services to the mentally ill has been constantly changing, reflecting current social trends, funding opportunities, and the prevailing theories of medical care delivery. Today, our bewildering array of mental health services can only be understood by looking at their historical origins. Therefore, of necessity, this chapter will present an historical framework that will include much of the historical information presented in Parts I and II.

It is the author's thesis that the current delivery of mental health services has not been planned; existing services are a result of historical, reimbursement, and political factors. As a result, while some logic can be perceived in their development, the reader is warned that this may more accurately reflect *post hoc* analysis rather than forward planning.

In looking at the way we deliver mental health services, it becomes clear that at times we are looking at models of delivery (e.g., community mental health centers [CMHCs]), at times ideological forces (e.g., prevention of mental illness), and at times pragmatic translations of social beliefs (e.g., institutionalization and deinstitutionalization). Five distinct but overlapping periods, phases, or eras in the evolution of mental health services in America have been identified (see Figure 1–1):

1. The institutional period
2. The alternatives to hospitals phase
3. The era of prevention
4. The era of the community mental health center and deinstitutionalization
5. The period of systems approaches

In the following sections of this chapter, these periods will be elaborated, giving their history, current state, problems, and suggested solutions that have led to the next era.

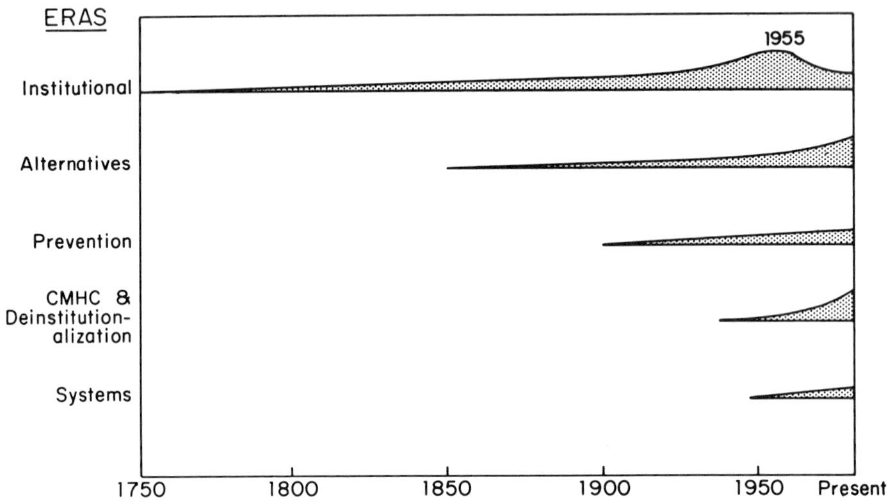

Figure 1-1 Chronology of phases in the development of mental health service delivery patterns in America.

THE PERIOD OF INSTITUTIONAL GROWTH

Historically, the delivery of mental health services in this nation has depended on their attachment to institutions, especially hospitals. Early in America's history, the mentally ill could be found in their own or relatives' homes, rooming with physicians, or wandering about the towns and countryside, often having been "dumped" over town or county lines.[1] The earliest institutions in America, jails, workhouses, almshouses, and poorhouses, while established to care for criminals, the needy, rogues and vagabonds, or the idle and disorderly, soon became the repositories for the mentally disturbed.[2–5] Such institutions were usually established by counties to care for their deviant citizens and frequently were used by several populations.

The Pennsylvania Hospital, which opened in 1752, was the first hospital to provide care for the mentally ill in a separate unit. The first hospital designed exclusively for the mentally ill, the public hospital was opened in 1773 in Williamsburg, Virginia. The first private hospital for the mentally ill, the Friends' Hospital opened in 1917 in Philadelphia. All were locally initiated facilities.

The first state hospitals opened in Massachusetts and New York in the early 1800s. They were well-intentioned replicas of locally developed, privately sponsored mental hospitals and followed the lead of those facilities in providing "moral treatment."[1,2] The states intended to further develop institutions, which were then the only models of care and treatment, rather than develop alternatives to institutional care. Their expansion in the mid-1800s, under the influence of Dorothea Dix, merely continued this belief in total institutions.

While care in these state facilities was periodically condemned throughout the 19th century,[1,6–10] the institutional model was not abandoned; rather, it was further expanded by universities with their psychopathic hospital units, by localities

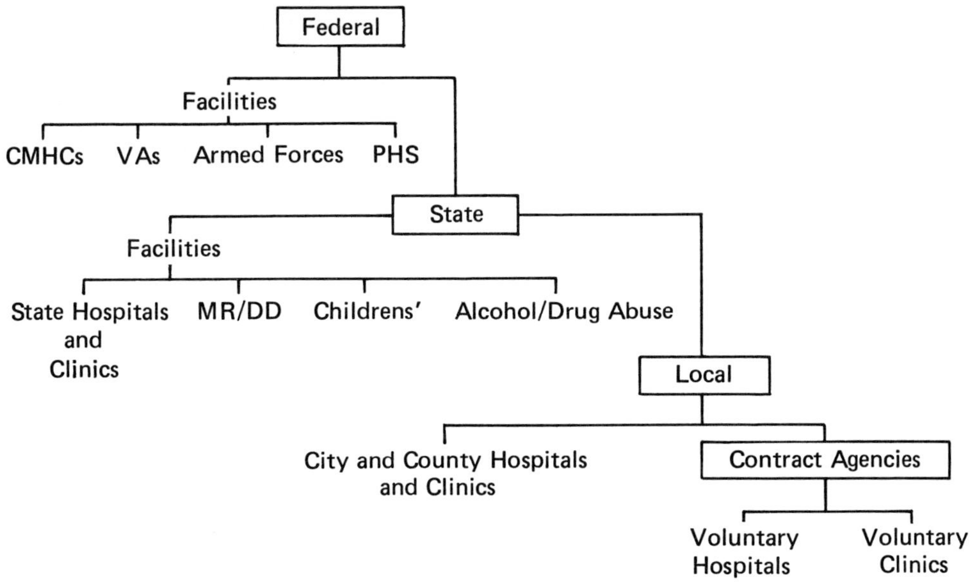

Figure 1-2 Levels of government funding.

with general hospital units, and by groups of individuals establishing private mental hospitals. The federal government then became a major developer of psychiat ric facilities and units during the 20th century, with Veterans Administration (VA) hospitals, public health service hospitals, and armed forces facilities.

The current array of psychiatric facilities in this country can be best appreciated by a theoretical table of organization (see Figure 1-2) in which each level of government (federal, state, county, or city) provides psychiatric services directly and contracts with locally based private or voluntary hospitals to provide such services. This leads to several problems, which will be discussed below.

Inherent in a mental health delivery system that depends heavily on institutions such as hospitals are the following problems:

1. The tendency to over hospitalize mentally ill individuals because beds are readily available.
2. The difficulty in providing follow-up treatment or aftercare to those who do not live close to the institution.
3. The phenomenal degree of fragmentation and lack of coordination with so many competing elements of the mental health system treating the same group of mentally ill individuals.
4. The lack of responsibility for care of some population groups perceived as:
   a. undesirable–e.g., unkempt patients
   b. unrewarding or difficult–e.g., chronic patients
   c. unremunerative–e.g., those without insurance or not eligible for Medicaid or Medicare
   d. unlike the caregivers–e.g., racial minorities.
5. The fact that it is an extremely expensive system for the taxpayer because of the lack of alternatives to hospital care.

6. The tendency for all its component institutions to preserve their turf and, indeed, to expand their empires.
7. The inability to provide services where they may be needed rather than where institutions are located.
8. The inherent conflict of interest between all levels of government both operating facilities and contracting with competing local hospitals for psychiatric services.

These problems have been known and identified for years, and as we shall see in the following sections, each phase in the delivery of psychiatric services has tried to address one or more of them. A search for alternatives to hospitalization and for adequate posthospitalization treatment were among the earliest problems addressed.

ALTERNATIVES TO HOSPITALS

While the program developed in the 13th century in the Belgian town of Gheel probably represents the oldest example of a large-scale alternative to hospitalization for the seriously and chronically ill, it was not until the mid-1800s that Americans tried alternatives to hospitalization. A farm program was begun by J. M. Galt in 1855, a cottage plan was developed in Kankakee, Illinois, in 1877, and a boarding-out program was initiated in Massachusetts in 1885.[11–13] These programs were intended to provide posthospital care for seriously and chronically ill persons in semistructured environments.

Aftercare, the attempt to return patients to their home environments while providing them with follow-up care in hospitals or clinics, gained support in the 1890s. Soon states were implementing widespread programs of aftercare treatment.[14] Further developments were the initiation of outpatient services in the voluntary and private sectors. The first private service was offered at the Pennsylvania Hospital in 1904, and a traveling clinic was initiated in New York State in 1909.[6] By 1927, there were 400 "mental clinics" in America, and universities had begun to establish "satellite" outpatient clinics.[15,16]

The initiation of outpatient treatment by institutions was followed by the development of the office-based practice of psychotherapy for ambulatory mentally ill persons. Spurred by the influence of Sigmund Freud, individual psychotherapy and psychoanalysis became more available as the 20th century progressed.[17] In addition, Joseph Pratt began the practice of group therapy in 1905.[18] Thomas Salmon's experience immediately before our entry into World War I ensured the importance of short-term crisis intervention. This approach stressed immediacy, proximity, and expectancy.[19]

By the mid-1900s, several developments in Europe continued this search for alternatives: the first day hospital opened in Moscow, Querido began a home care program in Amsterdam, and Bierer began a therapeutic social club in England.[21,22] By the 1950s, partial hospitalization programs, homecare programs, and psychosocial rehabilitation programs were all commonplace in this country[20,23]. In addition, the 1950s saw the introduction of halfway houses, vocational rehabilitation programs, and 24-hr emergency walk-in services.[20,24,25]

The services and settings shown in Figure 1-3, while not available in every

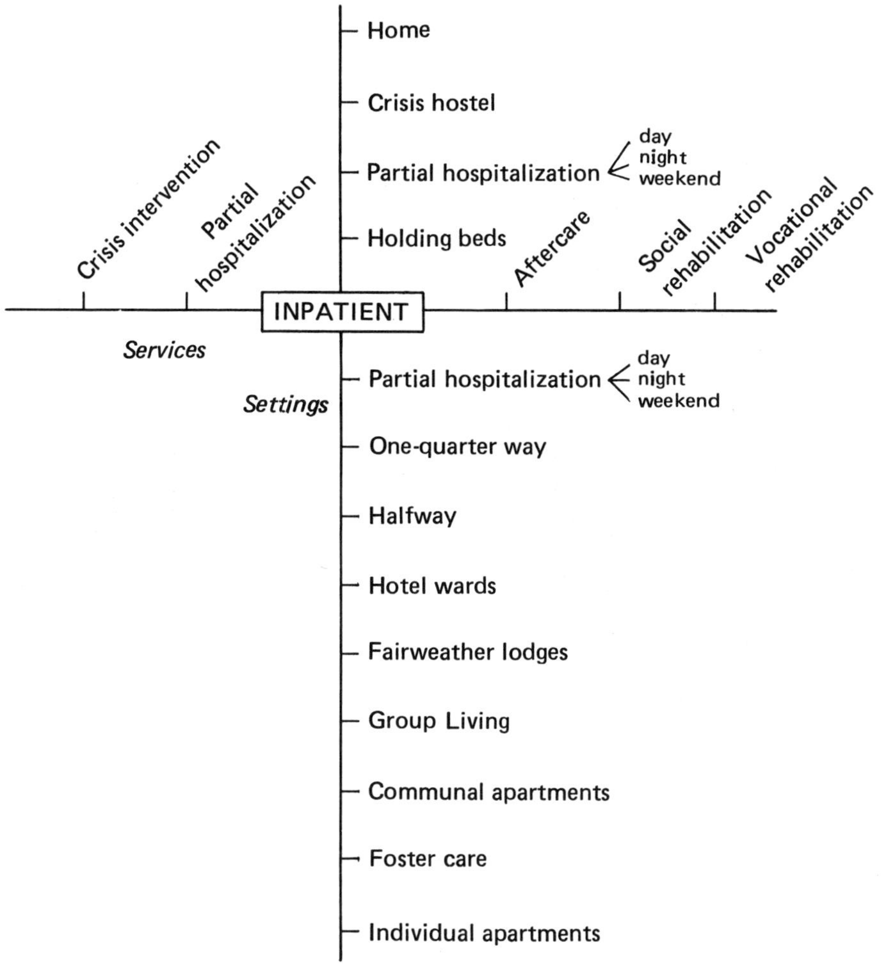

Figure 1-3. Setting and services for the mentally ill.

catchment area or county, demonstrate the range of alternatives that now exist for the mentally ill. The shifts in psychiatric care from 1955 to 1973 (Fig. 1–4) demonstrate the trend away from care that is totally institution based toward ambulatory and community-based alternatives.

The problems encountered during the period of alternatives to institutional care remain sizable: lack of adequate funding for nonhospital-based and even noninpatient services; the lack of definition of which mentally ill persons need which levels of care, treatments, and settings at what points in their illness and rehabilitation; the appalling lack of coordination between nonhospital-based elements in the system; the duplication in some instances of some services (e.g., outpatient departments) and the absolute lack of others (e.g., crisis hostels); the nonmedical, untraditional flavor of many such services; and the idiosyncratic view that each service has concerning its own mission in the absence of a comprehensive (systems) view of the entire universe of needs and care.

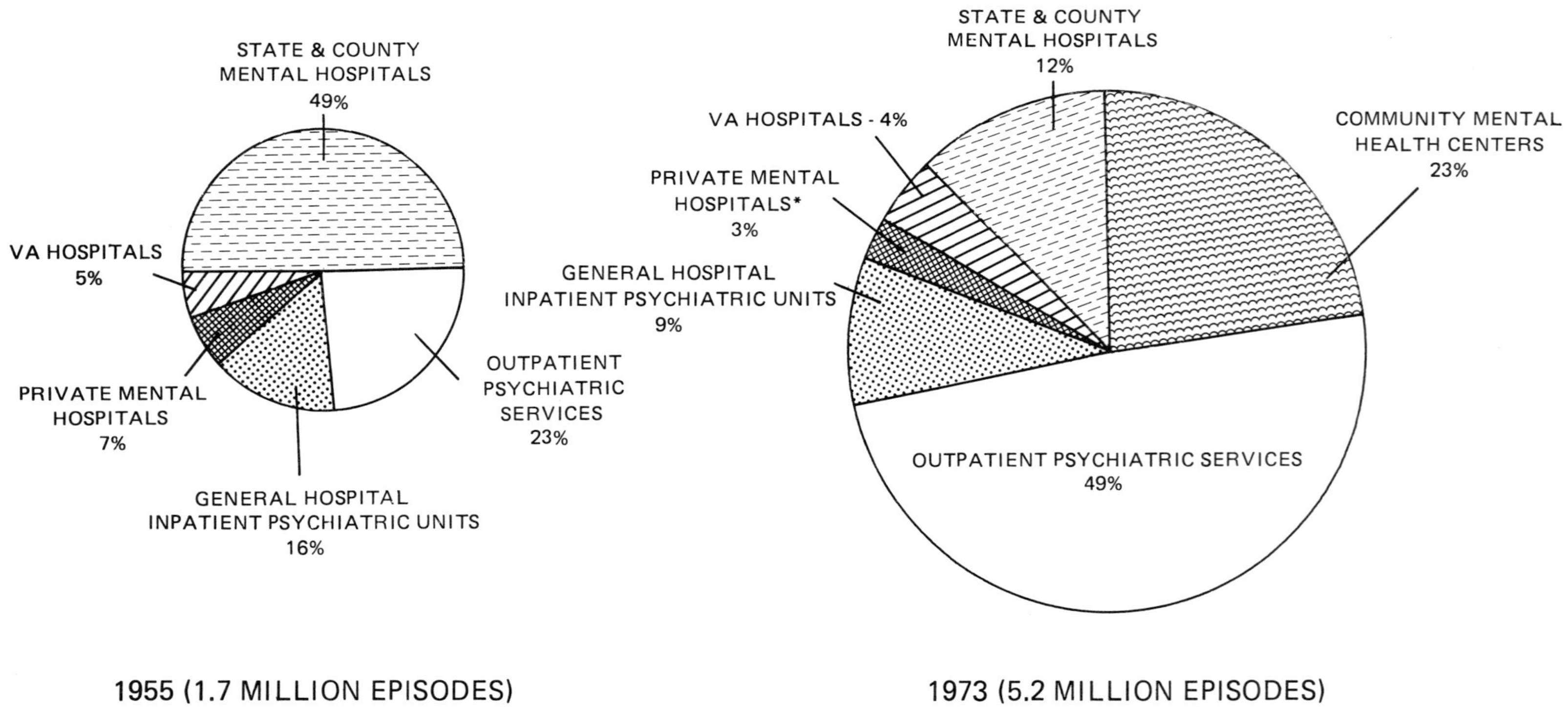

Figure 1-4. Percentage distributions of inpatient and outpatient care episodes in mental health facilities, by type of facility: United States, 1955 and 1973. From Kramer M: Psychiatric services and the changing institutional scene, 1950–1985. Rockville MD, US DHEW, 1977, DHEW Pub (ADM) 77–433.

The solutions to these problems remain incomplete, but with increasing attention to the prevention of mental illness after the turn of the century, some attempt to remedy the situation was attempted.

THE ERA OF PREVENTION

A public health approach to psychiatry was first advocated by Adolf Meyer soon after the turn of the century. Meyer stressed the importance of prevention of mental illness and public education as well as an integration of prevention, treatment, and aftercare.[26] The mental health movement, begun by Clifford Beers as an attempt to remedy the horrible conditions found in mental institutions, later directed its attention to the positive acquisition of mental health, never clearly defined or understood.[27] Likewise, another movement occurring after the turn of the century, the child guidance movement, also stressed prevention, early detection, and prompt treatment.[28]

People believed that mental illness was the result of environmental conditions, such as inadequate child rearing, slum conditions, and poor family background, rather than biological and hereditary influences. This idea exemplified the change in social attitudes from Social Darwinian to progressive thinking after the turn of the century.[17] Just as a belief in asylum-based care reflected Darwinian thinking, family-oriented intervention was consonant with progressivism. The culmination of the latter approach occurred in the 1920s with the concept that society's ills were the result of faulty mental health, which could only be cured through social engineering.[28]

Throughout the first half of the 20th century, leaders in the field advocated work with other professionals to promote mental health, e.g., nurses and social workers as well as families, legal authorities, teachers, clergymen, industrial and business executives, and recreation leaders.[29] During World War II, psychiatrists routinely provided consultations to other health care professionals in general (rather than mental) hospitals,[32] and during the Korean War command consultation (consulting with gate keepers and commanders) was widely practiced.[32] In addition to these preventive efforts, the previously mentioned work by Salmon, stressing early intervention, was followed by Lindeman's articulation of crisis theory and crisis intervention.[32]

But it was Gerald Caplan who brought together the existing knowledge and systematized the concept of prevention.[33,34] Caplan's own interest was principally to provide primary preventive techniques—those that would reduce the total occurrence of new cases of mental illness in the community (incidence). To do this, he advocated consultation to community care givers (e.g., social workers, public health nurses, teachers), especially at critical time periods (e.g., childbirth, bereavement, separation). He advocated four types of consultation: client-centered case consultation (working with care givers around specific cases they were treating); consultee-centered case consultation (working with professionals around their problems in handling cases in general); consultee-centered administrative consultation (helping administrators handle their programmatic problems, especially regarding group dynamics and interpersonal aspects); and program-centered administrative consultation (helping agencies improve their services without nec-

Table 1-1.
Caplan's Schema for Prevention of Mental Illness

Type of Prevention	Goal	Methods
1°	Reduction in the incidence of all mental disorders	1. Consultation to care givers 2. Education of community leaders 3. Social action
2°	Reduction in the duration of of those incidents of mental illness that do occur	1. Early detection and screening 2. Early diagnosis and referral 3. Prompt and effective treatment
3°	Reduction in impairment resulting from mental illness	1. Education to eliminate prejudice 2. Communication with social networks 3. Avoidance of hospitalization 4. Hospital–community proximity

essarily addressing problems posed by the administrator, as one would with a consultee-centered administrative consultation).

Caplan's schema (Table 1-1) demonstrates his articulation of the levels of prevention (primary, secondary, and tertiary) that could be used by psychiatry. It is clear now that while Caplan himself stressed primary prevention, feeling that secondary preventive services were abundant and represented an unnecessarily large portion of preventive efforts, he, among others, did not sufficiently recognize the necessity for tertiary prevention as the nation turned toward deinstitutionalization. It is also important to stress that while his schema did identify the ingredients for a complete preventive approach, his reputation as one interested solely in primary prevention, and especially in community consultation and education, is not completely accurate.

The current status of preventive psychiatry reflects the fact that too much emphasis was placed on primary preventive approaches in CMHC legislation, with inadequate attention given tertiary prevention during a time of unprecedented depopulation of mental institutions. This imbalance in preventive efforts has led, in part, to our current disastrous state.

Primary prevention was enthusiastically pursued without adequate scientific evidence of its efficaciousness, and its results are uncertain. Secondary preventive efforts have always been numerous in this country, and although fragmented and lacking good outcome studies, did not really suffer during this period. Tertiary prevention was neglected and clearly needs more emphasis today. The zeal for primary prevention at the expense of secondary and tertiary prevention made for heady times in many services and agencies. Staff, however, were often off lecturing "the community" while acutely and chronically ill persons went unserved. Nonmedical staff preferred dealing with less sick persons, and today few persons believe we are any closer to knowing how to prevent mental illness than in Meyer's time.

There are solutions to these problems. In the absence of more secure research as to the causes and prevention of mental illness, primary prevention must be de-emphasized. Increased attention must be paid to outcome studies to test the efficaciousness of secondary prevention along with a rededication to tertiary preventive efforts and research. The period to be described next, the CMHC movement and deinstitutionalization, represents a continuation of the preventive era rather than an attempt to answer its problems, although attempts to provide a balanced model of services have occurred.

COMMUNITY MENTAL HEALTH AND DEINSTITUTIONALIZATION

The roots of community mental health lie in many of the previous periods. The development of alternatives to hospitalization, new modalities of treatment, and preventive approaches were necessary for the introduction of this new philosophy of care, which was, at the same time, an approach to the delivery of mental health services. During World War II, an unprecedented interest in psychiatry and mental health developed. This was due to the identification of thousands of mentally ill inductees coupled with the use, for the first time, of psychiatrists throughout the armed services.[25,26]

The Mental Health Act of 1946 created the National Institute of Mental Health, whose purpose was to "apply the traditional public health approach . . . to the mental health field."[17,37] Money was appropriated specifically for "community programs" in addition to research. Programs were intended to provide screening, prevention, and outpatient treatment to prevent hospitalization, and permit early discharge from mental hospitals.[38] By the 1950s, the blueprints for what was to become the CMHC began to emerge from several quarters (Table 1-2).

In 1952, a blue-ribbon committee of the World Health Organization (WHO) spelled out what it thought the ingredients of a "community mental hospital" should be.[39] New York State, in 1954, passed a Community Mental Health Services Act that included a model for four essential services. The eventual list of five essential and five adequate services bears striking resemblance to the previous models.

The thrust of the CMHC model was not to be found merely in its elements but also in its attempts to deliver mental health services in a truly different way. The emphasis was on catchment area responsibility, community orientation, accessibility, comprehensiveness, and continuity of care. As Zusman has pointed out, the belief that the method of service delivery is as important as the service itself represented an entirely new theme in American psychiatry.[40]

Excesses inevitably evolved from these new or newly articulated features: community orientation became citizen control; catchment area responsibility became the "it's not my table" syndrome; comprehensive came to mean diluted; and prevention, as so often in the past, became interpreted as primary prevention. Most important, however, because of the not-so-subtle hidden agenda of closing state hospitals, government officials became blind to all but the CMHC model. It was not until the debacle of deinstitutionalization became apparent, in the mid-1970s, that American psychiatry took note of the problems of this model and the need to address the entire system, or nonsystem.

It became clear after a decade and a half of the CMHC movement that often the sickest patients were not receiving their share of attention; that medical and

Table 1-2.
Components of Community Mental Health Centers

		Regulations	
WHO Committee (1954)	New York State (1954)	CMHC (1965)	CMHC Amendment (1975)
	Inpatient	Inpatient	Inpatient
Outpatient	Outpatient	Outpatient	Outpatient
Partial hospital		Partial hospital	Partial hospital
		Emergency (24-hr)	Emergency (24-hr)
Community education	Consultation and education	Consultation and education	Consultation and education
		Diagnostic	
		Precare and aftercare	Screening patients for courts and agencies prior to state hospital
			Follow-up care
Rehabilitation	Rehabilitation	Rehabilitation	
Research		Research and evaluation	
			Transitional housing
			Services for elderly
			Services for children
			Services for alcoholics
			Services for drug problems

psychiatric care as well as 24-hr emergency services often were were not available in CMHCs; and that state hospitals had not been replaced and some patients would remain chronic despite the community psychiatry movement. Deinstitutionalization's faults cannot be laid solely on the doorstep of the community mental health movement. Certainly it was aided and abetted by the civil liberties movement, by the introduction of phenothiazines, and by the ability of states to shift almost 100 percent of the burden of funding the chronically mentally ill in state hospitals to predominantly federal-based funding following passage of Medicaid, Medicare, and supplemental security income (SSI) legislation in the 1950s and 1960s.[41] Community psychiatry's zeal in advocating for care close to home, the implication that prevention could stop the occurrence of chronicity, and the move to compete for the right to treat the less ill portion of the population nevertheless aggravated the growing problem of the deinstitutionalized and of those never institutionalized.

While deinstitutionalization began in 1955, when the state hospital population nationwide was over 560,000 (it is now less than 150,000), it was not until 1975, 20 years later, that psychiatry and government became truly concerned with the problem of providing services for the deinstitutionalized mentally ill. Since that time, the General Accounting Office, the Group for the Advancement of Psychiatry, and the American Psychiatric Association have all published major reports on the problem.[42–44] The lessons that are now apparent include the seemingly obvious fact that patients cannot be adequately treated in the community without a community support system, alternative living settings, and training in the skills of everyday living. As Elizabeth Boggs has demonstrated (Fig. 1-5), the interplay between services and relative independence of patients is a critical one and one that deserves attention if persons are to move to increasing levels of functioning and decreasing dependence.[44]

As discussed previously in respect to Figure 1-3, a range of alternatives must be made available if the patient is to be able to shift from one setting to another and to function at his or her highest level of functioning. In deinstitutionalizing thousands of severely and chronically mentally ill, insufficient attention has been paid to the need to teach the skills necessary to survive outside total institutions. For those returning to community life after 5, 10, 20, or sometimes 40 years of institutional care, these skills of everyday living were found to be more critical to community tenure than medication, medical care, or housing (Table 1-3).

The current state of this period of community mental health and deinstitutionalization is uncertain. While President Carter's Commission on Mental Health and Illness addressed the problems of CMHCs and deinstitutionalization at length and the mental Health Systems Act of 1980 was designed to partially remedy those problems, the recommendations have yet to be implemented.[26,47]

The problems that have emerged are rooted in the simplistic solutions proposed by the CMHC movement and its avoidance of the need to deal with the complexities of both real patients and existing mental health systems. While deinstitutionalization was not necessarily a bad idea, it was implemented with inadequate or absent community services and housing and with no glue to hold together the services needed by the chronically ill. It was bound to fail.

The solutions to these problems lie in looking comprehensively at the patient population and the Mental health system. Solutions will not emanate from

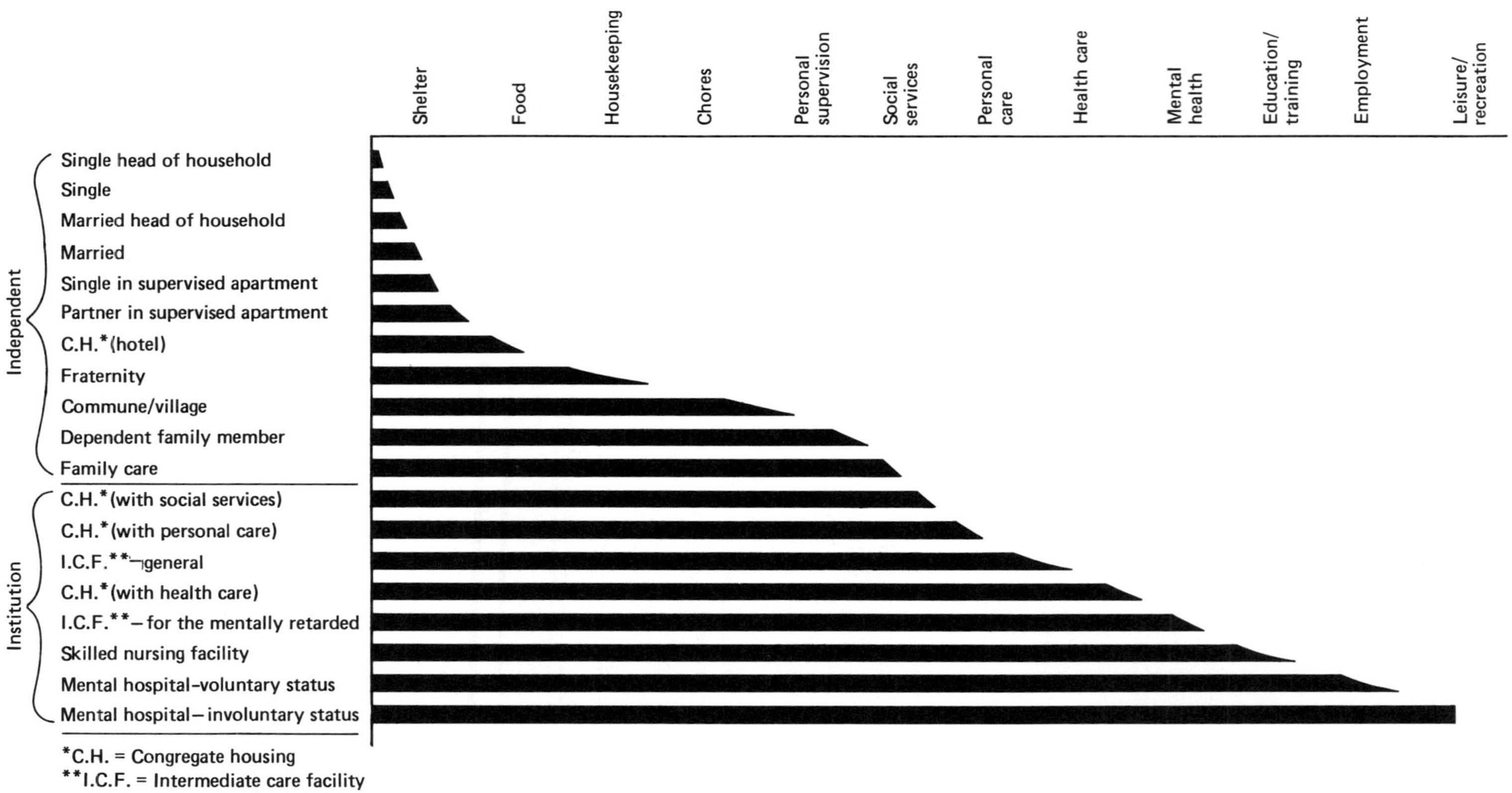

Figure 1-5. Needs and settings for the chronically ill. From Elizabeth Boggs, Ph.D., personal communication.

Table 1-3.
Skills of Everyday Living

In the home:	cooking
	cleaning
	personal hygiene
	dressing
	budgeting, bill paying, etc.
	telephoning
	writing letters
	child care
	caring for pets
	sewing
	gardening
	house cleaning
	fixing appliances
In the community:	shopping
	banking
	using laundromats, services
	making appointments
	transportation
	public transportation
	automobile
	conversing
Leisure:	hobbies
	exercise
	reading
	artistic
Work:	interviewing
	filling out forms
	promptness and reliability

embracing one simple model to deliver services or hoping that one particularly vexing subpopulation of the mentally ill will go away by shifting their place of residence. The problems of the severely and chronically ill cannot be solved with such a simple solution or a single model. Chronic patients' needs will be met only when the following multiple issues are addressed:

1. *Economic reform,* with adequate reimbursement of ambulatory, long-term, maintenance services.
2. *Administrative clarity,* with designated responsibility for the chronically ill, money moving from federal to local levels, and services being delivered by local entities with no inherent conflicts of interest, as now occur with federal, state, and city governments.
3. *Community education.*
4. *Training of persons now treating the chronically ill* or who are likely to do so, e.g., family practitioners, physicians in emergency rooms, and so on.
5. *Research* into what treatment works for which patients in what settings, into outcome, and into the maintenance and prevention of chronicity.
6. *Attaining continuity of care* through some form of community support system with case management.

Table 1-4.
Needs of the Chronic Mentally Ill

Housing	Income	Vocational	Rehabilitation	Medical-Psychiatric
HUD	SSI	HRA	HSA	MEDICAID/MEDICARE

7. *Reinvolving psychiatrists in the planning, implementation, and monitoring* of care of the chronically ill.
8. *Reversing discriminatory economic, housing, educational, vocational, and medical policies* concerning the chronic mentally ill.[44]

The stage is therefore set for the final era in modern history—that of a simultaneous systems and patient approach.

AN INTEGRATED SYSTEM FOR THE INDIVIDUAL PATIENT

Several attempts have been made to deliver unified services to individual patients. Efforts are being made to address the fragmentation of services evident in this country and the inability to meet the needs of the severely and chronically ill. A two-tiered conceptualization is necessary.

The needs of caregivers, especially hospitals, are traditionally given first consideration. This must be abandoned if a systems approach is to be taken. The systems approach recognizes that individual patients have individual needs and that these needs must be considered first (Table 1-4). Such an approach leads to the inevitable conclusion that there must be some way of connecting services and making them readily available to individual patients. One might also conclude that some mechanism must be found to allow patients to manipulate the system so that it more ideally satisfies their needs, rather than continue the practice of the system manipulating the patients.

A look at the existing system (Fig. 1-2) leads to the inevitable conclusion that it does not meet the requirements of a system.[48] An ideal system requires (1) a clear separation between planning and implementation (2) point responsibility for a specific population, with one person in charge and all services administratively responsible to one person (3) clinical integration at the lowest level of government (4) elimination of both competition between elements in the system for elite patients and neglect of undesirable patients (5) elimination of duplications and gaps in services (6) elimination of communication difficulties (7) tracking mechanisms for patients, and (8) a single funding mechanism.

A number of different attempts have already been made to attempt integration along these lines. Since 1973, there have been reports of regional attempts to unify county, state, and CMHC operations through *contracts* with service providers.[49–52] Such attempts divide up the labor, redistribute the finances equitably, enjoy shared staffing, and provide uniform entry and exit points for patients. Another method involves *legally encouraging* county-state cooperation and alteration in services.[53–55] In California, Lanterman-Petris-Short and Short-Doyle initiatives altered the funding formulae for counties, enabling them to move from 90 percent county-10 percent state, to 50–50 percent, and finally 10–90 percent funding in just two decades. This funding shift gave localities ample incentive to provide services and decrease their utilization of state hospitals, a situation that encouraged the development of crisis intervention services and alternatives to hospitalization. While this funding arrangement worked moderately well for California, with its traditionally strong county government, another such state/local sharing arrangement did not work in New York State. Here unified services legislation provided too few economic incentives for local control, and state hospitals have continued to retain the lion's share of the mental health dollar while only treating 1 out of 7 inpatient episodes and 1 out of 22 outpatient ones.[56] A third method has been through *agreement* to shift from state hospital to CMHC models.[57,58] Here attempts are made to equalize services and reimbursement and to provide comprehensive services through agreement, thus dividing the labor by apportioning the population. A fourth method attempts to move from state hospital to community programs through *policy articulation.*[59] This attempt has failed in most places because of an inability to fund adequately the two systems (state and community) during the overlapping period. A fifth method, frequently discussed but rarely attempted, would divide the population by enrollment in competing *health maintenance organizations* rather than by geographical division. A radical means of unifying the system is that carried out by Australia. Following a report by its Royal Commission in the 1950s, government "bought out" the private sector. This method could be used in the opposite manner as well. Finally, unification could be attempted by allowing the *marketplace* to decide where the patient chooses to spend his or her portion of the mental health dollar. This system could either be designed to provide all severely and chronically ill persons with vouchers for the purchase of services, or it could reimburse all providers equally. Either way, competition in the marketplace would determine the array of services "needed" by mental patients rather than their being determined by providers, government, or third-party reimbursers.

What can be learned from these admittedly incomplete attempts at providing a unified system of services? First, integration can work despite the fact it has only been attempted in isolated and unusual instances to date, and the best integration may be none at all (e.g., when there is only one setting in a region). Most examples in the literature occur in one region or county, while the rest of the state is not involved. Second, where integration has been successful, several factors seem important: legislative and community support; fiscal flexibility; individual leadership; equitable division of turf by geography, facility functioning, or patient population; joint appointment of staff; and involvement of the university. Third, a major obstacle to unification is the opposition of unions. Unions objection to unification include concern about administrative clarity (e.g., state versus local responsibility), differential salaries and benefits, as well as the threats that shifts in patterns may pose to local community businesses.

The period of the systems approach is currently in the planning phase. It is too early to tell whether serious attempts will be made to implement such a concept, but the alternative (continuing business as usual) may prove so unpalatable that some reform will result. Certainly future efforts must consider past problems in the delivery of services, especially those related to reimbursement, administration, and planning.

REFERENCES

1. Dain N: From colonial America to bicentennial America: two centuries of vicissitudes in the institutional care of mental patients. Bull NY Acad Med 52:1179–1196, 1976
2. Quen JM: Learning from history. Psychiatr Ann 5:15–31, 1975
3. Rothman DJ: The Discovery of the Asylum: Social Order and Disorder in the New Republic. Boston, Little Brown, 1971
4. Maxmen J, Tucker GJ, Lebow M: Rational Hospital Psychiatry: The Reactive Environment. New York, Brunner/Mazel, 1974
5. Quen J: Review of Rothman DJ: The Discovery of the Asylum: Social Order and Disorder in the New Republic. J Psychiatr Law 2:105–122, 1974
6. Caplan RB: Psychiatry and the Community in Nineteenth-Century America. New York, Basic Books, 1969
7. Quen J: Asylum psychiatry, neurology, social work, and mental hygiene: An exploratory study in inter-professional history. J. Hist Behav Sci 13:3–11, 1977
8. Fuller R: An account of the imprisonment and sufferings of Robert Fuller of Cambridge. Boston, (Privately printed.) 1833
9. Davis LC: A modern lettre de cachet. Atlantic Monthly, 21:588–602, 1868
10. Ray I: A modern lettre de cachet reviewed. Atlantic Monthly 22:227–243, 1868
11. Copp O: Further experience in family care of the insane in Massachusetts. Am J Insanity 53:361–5, 1907
12. Deutsch A: The Mentally Ill in America: A History of Their Care and Treatment from Colonial Times. Garden City, NY, Doubleday, 1937
13. Galt JM: The farm of St. Anne. Am J Insanity 11:352–357, 1855
14. A century of debate surrounding community care. Hosp Community Psychiatry 27:490, 1976
15. Jarrett MC: Mental clinics, in Davis MM (ed): Clinics, Hospitals and Health Centers. New York, Harper, 1927
16. Ewalt JR: The birth of the community mental health movement, in Barton WE, Sanborn JC (eds): An Assessment of the Community Mental Health Movement. Lexington, Mass, Lexington Books, 1975
17. Musto D: The community mental health movement in historical perspective, in Barton WE, Sanborn JC (eds): An Assessment of the Community Mental Health Movement. Lexington, Mass, Lexington Books, 1976
18. Pinney EL: The First Group Psychotherapy Book. Springfield, Ill, Thomas, 1970
19. Salmon T: War neuroses: "shell shock." Milit Surg 41:674–694, 1917
20. Becker A, Murphy M. Greenblatt M: Recent advances in community psychiatry. New Engl J Med 272:621–626, 674–679, 1965
21. Querido A: Early diagnosis and treatment services, in Milbank Memorial Fund: The Elements of a Community Mental Health Program. New York, Milbank Memorial Fund, 1956
22. Bierer J: The Marlborough experiment, in Bellak L (ed): Handbook of Community Psychiatry and Community Mental Health. New York, Grune & Stratton, 1964
23. Modlin H: Personal communication
24. Black B: Psychiatric rehabilitation in the community, in Bellak L (ed): Handbook of Community Psychiatry and Community Mental Health. New York, Grune & Stratton, 1964
25. Bellak L: The comprehensive community psychiatry program at city hospital, in Bellak L (ed): Handbook of Community Psychiatry and Community Mental Health. New York, Grune & Stratton, 1964
26. Meyer A: Organizing the community for the protection of its mental life. Survey 34:557–560, 1915
27. Beers C: A Mind that Found Itself. Garden City, NY, Doubleday, 1908
28. Caplan G, Caplan RB: Development of community psychiatry concepts, in Freedman AM, Kaplan HI (eds): Comprehensive Textbook of Psychiatry. Baltimore, William & Wilkins, 1967
29. Bassett C: Mental Hygiene in the Community. New York, Macmillan, 1933
30. Linn: Some aspects of a psychiatry program in a voluntary general hospital, in Bellak L (ed): Handbook of Community Psychiatry and Community Mental Health. New York, Grune & Stratton, 1964
31. Bushard BL: The U.S. army's mental hygiene consultation service, in Symposium on Preventive and Social Psychiatry. Washington, DC, Walter Reed Army Institute of Research, 1957
32. Lindeman ME: A community organizes for mental health programming. Am J Occup Ther 10:43–46, 1956
33. Caplan G: An Approach to Community Mental Health. New York, Grune & Stratton, 1961

34. Caplan G: Principles of Preventive Psychiatry. New York, Basic Books, 1964
35. Mora G: Recent American psychiatric developments (since 1939), in Arieti S (ed): Handbook of American Psychiatry. New York, Basic Books, 1959
36. Whittington HG: Psychiatry in the American Community. New York, International Universities Press, 1966
37. Mechanic D: Mental Health and Social Policy. Englewood Cliffs, NJ, Prentice Hall, 1969
38. Felix RH: Psychiatry in prospect. Am J Psychiatry 103:600–604, 1947
39. Glasscote R, Sanders, D. Forstenzer HM, et al.: The Community Mental Health Center: An Analysis of Existing Models. Washington DC, Joint Information Service, 1964
40. Zusman J: The philosophic basis for a community and social psychiatry, in Barton WE, Sanborn JC (eds): An Assessment of the Community Mental Health Movement. Lexington, Mass, Lexington Books, 1976
41. Talbott JA: Toward a public policy on the chronic mentally ill patient. Am J Orthopsychiatry, 50:43–53, 1980
42. Returning the Mentally Disabled to the Community: Government Needs to do More. Washington DC, US. General Accounting Office, 1977.
43. Committee on Psychiatry and Community: The Chronic Mental Patient in the Community. New York, Group for the Advancement of Psychiatry, 1978
44. Talbott JA (ed): The Chronic Mental Patient: Problems, Solutions and Recommendations for a Public Policy. Washington DC, American Psychiatric Association, 1978
45. Boggs E: Personal communication
46. Report to the President from the President's Commission on Mental Health, Supt of Documents, Washington DC, 1978
47. Public Law 96–398: The Mental Health Systems Act, US Congress, Washington, DC, 1980
48. Ginzburg E: Personal communication
49. Biegel A., Bower WH, Levenson AI: A unified system of care: blueprint for the future. Am J Psychiatry 130:554–558, 1973
50. Snow HB, Blackburn DP: Unifying state hospital and local services to prevent or shorten hospitalization. Hosp Community Psychiatry 24:487–489, 1973
51. Osberg JW: Unifying state hospital and community mental health systems through area programs. Hosp Community Psychiatry 23:105–108, 1972
52. Rollins RL, Stratas NE: The geographic unit as a phase in merging hospital and community programs. Hosp Community Psychiatry 25:378–380, 1974
53. Barter JT: Sacramento county's experience with community care. Hosp Community Psychiatry 26:587–589, 1975
54. Elpers JR: Orange county's alternative to state hospital treatment. Hosp Community Psychiatry 26:589–592, 175
55. Forstenzer HM, Miller AD: Uified services in New York State, in Zusman J, Bertsch EF (eds): The Future Role of the State Hospital. Lexington, Mass, Lexington Books, 1973, pp 281–300
56. Prevost J: Personnel communication
57. McAtee OB, Zirkle GA: The evolution of a state hospital into a human-services center. Hosp Community Psychiatry 25:381–382, 1974
58. Tyce FAJ: State hospitals as community mental health centers, in Talbott JA (ed): State Hospitals: Problems and Potentials. New York, Human Sciences Press, 1980 pp 181–192
59. Sills M: The transfer of state hospital resources to community programs. Hosp Community Psychiatry 26:577–581, 1975

Herbert C. Modlin, MD

2

A History of Mental Health Services Prior to World War II

Historically, society's efforts to cope with the mentally ill brought about their institutionalization both literally and figuratively. The financial and political origins of government involvement in medicine are traceable to the earliest public mental hospitals in the 1830s (see chapter 5). Psychiatry's gradually achieved status as a respectable medical specialty together with grudging public acknowledgment of the extent of mental illness as a fact of community life resulted in the present complex mental health delivery system. Grown with little planning or goals, it is referred to as "the mental health delivery nonsystem" by some cynics.

Jargon and concepts of the marketplace such as delivery system, consumer, provider, and cost containment are relatively recent additions to health and mental health vocabulary and practice. The frequent use of the terms "delivery of *health services*" and *mental health services* analogous to the delivery of other public services and goods is disquieting to professionals and is experienced as demeaning by those treating patients within a traditional context of a confidential medical practice. The very size and scope of the health system, however, which now consumes 10 percent of the gross national product, makes such a comparison with other megabusinesses inevitable. Once so identified, controlling government regulations are a predictable consequence.

Within the general medical system, the mental health subsystem is subject to as much (or more) institutionalization, bureaucratization, industrialization, and regulation as its parent system. Although there are overlapping functions and territorial blurrings, the present mental health system is composed of five subsystems: public mental hospitals, private mental hospitals, psychiatric units in general hospitals, private practice, and community mental health centers (CMHCs).

THE ASYLUMS

With hindsight, one can recognize the first institution for the mentally ill in America as a psychiatric unit in a general hospital.[1] The Pennsylvania Provincial Assembly, in approving the building of the Pennsylvania Hospital in 1751, specified that the hospital would care for "those ill in body and also those distempered Persons suffering various Disorders of Body and Mind."[1] When the hospital opened in 1756, the mentally ill were segregated in the basement, but in 1796 they were moved to a new wing above ground. In 1840, they were moved to Dr. Kirkbride's new hospital at the west edge of the city. The assembly appropriated 2000 pounds for the hospital, provided a like amount was raised by private subscription. From its inception, the Pennsylvania Hospital has remained a private institution. In 1791, the New York Hospital also established a basement mental ward and 50 years later moved the patients to a new institution in White Plains.[2]

The first asylum exclusively for the mentally ill was established in 1773. Various colonial legislatures were considering such an innovation, but the Virginia House of Burgesses acted to found the Eastern Lunatic Hospital in Williamsburg. These pioneering endeavors stood alone for several decades until influences from Europe stimulated a renewal of interest in the plight of the mentally ill.[2]

The new nation was apparently preoccupied with establishing its identity at home and abroad and with exploring the division of authority and responsibility and autonomy between federalism and states rights and between state and local governments. As the states defined their territories and responsibilities and developed bodies of laws appropriate to the perceived needs of each, their legislatures eventually gave some attention to the unfit. The random system of local poor farms and almshouses of colonial America in the 1800s was deemed inadequate and induced the rise of state-endorsed and supervised poorhouses, particularly in Massachusetts and New York during the decade of almshouses.[3]

Meanwhile, the seminal work of Philippe Pinel in France and Thomas Willis and William Tuke in Great Britain ushered in the era of moral treatment of the insane. The success of that movement and its ready acceptance in America was based on several principles: (1) the decline in the belief in witches and demons in favor of specific social and physical explanations of mental illness; (2) the acceptance of criteria for recognizing and classifying certain types of social misfits as mentally ill; (3) approval of a medical model, i.e., insanity, becoming the business of physicians; (4) the demonstration that insanity was curable; (5) the view that the mentally ill differed from the physically ill and required separate institutional surroundings and treatment methods.

The decade of almshouses was superseded by the cult of curability; between 1833 and 1843, public mental hospitals opened in nine states. In addition, the example of William Tuke's York Retreat influenced the construction of four private hospitals: the Friends Asylum in Philadelphia, 1817; McLean Hospital in Boston, 1818; Bloomingdale Asylum in New York, 1821; and the Hartford Retreat in Hartford, Connecticut, 1824.[2]

Moral treatment, which lasted until the 1860s, was based on the etiological assumption that all men are indeed created equal and that insanity is caused by unfortunate, stressful life events and circumstances. Moral treatment became virtually synonymous with asylum residence since relief from a noxious environment was believed central to an effective treatment regime. Expensive institutions were erected, staffed, and maintained. Since insanity was, in effect, thrust upon unfortunate victims, therapeutic reversal was obviously possible and cure reasonably expected from proper ministrations. That optimistic estimate resulted in unrealistic expectations and overselling of the system.[3]

Originally, the asylums were administered by humanitarian laymen, although physicians were hired part time or full time for tending physical illness and prescribing purging, emetics, and bloodletting. The first medical superintendents were Dr. John Galt at Williamsburg and Dr. Samuel Woodward at Worcester. The shift to administrative physicians became popular, and 13 such professionals convened in 1844, to form the Association of Medical Superintendents of American Institutions for the Insane, the forerunner of the American Psychiatric Association.

Moral treatment arose in an era of general social reform and in practice was a clear improvement over the care accorded the insane in almshouses. For example, Worcester Hospital, opened in 1830 with Dr. Woodward as medical superintendent, housed 120 patients in a homelike setting, and provided occupational therapy, amusements and games, a religious atmosphere, and a humane attitude toward inmates. Annual reports documented a high recovery rate, and the hospital became a model for other institutions. Patients and staff shared similar ethnic, religious, and cultural values. The small number of patients potentiated close relationships: Dr. Woodward knew every patient by name. The funds required from the legislature were only a modest part of the total state budget. In recognition of his achievements, Dr. Woodward was elected first president of the association.[4]

Two levels of care existed from the beginning: private hospitals for those who could pay and public hospitals for those who could not. Due to general acceptance of both kinds of institutions by society, the insane were removed from the jurisdiction of the poor laws and the criminal laws. A large body of new legislation was enacted for regulating commitment procedures, admission, administration, and funding of institutions; fixing of responsibility for payment; determining criminal responsibility; protecting property rights of the mentally disturbed; and providing for guardianship. Each piece of legislation spawned a plethora of associated executive regulations.[3]

In spite of the advances noted, the fate of the insane was far from remedied, as Dorothea Dix discovered in the 1840s. When that remarkable woman focused concerned attention on the mentally ill, she was able to document that the majority were still incarcerated, caged, and chained in jails and almshouses. Her single-minded solution to the distressing situation was more and better state hospitals. Her crusade to improve the lot of the mentally ill rested primarily on the conviction that they must be accepted as wards of the state. The crusade's success depended on persuading legislatures to assume that legal, administrative, and fiscal responsibility. Her success was realized in state after state and later in Canada and Europe.[4]

From the clarity of hindsight, Dorothea Dix's success was one factor that led to the demise of moral treatment and the advent of the custodial era. The manifest need for more beds was engendered, particularly, by a tidal wave of immigrants in the 1840s as well as an increase in the native population. New hospitals were quickly filled to overflowing. The Worcester census doubled by 1860. A new 500-bed hospital opened in 1877 and housed 811 patients by 1890 and 1100 by 1900. In the late 1860s, curability was abandoned as a myth in the face of the accumulating mass of institutionalized chronically ill. All those factors led to one result: overcrowding. The reduced effectiveness of treatment caused by overcrowding resulted in an increased length of stay and decreased discharges, which produced more overcrowding. When another factor, a ubiquitous scarcity of subsidizing tax dollars, was added, the era of custodial treatment became entrenched for a long continuation; vestiges are still with us in the 1980s.

It should be noted that lamentable public mental hospitals were part of a general social reality, not alone the lot of the mentally ill. Jails, penitentiaries, orphanages, and almshouses were concurrently overcrowded and underfinanced. In the last half of the 19th century, the principle of segregating the unfit of all sorts in walled institutions was firmly established and approved by the public, professionals, and government.[5]

The latter half of the 19th century was the Dark Ages for the mentally ill in America. Since the custodial era in asylums was a consequence largely of overcrowding, an inevitable accompaniment was understaffing. The overworked physicians had little time or inclination for leisurely observation and systematic recording, much less clinical investigation and research. The pages of the *American Journal of Insanity* presented their major concerns: architecture, financing, farm management, inmate labor, and various administrative matters. Most of the asylums were geographically and functionally isolated from the growing and changing communities; most of the medical staffs were ideologically and functionally isolated from the mainstream of medicine. Caplan describes the rise of what she terms the Guild, the Association of Mental Superintendents, founded in 1844.[3] The association was close knit and strongly supportive of its own members. It defended them against pressures exerted by state legislatures, the press, and the public. It became effective in lobbying for entrenched practices. It tried to make psychiatry a distinct specialty, an exclusive domain; it also attempted to exclude nonmembers from the care of the insane and to prevent their appearing in court.

Not only penurious legislators, territorially entrenched superintendents, and an indifferent public but also developments in medicine and science contributed to the prolongation of custodial treatment. Dramatic advances in neurology and neuropathology directed attention to degenerative diseases of the brain and spawned a number of organic hypotheses to explain varieties of dementia. That scientific trend resonated with social theory. Several authorities on the period refer to Social Darwinism, a concept analogous to Darwin's biological ideas of natural selection and the survival of the fittest. When combined with therapeutic pessimism, Social Darwinism indirectly espoused the perpetuation of the asylum as a proper sanctuary for unadaptable social failures. Insanity was obviously a manifestation of biological degeneration resulting from allowing defective stock to reproduce. Attempts were made to differentiate the curable and incurable, and most of the latter became asylum residents. The newly popularized science of heredity was invoked to justify isolation of the insane and to discourage their propagation, even to the point of sterilizing them.[5]

Criticisms and exposés of asylum practice emerged bit by bit. Prevailing commitment procedures were questioned and denounced. Abuses common in the commitment process were exposed by Mrs. Elizabeth Packard's activities and her book *Modern Persecution.*[6] Mrs. Packard was committed by her minister–husband but succeeded in obtaining her release after 3 years. She embarked on a crusade in the 1860s and 1870s to convince state legislators to enact commitment laws more protective of the rights of patients and to guard against railroading of family members by relatives. She persuaded the Illinois legislature to require a jury trial for commitment and influenced similar kinds of legislation in Massachusetts, Iowa, and other states.[5] Unfortunately, as with Dorothea Dix, unforeseen consequences followed the success of her project. The commitment procedure became criminalized: the accused had charges read against him, was cross-examined by a prosecuting attorney, was tried, and became subject to a verdict.[2]

Criticisms mounted as the deplorable conditions in many asylums surfaced. Enterprising reporters had themselves admitted as patients and wrote scathing stories of brutality and neglect of inmates: starvation, cruel restraints, beatings, and even murder. Several murder trials of asylum employees provided opportunity for more unfavorable publicity. Fuel was added to the fire by revelations of dishonest practices by some superintendents who pocketed money in dealings with contractors for food, supplies, and services, leading to legislative inquiries.[3]

By the 1880s, a reform movement was clearly evident as censure swelled. The medical profession, particularly neurologists in private practice and academic positions, faulted the isolation of psychiatrists from medicine as well as from the community. The type of training and other required qualifications of psychiatrists were questioned. In the community, formal organizations of citizens such as the National Association for the Protection of the Insane, the Anti-Kidnapping League, and the Lunacy Reform Association became active. The Guild evaded, denied, and counterattacked, but dissension within its own ranks occurred because some of its members listened to these complaints.

In 1894, at its 50th anniversary meeting, the Guild, now the American Medical-Psychological Association, invited the prominent neurologist S. Weir Mitchell to present a critical analysis of the psychiatric profession and psychiatric institutions. He accepted the invitation literally and delivered a forthright polemic on their many deficiencies, including understaffing, untrained auxiliary personnel, insipid food, work exploitation of patients, unnecessary use of restraints, and absence of recreational facilities. His main attack was on the doctors for maintaining a contented, calm, and comfortable assurance in splendid isolation from medicine and the public. He accused them of indifference to research and expanding clinical knowledge; disinterest in continuing their personal growth and exercising intellectual curiosity; negligence in teaching the public regarding the real nature of mental illness and the needs of their patients; and failing to confront legislatures to demand a hearing of their requirements for personnel, equipment, and institutional improvement.

By 1900, many potential changes in the care of the mentally ill and the attitudes of psychiatry had begun to form. In large part, the history of psychiatric institutions and the development of mental health care systems in the 20th century is a record of efforts to find alternatives to public mental hospital care.

THE HOSPITALS

Although the late 19th and early 20th century was a period of continued criticism of the asylums and of emerging tentative reforms, the need for hospitalization of the overtly mentally ill was not questioned. The psychotic patient was a main concern of both medicine and society; expulsion of those misfits from the community was accepted practice. The progressivism of the times thus included attempts to improve asylum conditions and practices. Two examples are of current interest in that although they waxed and then waned into oblivion, they presaged later events.

Tent treatment at Manhattan State Hospital on Ward's Island started in 1901 due to apprehension over an outbreak of tuberculosis among the patients. Groups of 20 were assigned for the summer to large tents on the grounds. Spectacular improvement in mental functioning and social behavior resulted. Nontubercular patients were moved into tents with similar results. On return to the hospital wards in the fall, many relapsed. By 1905, 200–300 patients were "tented" each summer. Articles about the novel treatment appeared in the *American Journal of Insanity,* and other hospitals quickly initiated a like procedure. Two 35-bed frame camp buildings with removable sides to admit summer's fresh air and sunshine were constructed on Ward's Island. They soon housed 50 patients with no increase in staff. The familiar ward regimentation prevailed, and the expected improvement in patients failed to occur. The deleterious effects of what later would be labeled "hospitalism" existed but were not recognized.[3]

In a similar vein, a cottage system, another European import, developed at McLean Hospital and was copied in the early 20th century by several state hospitals.[2] Separate buildings housed 50–60 such patients, who were partially self-sufficient. Their kitchens, dining rooms, and living rooms simulated a homelike atmosphere, but the minimal staff, regimentation, and lack of therapeutic programs canceled these potential benefits. The possibilities of what later would be labeled halfway houses were thus discovered but not implemented. There were, however, alternatives to the asylum that fared better; a discussion of these alternatives follows.

The Psychopathic Hospital

Along with many experiments, some successful, some abortive, around the turn of the century, the concept of the psychopathic hospital was imported from Europe, where it had prospered, particularly in Germany. The American hospitals were usually associated with a medical school, general hospital, or state hospital system located in urban areas.

The first such institution was Pavilion F at Albany State Hospital in 1902, followed shortly by one affiliated with the University of Michigan. The Boston Psychopathic opened in 1912, and a few years later similar hospitals operated in Iowa and Colorado. In 1895, the New York State Hospital system had started the Pathological Institute, headed by a neuropathologist and devoted primarily to research. Some years afterward, under its second director, Adolf Meyer, it was renamed the Psychiatric Institute and admitted patients for treatment.

Those institutions provided short-term inpatient as well as outpatient care for acute cases. They were also research and teaching centers and often were headed by a neuropathologist. The expectation was that a well-staffed hospital providing the most modern treatment could return improved patients to the community after a relatively short stay and maintain their improvement with appropriate aftercare. The result would be decreased admissions to the asylums.

Ironically, the reverse occurred. Convenient access of large populations, liberal admissions policies, and community consent flooded the psychopathic hospitals with patients who were not promptly responsive to brief treatment. The hospitals became diagnostic and referral units, "the front door to the asylums."[7] Furthermore, asylum superintendents, true to form, fought the innovation, complaining to state legislators that it deprived them of their "best" patients—those who could return to the community. In addition, the chronically underfunded and understaffed asylums relied on patient labor. Moreover, since the asylums received state funds based on patient census, the superintendents feared a loss of income.

One possible alternative to the asylums thus proved ineffective. The half-dozen psychopathic hospitals surviving today have a mission far different from that originally conceived. They are affiliated with medical schools and are prestigious training and research centers.

Private Hospitals

A number of the first charitable private hospitals developed in the early 19th century have survived and thrived. In particular, those on the eastern seaboard—the Pennsylvania Hospital, Philadelphia; McLean Hospital, Boston; Butler Hospital, Providence; New York Hospital, White Plains; Sheppard and Enoch Pratt Hospital, Baltimore—became bastions of enlightened patient care, innovative practices, research, and training. Most of the hospitals were affiliated with medical schools; their staff members became professors and department chairmen, many of whom became presidents of the American Psychiatric Association. Rothman points to the Pennsylvania Hospital as a shining example of excellence in the midst of widespread deterioration of care in the asylums. The chief advantage the Pennsylvania Hospital enjoyed, its ability to refuse state financial aid, allowed it a selective intake policy; in contrast, the public hospitals had to admit any community nuisance or embarrassment sent by the courts. Under Dr. Thomas Kirkbride's direction, it restricted the admission of committed chronic patients to a small percentage of the patient census and maintained uncrowded wards, a high staff–patient ratio, minimal use of restraints, and an active daily treatment program.[5]

The growth in numbers of private hospitals in the 19th century was imperceptible. Late in the century, a number of sanitariums, stimulated by the popularity of S. Weir Mitchell's famous rest cure for the nervous, asthenic, hypochondriacal, and hysterical, catered to the paying nonpsychotic public and became havens for the disabled neurotic. Mitchell advanced the theory of nervous exhaustion, and advocated enforced rest and isolation in the sanitariums based on the principle of recharging rundown batteries.[14] Many sanitariums declined in popularity as the rest cure proved less than curative of chronic conditions. A survey by Kano and Glasscote revealed that of the 170 private psychiatric hospitals operating in 1965, only 21 had opened their doors prior to 1900, and half of those were the old, established eastern institutions.[8]

In the 20th century, slow but steady community recognition of various mental disorders led to a gradual increase in small private mental hospitals, commonly of about 50 beds. In the period 1910–1940, one or two new hospitals opened yearly, usually contiguous to population centers. After World War II, a combination of factors led to rapid expansion; 35 new hospitals opened between 1945 and 1955. The factors influencing this growth included acknowledgment of the military statistics showing mental illness to be prevalent in all social classes; utilization of individual and group therapies based on psychoanalytic principles; acceptance of milieu therapy as a valid treatment modality; and increasingly profitable private hospital operations made possible through the advent of third-party payers.

After the postwar boom, the number of private hospitals leveled off. There were 165 in 1964 and 158 in 1971.[9] In the past 10 years, a mild annual increase in numbers (183 in 1976) has resulted from the opening of chains of proprietary hospitals owned by business organizations and corporations.

Although an established segment of the current mental health delivery system, private psychiatric hospitals (see Chapter 7) handled only 3 percent of the total patient-care episodes in mental health facilities in 1975; there were 130,000 admissions for that year. As in private office practice generally, over 90 percent of patients in psychiatric hospitals are Caucasian, and 80 percent are between 18 and 64 years old.[9]

Psychiatric Units in General Hospitals

Although the Pennsylvania and New York hospitals at first admitted mental patients to special wards, in response to the trend of the 1940s, they built separate institutions for the insane some miles from the general hospitals (see Chapter 6). Greenhill notes that the history of psychiatric units apparently begins with the Albany General Hospital in 1902, although detention wards operated at Bellevue Hospital in New York City from 1789 and in 1890 at the Philadelphia General Hospital.[10] A second "legitimate" unit opened in the Henry Ford Hospital, Detroit, in 1923. In 1924, Menninger reported being able to find only half a dozen 10–12 bed units in the country.[11] In 1933, the Rockefeller Foundation provided financial incentive for the development of psychiatric units in university hospitals. These units served as a pattern for general acceptance of the contention that a general hospital should serve all the medical needs of its community. The movement grew slowly, however, and in the 1940s only 40 such units functioned. One factor hindering wide acceptance was that psychiatric units were less remunerative than medical and surgical for each square foot of required hospital space.

The explosion of interest in psychiatry and the mentally ill following World War II was reflected in a rapid increase in psychiatric wards. In a 1956 survey, Bennett et al. reported 279 general hospitals with at least a 15-bed unit and another 50 hospitals admitting psychiatric patients for temporary custody.[12] Of the total 163,000 beds in all general hospitals, 23,000 were earmarked for psychiatry. Bennett noted, however, that over one-third of the 73 four-year medical schools had no psychiatric unit in their university hospitals.

In the postwar era, the Veterans Administration assigned 25 percent of its general hospital beds to psychiatric and neurological patients. The Joint Commission Report of 1961 strongly advocated short-term units in all community hospitals. The movement caught on, particularly because of the mushrooming number of psychiatrists entering private practice with a need for short-term inpatient facilities. By 1963, there were 500 such units; the number climbed to 614 in 1967 and 870 in 1976, treating nearly a million patients annually.[9]

General hospital psychiatric units have become significant purveyors of mental health services, providing 14 percent of the 6.7 million patient-care episodes recorded for all mental health facilities in 1976. Although some units are affiliated with community mental health centers, most of them are part of the private not-for-profit sector of mental health care. As is true of private psychiatric hospitals, the bulk of patients are white (87 percent) and between ages 18 and 64 (85 percent).[9]

PRIVATE PRACTICE

Although not a well-defined subsystem, private practice is a functionally important segment of the current mental health delivery network. It includes private office practice and, for many practitioners, utilization of general hospital psychiatric beds for short-term treatment of their patients. In several respects, its practice differs markedly from that in the public sector.[13]

In the asylum period, "nervousness," recognized as a dysfunction afflicting women chiefly, was accorded little attention. Since such a condition was neither physical disorder nor insanity, it was not really the province of either the general physician or the alienist. The overt psychoneuroses were medical curiosities, like, for example, *grand hysterie* in Charcot's Clinic.[14]

Within the framework of evolving neurological knowledge during and after the Civil War, many nonorganic disorders simulating neurological symptoms constituted a significant proportion of neurological practice, and by 1880, "neuropsychiatrists" appeared occasionally in the medical literature. S. Weir Mitchell's espousal of "nervous exhaustion" provided a plausible medical explanation for neurasthenia, psychasthenia, hypochondriasis, and so forth, and those conditions became legitimate medical concerns.

The developments in private practice and the separation of psychiatry from neurology are historically obscure. Little data seem documented on which to base conclusions. By the 1920s, there were separate departments of psychiatry and neurology in many medical schools, although the faculty regularly held appointments in both specialties. Generally, the practitioners were neuropsychiatrists. The influence of Meyer and Freud strengthened interest in the neurotic, and varieties of psychotherapy became respectable treatments. In addition, six psychoanalytic institutes had opened prior to World War II.

The war experience produced an explosion of interest in psychiatry. The now-familiar statistics are impressive: one-third of induction station rejections were for neuropsychiatric reasons; one-third of military medical discharges were based on neuropsychiatric diagnoses.[15] To meet the pressing need for military psychiatrists, 90-day crash courses were devised for new medical officers, particularly pediatricians and obstetricians, who functioned creditably as psychiatrists for the duration of the war. Many became intrigued, and of the several thousand course graduates, about half chose to enter careers in psychiatry after discharge.[15] For example, in 1946, the Menninger Clinic received 700 applications for residency training.

The few studies available for the past 30 years indicate no shift in the percentage of psychiatrists in private office practice—about 55 percent of the total.[16–18]

The numbers of patients seen have also remained steady, but the percentage of patient episodes occurring in private offices has declined from 50 percent to 13 percent of all patients seen in mental health facilities.[9] The shift is attributable to (1) the surging increase in CMHCs and free-standing clinics and (2) the numbers of clinical psychologists, psychiatric social workers, and psychiatric nurses functioning as primary mental health care givers.

In reviewing the overall development of mental health delivery systems in the past 175 years, their present complex functioning and wide distribution, and their ability to serve the public effectively, it should be noted that the majority of mentally ill persons are not treated in mental health facilities. Of those patients presenting mental disorders in 1975, 73 percent received care solely in the general medical sector; 19 percent solely in the mental health sector; and 8 percent in the two sectors combined.[9] Planners, in considering manpower distribution, professional training, financing, and government regulation, need to keep in mind that only a minor portion of psychiatric practice is conducted in mental health facilities.

COMMUNITY MENTAL HEALTH CENTERS

Although this historical account of mental health systems stops with World War II, all the ingredients subsequently dropped into the stew pot of CMHCs were available before 1963 and awaited only an imaginative chef. (See Chapter 2.) This section will recount briefly developments in psychiatry, social work, sociology, government, and public attitudes that made the creation of mental health centers possible. He who delves into the bypaths of history finds records of hunches, ideas, philosophies, prognostications, and actions that at the time came to little but resurfaced years later to influence events and accomplishments. This brief account will not include an exposition of community psychiatry or the community mental health movement except as those concepts pertain directly to the emergence of the centers as a significant segment of the present mental health delivery system.

The Mental Hygiene Movement

In 1908, Clifford Beers' book *A Mind That Found Itself* provided the blueprint for a mental hygiene structure and the solid edifice obtaining today.[19] Beers suffered 3 years in the asylums of the time, experiencing the usual beatings, chokings, strait jackets, and reviling attitudes at the hands of his keepers. Unlike many of his fellow inmates, he made a complete recovery and, unlike most other critics, possessed the determination and ability to effect change. Moreover, unlike his illustrious predecessors Dorothea Dix and Elizabeth Packard, he did not limit his philippic to exposé and need for reform in the hospitals alone. He had first-hand evidence that mental illness was curable and convincing professional opinions that early recognition and treatment of his illness probably could have obviated his hospitalizations.

Beers was thus able to obtain the help and influence of William James, who wrote the book's introduction. Adolf Meyer suggested "mental hygiene" for reference to the Beers movement. Enlisting psychiatrists, educators, businessmen, and friends, Beers launched the Connecticut Committee for Mental Hygiene in 1908 and a year later the National Committee for Mental Hygiene in New York.

The importance of the mental hygiene movement to the subsequent development of CMHCs was in its championing (1) prevention, (2) child guidance clinics, (3) research into the social influences on mental breakdown, (4) community adaptation to and integration of formerly hospitalized persons, (5) application of mental hygiene principles in schools, prisons, and industry, and (6) public education.

Prevention

Prevention, both primary and secondary, was a central intent of the movement, to be pursued by study, surveys, research, dissemination of knowledge, contributions from government, and Committees for Mental Hygiene in every state to involve its community members. Adolf Meyer's belief that prevention was realizable patterned the committee's program. As early as 1908, Meyer was speaking and writing about prophylaxis.[20] He emphasized that aftercare of former hospital patients meant more than providing them decent boarding homes; it meant jobs, organized social contacts, and integration into community life, too, as methods of preventing recurrence of their illness.

Clinics

One of the first outpatient psychiatric clinics was established at the Pennsylvania Hospital (about 1885), at the site of the general hospital, not at Dr. Kirkbride's institution.[1] The general hospital served in part a ghetto population in the central city and made available to the poor services similar to those provided by the privately practicing neuropsychiatrists. The clinic concept developed rapidly in many urban hospitals serving low-income patients, particularly in Boston, Philadelphia, New York, and Baltimore.

The child guidance movement arose from concerns of the early juvenile court judges for the neglected and abused, as well as the delinquent, children they encountered. The Institute for Juvenile Research opened in 1909 as an adjunct of the Chicago court. Dr. William Healy, the first director, moved to Boston in 1917 to head the new Judge Baker Child Guidance Clinic.[2] Both Beers and Meyer considered preventive treatment of children important. National Committee surveys of school children documented need. When Dr. Thomas Salmon became director of the National Committee, he reported that the number of facilities compared to the need was grossly inadequate. In 1922, the Commonwealth Fund financed a 5-year demonstration program, and child guidance clinics sprang up throughout the country. Deutsch estimates that in the mid-1930s the 159 child guidance clinics comprised over one-third of all the nation's psychiatric clinics.[2]

Government

Among Adolf Meyer's signal contributions to present-day practice was his emphasis on the relevance of patient–environment interaction to the causes of mental breakdown as well as to its treatment. He advocated a number of the tenets and components of modern community psychiatry programs and in that sense was a proponent of public health psychiatry.[20] He urged attention to the importance of the social environment; integrated programs of prevention, treatment, and aftercare; participation of the family physician; organization of care within geographical districts (catchment area); and education of the public.

Proliferation of public assistance programs during the Great Depression indicated a changing public attitude toward citizens in trouble, a change by the government from reluctantly doling out tax dollars to accepting responsibility for innovative programs. Following passage of the Harrison Narcotics Act in 1914, the Public Health Service organized a narcotics division and later a hospital for treatment of drug addicts. In the 1930s, the division expanded into the Division of Mental Hygiene, and psychiatrists became public health officers. In 1946, the Mental Health Act changed the division to the National Institute for Mental Health (NIMH), with a public health psychiatrist, Dr. Robert Felix, its first director. Subsequently, NIMH became the agent for the development of CMHCs.

Social Work

The beginnings of social work in the United States are traceable to the settlement house movement of the late 19th century in the urban immigrant ghettos. The volunteer and salaried workers became self-taught professionals as they struggled to improve the lot of their clients and assist their coping with daily crises. "Social worker" and "caseworker" entered the vocabulary. By 1911, Adolf Meyer was publishing material regarding social casework and its relevance to psychiatry. The publication of Mary Richmond's *Social Diagnosis* in 1917 was a landmark for the profession.[21]

Psychiatric social work began at the Boston Psychopathic Hospital in 1913 through the collaboration of Dr. Ernest Southard and Miss Mary Jarrett. They initiated a small training program, and their book in 1922 gave impetus to interprofessional collaboration.[22] Their educational program prospered, and in 1919 Miss Jarrett became head of the first graduate social work school at Smith College. Subsequently, social work discovered Freud and Rank; emphasis turned from social diagnosis to social casework and therapy, and the basis for the current prominence of social workers in CMHCs evolved.

At the same time, sociological studies provided a theoretical base for social work practice as exemplified by Lawrence K. Frank's publications in the 1920s and 1930s.[23] He defined society as the patient as well as a causative agent, through social imbalance and social injustice, of mental illness, crime, and prostitution.

Crisis Intervention

In 1917, the surgeon general of the army organized the first military department of psychiatry and neurology and borrowed Dr. Thomas Salmon from the National Committee as consultant to the American Expeditionary Force in Europe. In postwar publications, Southard described the value of short-term crisis intervention, stressing immediacy, proximity, and expectancy—immediate treatment close to home with the expectancy of recovery.[24] These and other useful lessons from World War I were lost and had to be rediscovered in the next war.[15]

Crisis intervention as currently practiced in civilian life was strongly influenced by Eric Lindeman and, later, Gerald Caplan in Boston. The Coconut Grove night club fire in 1943 inundated hospitals and morgues with victims, and Lindeman discovered the need to work not only with victims but also with bereaved and disrupted families.[25] The tragedy led to an experimental Human Relations Service in Wellesley, a direct forerunner of mental health centers.

Mental Health Consultation

The mental hygiene movement, concerned as it was with community living, community adjustment, and prevention of mental illness, gravitated naturally to interest in community institutions other than hospitals and clinics. Out of its involvement in juvenile courts and delinquency came a concern with the plight of incarcerated criminals. The National Committee sponsored establishment of a psychiatric clinic at New York's Sing Sing Prison headed by Dr. Bernard Glueck. At several other large penitentiaries, similar clinics originated for diagnosis and treatment of mental illness and focused concern additionally on intramural adjustment of all inmates and later parole adjustment to reduce recidivism.[2]

In the years after World War I, Dr. Southard applied mental hygiene principles to problems in industry, pointing out that it is possible to promote workers' contentment and efficiency by helping them with personal problems, proper job fit, interpersonal relations on the job, management of stress and fatigue, improved work environment, and so on. In the Great Depression, this insight atrophied but was revitalized after World War II, particularly by Dr. William Menninger. As chief psychiatrist for the army, Menninger became convinced of the mental health significance of leadership, role performance, group cohesion, belonging, and group morale[15] and found in industrial organizations obvious parallels to the military experience.

REFERENCES

1. Morton T: The History of the Pennsylvania Hospital (rev. ed.). Philadelphia, Times Printing House, 1897
2. Deutsch A: The Mentally Ill in America. New York, Doubleday, 1937
3. Caplan R: Psychiatry and the Community in Nineteenth Century America. New York, Basic Books, 1969
4. Morrissey J, Goldman H, Klerman L, et al: The Enduring Asylum: Cycles of Institutional Reform at Worcester State Hospital. New York, Grune & Stratton, 1980
5. Rothman D: The Discovery of the Asylum. Boston, Little, Brown, 1971
6. Packard E: Modern Persecution. Hartford, Case, Lockwood and Brainard, 1882
7. Rothman D: Deinstitutionalization and state mental hospitals: We can't have both. In ADAMHA News, vol 6, No 16, Aug 6, 1980. Washington, D.C., US Dept of Health and Human Services
8. Kano C, Glasscote R: Private Psychiatric Hospitals. Washington, D.C., American Psychiatric Association, 1966
9. Vischi TR, Jones KR, Shank EL, et al: National Data Book. Washington, D.C., U.S. Dept of Health and Human Services, 1980
10. Greenhill M: Psychiatric units in general hospitals: 1979. Hosp Community Psychiatry 30:169–182, 1979
11. Menninger K: Psychiatric units in general hospitals. Mod Hosp 23:1–4, 1924
12. Bennett A, Hargrove E: The Practice of Psychiatry in General Hospitals. Berkeley, University of California Press, 1956
13. Modlin H: Organizational changes in mental health delivery systems: The private sector. Bull Menninger Clin 40:144–150, 1976

14. Gerty F: The private psychiatric hospital. I. Phases of development, in Talkington P, Bloss C (eds): Evolving Concepts in Psychiatry. New York, Grune & Stratton, 1969
15. Menninger W: Psychiatry in a Troubled World. New York, Macmillan, 1948
16. Survey of Mental Health Needs in Kentucky. Louisville, Kentucky Association for Mental Health, 1972
17. APA Task Force Report #6: The Present and Future Importance of Patterns of Private Psychiatric Practice in the Delivery of Mental Health Services. Washington, D.C., American Psychiatric Association, 1973
18. Knesper D, Carlson B: An analysis of the movement to private psychiatric practice. Arch Gen Psychiatry 38:943–949, 1981
19. Beers C: A Mind That Found Itself. Garden City, NY, Doubleday, 1939
20. Meyer A: Collected Papers, vol 4. Baltimore, Johns Hopkins Press, 1952
21. Richmond M: Social Diagnosis. New York, Russell Sage Foundation 1917
22. Southard E, Jarrett M: Kingdom of Evil. New York, Macmillan, 1922
23. Salmon T: Future of psychiatry in the army. Milit Surg 47:200–207, 1920
24. Frank L: Society as the Patient. New Brunswick, NJ, Rutgers University Press, 1948
25. Lindeman E: Symptomatology and management of acute grief. Am J Psychiatry 101:141–148, 1944

David F. Musto, M.D.

3

Recent Developments in Federal Legislation

The federal government first supported medical care in an organized manner after World War II when it began to subsidize hospital construction, scientific research, and the training of health professionals.[1] Some of the most significant steps, however, were taken in the 1960s and 1970s when the federal government commenced organizing the delivery of health care, attempting to ensure equitable availability to hospitals and physicians, and to provide health care to all the disadvantaged and elderly through Medicare and Medicaid.[2] The enormous costs of the newly planned and broadly distributed health care, however, led to serious and difficult problems for federal and state governments. By 1981, the debate over increased health care costs and governmental organization of service delivery had grown intense as economic conditions worsened and an administration antagonistic toward "excessive" controls was installed in Washington, D.C. The outcome is unclear.

With the massive development of governmental control and subsidy of medical care during the nearly four decades since World War II, psychiatry as a discipline and as a profession has undergone an uneven development. Psychiatry has both benefited from being perceived as something more than mainstream medicine—as when Congress provided large sums for the mental health centers program, which some thought would cure "sick communities"—and has suffered a loss of prestige and support when it has been perceived as something less than mainstream medicine—as when reimbursement for psychiatric care is criticized as payment for unproved methods and vague illnesses lacking a specific cure.

As psychiatry moved away from an organic basis in the late 19th century and became infused with dynamic theories and therapies, the gap between traditional and avant-garde medical care widened. Psychotherapy of one form or another was characterized by verbal communication; few drugs existed that were effective for psychoses or neuroses. Persons with emotional disorders who were thought inappropriate for psychotherapy or unable to afford private care were housed in large state hospitals under often discouraging conditions. Until World War II, the vast majority of patients cared for by psychiatrists were in mental hospitals, and the dynamic theories were more discussed and written about than practiced.

WORLD WAR II

During the war, psychiatrists impressed military and civilian authorities in two prominent roles: as gate keepers at induction centers and as therapists for those inductees who suffered breakdowns while in the service, especially during battlefield stress. As gate keepers, psychiatrists kept out of the armed services hundreds of thousands of able-bodied but emotionally suspect draftees. The magnitude of the number rejected as unfit for service astounded military leaders, and although the admirals and generals could have, in turn, rejected the psychiatrists' judgments, they were profoundly impressed by this display of professional knowledge. In retrospect, the gate keepers' criteria seem to have been excessively rigid and overly responsive to any hint of emotional disorder in the draftee's past. The British army, which had a very low rate of initial rejection for service based on psychiatric examination, had about the same battlefield breakdown rate. If the American examiners exercised extreme caution in their necessarily brief evaluations at induction centers, the fact was not soon appreciated, and the effect was to enhance the credibility of the small profession.[1,3]

The second boost in prestige occurred closer to the fighting. An example of this was quick treatment near the battlefield, using sodium pentothal to relax the patient and permit expression of his fears and trauma. This treatment both returned many soldiers to the front and appeared to prevent long-term invalidism. Here psychiatry's contribution was manifest, but the conclusion drawn from it by some prominent leaders of the profession, that such quick and intensive intervention could be as effective in civilian life, was, in retrospect, rather optimistic. American psychiatry, still a small part of American medicine, emerged from World War II possessing much greater prestige than it had ever before enjoyed. The profession's knowledge was arcane but powerful, and the lessons of the war were waiting for application to civilians hitherto denied psychiatric expertise.[4]

The extensive legislation regarding medical and psychiatric services that began in the 1940s originated within the profession largely from two sources, the Public Health Service, from which the National Institute of Mental Health (NIMH; 1949) would be separated, and those members of the profession who had become managers of substantial psychiatric services in the armed services, such as Francis Braceland and William C. Menninger, who would become the new, aggressive leadership of the American Psychiatric Association.[5]

The image of psychiatry and the other mental health professions increasingly rose in the esteem of health reformers and public-spirited activists, so that every effort to increase mental health services and research efforts received strong support in the media and before Congress. Advocacy of mental health legislation, especially at the federal level, acquired a public lobby with a dedication and effectiveness never before witnessed. Repeatedly, the official requests for NIMH annual budgets were increased by Congress with the active encouragement of lay advocates.

NATIONAL INSTITUTE OF MENTAL HEALTH

In general, until the early 1960s, the increases in budgets relating to mental health in the Department of Health, Education, and Welfare (HEW) provided more aid to research and training. The goal was more help rather than control of ongoing treatment within the states. The federal government had been prevented by conservative leaders at NIMH's inception from an active role in routine treatment of the mentally ill. Senator Robert Taft, Sr., for example, held that the federal government had no right to become involved in direct patient care, a route Senator Taft and his colleagues believed might be a subtle step toward socialized medicine.[6]

As the 1950s progressed, the amount of state funds allocated to care of the mentally ill continued to grow, with the result that in some states a crisis appeared in the fiscal future. Among leaders of the profession as well as investigators of community and social disorders, the conviction had been growing that discoveries about the social context, even the social cause, of individual mental illness now permitted reasonable and direct interventions in society to treat large numbers of the emotionally disturbed. In this mixture of desperation and hopefulness, the Joint Commission on Mental Illness and Health was authorized by Congress in 1955 (Public Law 84-182).[7]

JOINT COMMISSION ON MENTAL ILLNESS AND HEALTH (1956–1960)

After 5 years of studies and gradual consolidation of popular support, at the close of 1960 the Joint Commission published its final report, *Action for Mental Health.*[8] This report to Congress and the public remains valuable reading even now, representing thoughtful analysis of the issues. The Joint Commission carried the argument for funding treatment a step beyond the limits originally set upon NIMH: the Joint Commission recommended that the federal government undertake responsibility for much of the care of those in mental hospitals, thus relieving the states of a great and growing burden. A poll taken in 1958 indicated that next to education, the American public was most willing to be taxed for care of the mentally ill.[9] The time seemed ripe for an advance in the area of financial support for treatment. The Joint Commission did not place much hope in prevention of mental illness; the subject was so complicated and uncertain that keeping an open mind was thought to be the best approach.

The Joint Commission did recommend smaller state hospitals, with a maximum of a thousand beds, and the wider distribution of mental health clinics. Perhaps the greatest accomplishment of the Joint Commission and its leadership was the consolidation of support for a new era in the care of the mentally ill among many national groups as well as among the professionals themselves.

Within the federal government, the NIMH assumed the lead in preparing a program based on the final report. President Kennedy's personal interest in the topic—he is said to have read *Action for Mental Health* with care and interest—assured development of a plan within the executive branch; sympathetic chairmen of key congressional committees such as Senator Lister Hill made it likely that the plan would receive a friendly hearing. The final result of the administration's deliberations was embodied in President Kennedy's message to Congress of February 5, 1963 regarding mental illness and mental retardation.[10] It called for the establishment of community mental health centers (CMHCs) and represented a major shift in care of the mentally ill that President Kennedy had envisioned.

COMMUNITY MENTAL HEALTH CENTERS

President Kennedy expressed optimism about treatment for mental illness utilizing contemporary methods. "If we apply our medical knowledge and social insights fully," he declared, "all but a small portion of the mentally ill can eventually achieve a wholesome and constructive social adjustment." He was confident that "a concerted national attack on mental disorders is now both possible and practical." The key to success would be CMHCs, where it would be "possible for most of the mentally ill to be successfully and quickly treated in their own communities and returned to a useful place in society." The major emphasis would be on the prevention of mental illness, which was "far more economical and . . . far more likely to be successful." The centers, "ideally . . . at a community general hospital," would receive federal construction funds; and as a compromise between full, permanent payment of staff costs and no payment, the president recommended federal aid at 75 percent of staff costs for a 4-year period. The state hospitals, destined to play a "valuable transitional role," required $10 million in federal aid to improve existing care; moreover, professional manpower had to be increased from the 45,000 existing in 1960 to 85,000 in 1970.

Neither the funding level envisioned in Kennedy's message nor the idea of federal staffing grants survived the 1963 session of Congress. The Community Mental Health Centers Act that President Kennedy finally signed on October 31, 1963 (Public Law 88-164) provided for a 3-year construction program (between July 1964 and July 1967) of $150 million, to permit funding of about 145 centers. States were encouraged to proceed with their planning efforts while the administration made further attempts to appropriate staffing monies. The staffing grants finally did emerge, but not until the summer of 1965, when President Lyndon Johnson signed amendments to the Community Mental Health Centers Act authorizing $73.5 million for this purpose (Public Law 89-105).

In 1970, Congress extended the CMHC program through fiscal year 1973 (Public Law 91-211), with significant modifications in several areas.[11] The federal share of construction costs of a center could not exceed two-thirds; however, in poverty areas, that share could be 90 percent. Special aid was also given for staffing costs in poverty areas, and such centers could begin without the five "essentials" for a center (inpatient, outpatient, partial hospitalization, emergency, and consultation and education services) and were given 18 months to achieve full operation. In addition, provision was made for special care of narcotics addicts and alcoholics and for services to children and adolescents. Reflecting an awareness that local resources could not easily pick up costs after 51 months, the previous limit for federal staffing support, the limit was extended to 8 years.

As the CMHCs began to be established, it became obvious that states and localities could not easily assume full funding of CMHCs. After Richard Nixon became president, it also became clear that many members of his administration wanted to phase out the CMHC program. This opposition may have arisen from an underlying antagonism toward psychiatry, as the medical director of the American Psychiatric Association suspected.[12] The ostensible reasons, though, were fear that an open-ended commitment by the federal government to mental health care would become too large a drain on tax resources and—a rather ingenious argument—that the CMHC program was intended as a demonstration program, that it had been outstandingly successful, and therefore it was now time to stop federal support and let state and local governments seize the opportunity to care more efficiently for the mentally ill. Here administration spokesmen attempted a form of bureaucratic jujitsu, agreeing with all the wonderful claims for CMHCs put forth by mental health professionals and their lay allies and then concluding that the program's federal support should be ended.[13]

The administration intensified its attacks on CMHCs as fiscal year 1973—and CMHC funding—approached an end. Criticism came from other quarters as well. For example, the Ralph Nader report on mental health services in America, *The Madness Establishment* (1974), found CMHCs responsible neither to the NIMH nor to the consumers and citizens in the community they allegedly served.[14] In this atmosphere, supporters of the CMHCs program were happy simply to sustain the program through continuing resolutions of Congress. At one point, in late 1974, a major expansion of the program (Public Law 93-45) was approved by the Democratic Congress but successfully vetoed by President Ford. In 1975, a newly elected Congress resumed efforts to enact a comprehensive program of health services, including CMHCs. As a compromise with the administration, the total sum of the second bill was about a half billion dollars less than that vetoed by President Ford. Specifically, CMHCs received an authorization for Fiscal Years 1976 and 1977 of about $218 million, a reduction of about a third. Again, the bill was vetoed, but Congress passed the bill over the veto in July 1975 (Public Law 94-63).

The amendments to the Community Mental Health Centers Act (Title III of Public Law 94-63) expanded the original five "essentials" to include, if not otherwise available, services to children and the aged and provide aftercare, transitional halfway houses, screening of potential state hospital patients, and services for alcohol and drug problems.[15] Centers were also required to be governed by a board of community residents if they received funds under this amended act for the first time. In response to criticisms that the centers were rarely evaluated for effectiveness of care, new requirements were written into the act to help ensure that adequate medical records were kept. The act was extened in 1978, concomitant with a new federal effort to study and evaluate mental health services. In that year, President Carter established a Commission on Mental Health to gather information and opinion on the range of issues involved in the care of the mentally ill.[16] From the voluminous findings and the final report of April 1978 came the basis for a further revision of the mental health centers bill, which was signed by President Carter on October 7, 1980 (Public Law 96-398).[17]

Under the new formula, 1981 funds would go to existing centers, but starting in 1982, the bulk of the money would be distributed in the form of grants to the states, targeted for certain "underserved" groups such as the elderly, severely disturbed children and adolescents, and the chronically mentally ill. Grants were also provided for programs emphasizing the prevention of mental illness and rape as well as services to rape victims. This legislation strengthened the authority of states over community mental health programs, which previously had dealt directly with the federal government. In addition, a "bill of rights" for mental patients was recommended to the states.

It became clear after nearly 20 years that the mental health centers program never reached the levels of success so eagerly anticipated by its proponents. One of its strongest advocates, the American Psychiatric Association, established a task force to examine it in 1971. Among other recommendations it made was a pointed suggestion that evaluation of the centers' impact on mental illness had been delayed long enough.[18] Criticisms have been made repeatedly that the program, intended for all the mentally ill, had overlooked children, adolescents, the elderly, and those discharged from state mental hospitals. Furthermore, the distribution of CMHCs has been faulted for being uneven and the operation of individual centers as free from reasonable control from above. The Nader report was particularly severe on this aspect of the program. Nevertheless, the ultimate wisdom of treating persons near their home, avoiding as much as possible new admissions to a state hospital, and the attraction to legislators of a program about which the disparate and highly competitive mental health professions could reach substantial agreement have all sustained the CMHCs. In spite of severe attacks, the program remains similar in many respects to that which President Kennedy enunciated in 1963.

One of the most serious central problems facing the CMHC in recent years has been sustaining staff and facilities on funds received only from the federal and local governments in the absence of third-party payments from medical programs like Medicare and Medicaid. Steps have been taken to obtain some of this general funding, and a specific requirement has been made in CMHC legislation that the centers do their best to obtain all appropriate reimbursement from these funds. (Public Law 94-63, Section 206).

MEDICARE AND MEDICAID (1965)

Certainly the greatest change in health care delivery in the history of the United States has been the provision of medical care by means of Medicare for the elderly and Medicaid for the disadvantaged. The controversy over federal health plans began in earnest in the 1930s when President Franklin Roosevelt anticipated some form of health insurance under the Social Security system (1935).[19] His plan was aborted following pressure from the American Medical Association (AMA) and others who feared excessive governmental interference in the delivery of health services. In 1945, immediately following World War II, President Truman reopend the debate with his proposal to establish national health insurance (NHI). Still, there continued to be strong opposition to a large-scale federal health program until the mid-1960s. It is possible to claim that the CMHC legislation of 1963 represented the first major step toward the Medicare and Medicaid programs of 1965. In this light, the AMA perceived the CMHC acts as the opening wedge and fought strongly against its staffing provisions. Staffing funds and the larger health plans were both delayed until the 89th Congress, the most Democratic dominated session since the Great Depression. When President Johnson signed Public Law 89-97 on June 30, 1965, a new era had begun in American medicine.

Part A of Title XVIII of the Social Security Act (Medicare) is often termed "compulsory" health insurance, as those who pay social security contributions during their working lifetimes cannot opt out of the health insurance payments. Part B of that title provides supplementary medical insurance, chiefly for physicians' bills is voluntary, and is paid for by monthly contributions only from the elderly.

Medicaid, Title XIX of the Social Security Act, has been a catchall provision for medical services to the indigent, paying for out-of-hospital and nursing-home care as well as some gaps in Medicare for the indigent aged. Both plans have dramatically raised federal expenditures for medical care and nursing homes and are now under close scrutiny in the search for ways to curb or cap the rapidly increasing costs. Some of the increased costs are the result of the improved health of the aged and indigent. Infant mortality has dropped, and the average life span has increased beyond the age of 65 since the two programs were instituted, so now there are more persons to be cared for.[20] Another impact on mental health services has been the shift of many elderly citizens from state mental hospitals to nursing homes, reducing the census in mental hospitals.

Besides Medicare and Medicaid, several federal programs dating back to 1946 have continued to have an impact on health care. These include the Hill-Burton hospital construction program established in 1946, supplemental security income (SSI), and monitoring programs such as professional standards review organizations (PSROs) and health systems agencies (HSAs), all intended to fill gaps or curb costs.

HILL-BURTON ACT OF 1946

The Hill-Burton legislation, passed shortly after World War II, was intended to promote the construction of general hospitals in rural areas. Federal subsidies, limited to one-third of construction costs, were channeled through specially established Hill-Burton agencies, usually the state health department. Nearly $3.2 billion of federal funds were expended through the program between 1946 and 1968.

By 1965, the program had been expanded to include community health facilities and modernization of hospitals and to aid urban as well as rural installations. Hill-Burton funds were disbursed for over two decades to those who requested them and met certain construction standards; there was no requirement that hospital delivery systems change or that overall policies for hospital distribution be developed and followed.[21]

With the expansion of health care through Medicare and Medicaid came increased medical costs. In the early 1970s, the federal government took steps to gain some control over hospitals as well as individual providers such as physicians and ancillary professions. To attain authority over hospitals, HSAs were proposed for each state, while physicians' fees and hospital admission practices were targeted for scrutiny by PSROs.

Both of these have attracted considerable controversy over their effectiveness, or lack thereof, in accomplishing stated goals and over the point at which control turns into excessive federal interference. Powerful groups such as the American Hospital Association and the AMA have attempted to mold legislation so as not to encroach on what they consider essential processes of both institutions.

HEALTH SYSTEMS AGENCIES

On January 3, 1975, President Ford signed legislation (Public Law 93-641) revising the direction of the nearly three-decade-old Hill-Burton hospital construction program. New construction now would be limited to areas of recent population growth. In addition, the program was to concentrate on hospital modernization. This legislation also established a new national network of planning agencies, HSA's, charged with the task of preventing unnecessary development of hospitals, establishing priorities for development of needed facilities and services, and monitoring uses of federal funds in their particular areas.[21] Controversy has followed the program ever since. Conservative critics of federally inspired health planning were especially concerned that competition would be as stifled as it was in public utilities. Others also warned that it would be difficult to achieve innovation as well as reduction in costs.

PROFESSIONAL STANDARDS REVIEW ORGANIZATIONS

Equally controversial is another federal plan designed to bring some order and efficiency into the care received by Medicare and Medicaid patients. Enacted in 1972 (Public Law 92-603), this program gave physicians until January 1, 1976 to organize themselves into 200 review areas. Initially, the PSRO system was strongly attacked by the AMA leadership for interfering in the doctor–patient relationship; later, however, the AMA came to hail it as a "successful cooperative venture between government and the medical profession." On the other hand, the federal government and Congress have had second thoughts about the value of PSRO's. The Congressional Budget Office argued in 1979 that there were "no net savings" in PSRO reviews of Medicare during 1977, the latest year in which data were studied. At one point, President Carter even recommended that the program be terminated. It has survived, though, while the conflict over any savings from it has continued. Proponents stress that even if the savings are small, improving the quality of medical care and raising physicians' consciousness about the appropriateness of certain treatments and procedures are worth the cost (about $150 million each fiscal year). Again, conservative critics of federal activity in health care find PSROs cumbersome, enmeshed in reporting, and relying for their justification on the assurance of quality medical care, which is very difficult to measure.[23]

The creation of these cost-containment procedures and plans as well as arguments to scrap them arise from the enormous growth in health costs. In 1940, the percentage of the gross national product (GNP) expended on health was 4.1

percent. It had grown to 5.2 percent by 1960; 7.2 percent by 1970; by October 1977, it had reached 8.8 percent.[24] The Medicaid program is one cause for the increase in GNP devoted to health care. In 1967, the first full year of implementation, total federal and state costs were $1.9 billion. By 1979, the total reached $21.7 billion, with the states paying $9.9 billion of that amount.[25] The states have suffered serious financial problems not just because costs are rising but also because most are prohibited from deficit spending, i.e., their annual budgets must balance (unlike the federal budget). When medical costs rise, other programs must be reduced.

Efforts to provide adequate mental health services to previously underserved populations ushered in many of the great programs that now dominate health care delivery in the United States. Mental health services may have had an easier time obtaining federal support because they were usually considered to be more than a local responsibility; and mental illness seemed a strange and catastrophic event, relegating the sufferer to a long stay in an isolated state hospital.

Therefore, some of the criticisms of a national health insurance program could not be made as easily against mental health care at the community level.

Still, as general health care systems began to develop, the question of where the mental health professions fit in remains. Some of the same reasons that allowed the CMHC program to be perceived as not in the medical mainstream continue to complicate the provision of psychiatric care to those who would benefit from it. The outcome of current controversies over health care and costs will profoundly affect the practice of psychiatry and other health professions, but the ultimate result is still uncertain.

REFERENCES

1. Musto DF: Whatever happened to 'community mental health'? Public Interest 39:53–79, 1975
2. Stevens R, Stevens R: Welfare Medicine in America; a case study of Medicaid New York, Free Press, 1974
3. Menninger WC: Lessons from military psychiatry for civilian psychiatry. Mental Hygiene 30:571–589, 1946
4. Ridenour N: Mental Health in the United States: A Fifty-year History. Cambridge, Mass, Harvard University Press, 1961, pp 51–61.
5. Musto DF: A short history of orthopsychiatry, in Shore MF, Mannino FV (eds): Mental Health and Social Change: 50 Years of Orthopsychiatry. New York, AMS Press, 1977, pp 10–11
6. Brand JL: The national mental health act of 1946: a retrospect. Bull Hist Med 39: 231–244, 1965
7. Ewalt JR: Birth of the community mental health movement, in Barton WE, Sanborn CJ (eds): Assessment of the Community Mental Health Movement. Lexington, Mass, Lexington Books, 1977, pp 13–20
8. Joint Commission on Mental Illness and Health: Action for Mental Health. New York, Basic Books, 1961
9. Ridenour, Mental Health in the United States, p 137
10. Kennedy JF: Message from the president of the U.S. relative to mental illness and mental retardation. Document No 58, Rept, 88th Cong, 1st sess February 5, 1963
11. Congressional Quarterly Almanac, 1970. Washington, DC, Congressional Quarterly, Inc. 1971, pp 188–189.
12. Sabshin M: Politics and the stalled revolution. Psychiatr Ann 7:541–542, 1977
13. Congressional Quarterly Almanac 1973. Washington, DC, Congressional Quarterly, Inc. p 490; 1974, p 415
14. Nader R: Preface, in Chu FD, Trotter S (eds): The Madness Establishment. New York, Grossman, 1974, p xxiii
15. Congressional Quarterly Almanac, 1975.

Washington, DC, Congressional Quarterly, Inc., pp. 591–593
16. President's Commission on Mental Health: Report to the President, vol. 1. Washington, DC, Government Printing Office, 1978
17. Congressional Quarterly Almanac, 1980, Washington, DC, Congressional Quarterly, Inc., pp. 430–434
18. A.P.A. Task Force on Community Mental Health Centers: Research aspects of community mental health centers. Am J Psychiatry 127:993–998, 1971
19. Burrow JG: AMA: Voice of American Medicine. Baltimore, Md, Johns Hopkins Press, 1963, p 194ff
20. Weintraub B: Don't throw out the baby with the Medicaid-Medicare bathwater. *New York Times,* 12 July 1981, pp 22, Sect E.
21. Stevens R, Stevens R: Welfare medicine pp 43–44
22. Congressional Quarterly Almanac, 1974, Washington, DC, Congressional Quarterly, Inc., pp. 405–407
23. Demkovich LE: The physicians' peer review program—does it cost more than it saves? National Journal 12:733–736, 1980
24. Zelten RA: Consequences of increased third-party payments for health care services. Ann Am Acad Pol Soc Sci 443:29–30, 1979
25. Demkovich LE: For states squeezed by medicaid costs, the worst crunch is still to come. National Journal 13: 44–49, 1981

SUGGESTED READINGS

Barton WE: Administration in Psychiatry. Springfield, Ill, Thomas, 1962

Feldman S: The Administration of Mental Health Services. Springfield, Ill, Thomas, 1973

Feldman S, Goldstein C, Offutt J: Mental Health Administration: An Annotated Bibliography. Washington, DC, Dept. Health, Education and Welfare, Government Printing Office, 1978

PART II

Psychiatric Services

Seymour R. Kaplan, M.D.

4

The Formal Structures of Psychiatric Institutions

The formal structures of psychiatric organizations with a particular focus on a comparison between public psychiatric institutions and psychiatric services in the private voluntary institutions will be discussed in this chapter. Figures of representative organizations will be used to illustrate graphically their formal structures. Although the administration of psychiatric institutions involves complex processes that are not indicated by the institutions' formal structures, structures are the foundation for the variety of informal arrangements that constitute the decision-making processes of the institutions' psychiatric services. The illustration of governance structures will be considered first.

GOVERNANCE STRUCTURES

Governance structures are defined by this author as the external "bodies" (state, county, or municipal legislatures and their delegated agencies in the public sector and chartered boards in the private sector) that are legally authorized and responsible for the hospitals, departments, clinics, or centers that they sponsor to operate psychiatric services; they are not, in this context, regulatory, monitoring, or accreditation agencies.

The governance structures of public psychiatric organizations have characteristic differences from the governance structures of private psychiatric organizations. Private organizations, in turn, have a different governance structure if the services are proprietary (for profit) or voluntary (not for profit), and if the services are in general hospitals or in psychiatric hospitals. There may be other differences in the governance of public or private psychiatric organizations if, for example, they have an affiliation with a university medical center. Figure 4-1 illustrates the relationships of the governance structures of the Department of Psychiatry of the Albert Einstein College of Medicine, which, in 1970, had contractual authority over the psychiatric services (or over the academic appointment of psychiatric professionals) of two muncipal general hospitals (the Bronx Munici-

The figures in this chapter are reprinted from Kaplan SR, Roman M: The Organizational Delivery of Mental Health Services: The Lincoln Hospital Experience. New York, Praeger Publishers, 1973. With permission.

pal Hospital Center and the Lincoln Municipal Hospital); of two community mental health centers (the Lincoln CMHC and the Sound View Throgs Neck CMHC); of two state hospitals (the Bronx Psychiatric Center and the Bronx Children's Psychiatric Center); and of a private voluntary general hospital (the Montefiore Hospital and Medical Center). Except for private proprietary psychiatric hospitals, Figure 4-1 contains examples of the major institutional structures under which psychiatric services are provided.

Governance of Public Psychiatric Institutions

The governance bodies of public psychiatric institutions are the state, county, or municipal legislatures whose policies are implemented by their respective delegated agencies. The directors of these agencies (commissioners) are political appointees of the elected executive (governors, county executives, mayors) of the political areas over which the legislative bodies have authority. A number of collateral governmental agencies, in addition to a mental health agency, may have authority in the implementation of legislative policies that affect psychiatric services. There are top-level state agencies whose authorization is required for the allocation of specific budget appropriations to state psychiatric hospitals, e.g., for specific personnel lines, for funds for facility maintenance, and for the purchase of supplies.

The authority of state agencies over state psychiatric hospital budgets has become more complex in the last 10 years. For example, the functions of the commissioner of mental health of the New York State Department of Mental Hygiene, as illustrated by his line of authority in Figure 4-1, was relatively uncomplicated and comprehensive in policies concerning state psychiatric hospitals. The major other body that exerted informal influence over policies was the group of state hospital directors (previously called superintendents); that was in 1970. There no longer is a Department of Mental Hygiene. (It is now subsumed under a tripartite body with separate authority over programs for the mentally retarded, for substance abuse, and for psychiatric services).

More importantly, the State Office of the Budget has major policy authority over financial matters concerning psychiatric institutions, and the authority of the director of state mental hospitals (now state "psychiatric centers") has been radically altered by changes in the standards and in the methods by which they are appointed. The residual authority for state hospital policies now rests, for the most part, with the director of the Regional Offices of the State Department of Mental Health that have since been established.

In other states, the authority of mental health commissioners has been subsumed by subordinating their offices (and offices of other state commissioners), under the umbrella of the office of a secretary of public welfare or public services. In these states, budget and personnel offices for various public agencies are under the authority of the secretary, who usually also has the direct or indirect authority in the appointment of the commissioners.

The function of the commissioner of mental health for New York City regarding the operation of municipal public mental health services in 1970 (Figure 4-1) was similar to the subordinate role of state commissioners to an umbrella agency. At the time, the New York City Department of Mental Health, as well as the Department of Hospitals and the Department of Health and their respective commissioners, were subordinate to the New York City Health and Hospitals Corporation and its president. There was an additional state-level authority over

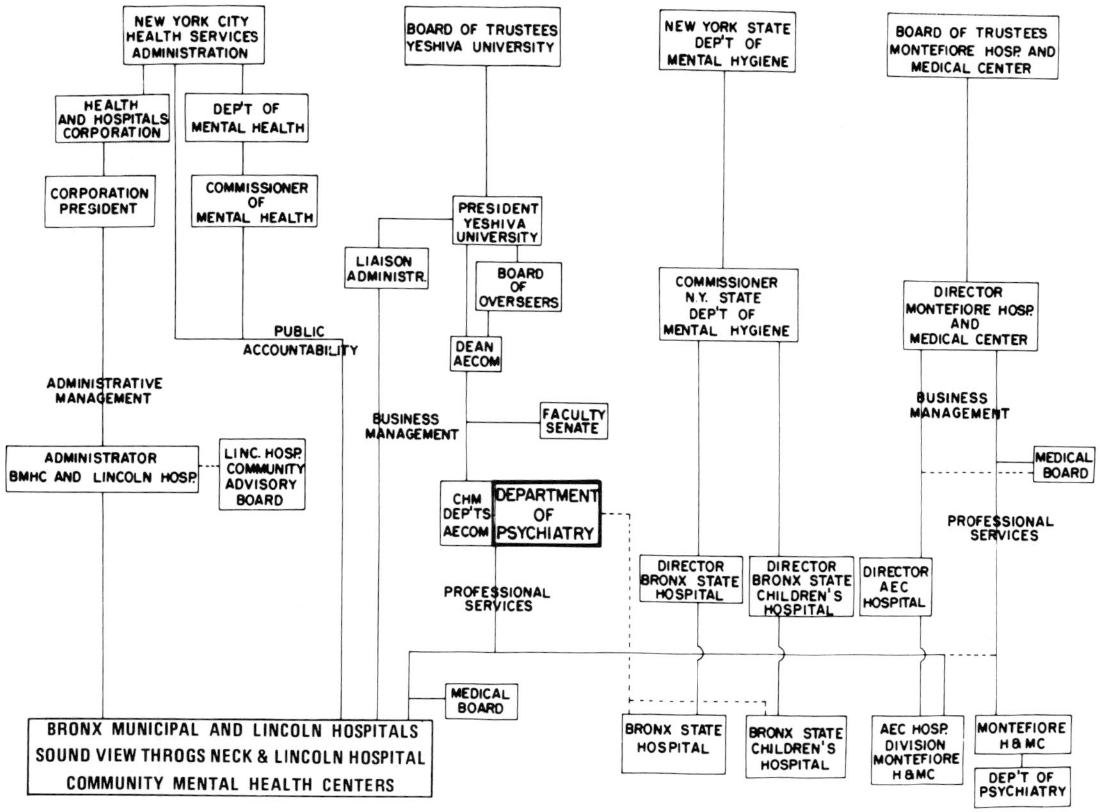

Figure 4-1. Structural relationship of public and private institutions and boards to the department of psychiatry of the Albert Einstein College of Medicine (1970).

the New York City Department of Mental Health due to the separate arrangement for state matching funds for the city's psychiatric services. This authority now is exercised by the director of the Regional Office of the State Department of Mental Health for the area that includes New York City.

The boards of directors (governors) of state (city, county) psychiatric institutions, whose members are appointed to the boards, function in an advisory capacity. Although the influence of the boards on the governance of public psychiatric institutions varies, often dependent on the informal political contacts of its members, generally their presence is not evident except when a crisis gains the attention of the public media.

Governance of Private Voluntary (Not-For-Profit) Psychiatric Institutions*

By contrast, the boards of directors (trustees) have a central role in the governance of private voluntary psychiatric services, as illustrated in Figure 4-1 by the unilateral authority of the board of trustees over the Montefiore Hospital and Medical Center. As in the instance of Montefiore, the majority of private voluntary psychiatric services in this country are in general hospitals (see Chapter 5), although there are a number of well-established voluntary psychiatric hospitals (see Chapter 7).

Private voluntary hospitals are authorized to provide services under a charter granted by the state legislatures. The charter requires the formation of incorporated boards whose bylaws must include procedures by which the boards will oversee the operations of the hospitals. The bylaws should contain information concerning the membership of the boards of directors, the procedures for the selection of the chairmen and other officers of the boards, how often they will meet, and the arrangements for maintaining records of the boards' proceedings. The boards of directors also are responsible for the formation of medical boards, composed of physicians who utilize the facilities of the hospitals.

The actual exercise of the authority granted by charters over the operations of the hospitals varies. In some instances, the members of boards of directors take an active role in the formulation of hospital policies. In other instances, they defer to the decisions of the directors of the hospitals, who are appointed by the boards of directors. The members of the medical boards may also exercise influence over hospital policies. Their authority is enhanced in areas in which a surplus of beds makes the financial stability of the hospitals dependent on the utilization of their facilities by the attending physicians.

In summary, Figure 4-1 has been presented to illustrate the governance of public psychiatric institutions, which involves complex multiauthority superordinate structures. Figure 4-1 also has been used to illustrate that the governance of private voluntary psychiatric institutions (or of psychiatric services in general voluntary hospitals) is under the unilateral authority of a state-chartered board of trustees (directors). In the following section, the formal (internal) administrative structures of the business and medical services of public and private psychiatric institutions will be graphically illustrated.

* The governance of private proprietary (for profit) psychiatric institutions is discussed in Chapter 7. They have provided a small percentage of psychiatric services until recently, but the devlopment of private-for-profit hospital chains may change this situation.

ADMINISTRATIVE STRUCTURES

Administrative Structures of Public Psychiatric Institutions

The Administration of the Business Office

The structures for the administration of the business affairs in the typical state psychiatric hospital reflect the structure of the governance bodies and their delegated state agencies. The conduct of business activities, e.g., salary levels, personnel and labor–management practices, and plant and facility maintenance work, must directly conform to the policies of the governance bodies and to the standards established to implement the policies by the delegated state agencies. The structures for the internal administration of business affairs in the state psychiatric hospital, therefore, are organized to meet the payroll, personnel, and facility maintenance regulations of the external policy-making structures. The traditional pyramid structure of bureaucratic organizations is used in Figure 4-2 to illustrate the administrative structures of the business office in a typical state psychiatric hospital.

The Administration of Professional Services

In Figure 4-2, the administrative structures for psychiatric services are also represented by the bureaucratic pyramid structure. Although the directors of state psychiatric hospitals have some discretionary authority over specific psychiatric services and the allocation of staff to the services, decisions of the legislative bodies and their delegated state agencies dictate overall policies about the number and type of patients admitted to state hospitals; the overall number and type of medical and ancillary staff to be allocated to each hospital; and the extent of aftercare services provided patients upon discharge. These constraints, along with mandated medical legal procedures, result in the hierarchical organization of medical and ancillary staff, illustrated by Figure 4-2.* Moreover, since medical staff members are salaried, they do not have the autonomy of the attending medical staff in private voluntary psychiatric institutions.

Administrative Structures of Private Voluntary General Hospitals

The Administration of the Business Office

The structures for the administration of the business affairs in the larger private voluntary general hospitals in recent years also have taken on the characteristics of bureaucratic pyramid structures, although for nonbureaucratic reasons. Max Weber introduced the bureaucratic concept in response to the need for orderly and standardized methods of conducting the routine daily business operations in large

*Variations of this structure in public psychiatric services may occur when there are other governance bodies, such as a university medical center, that are able to influence the arrangements of some of the medical staff. As illustrated in Figure 4-1, the Department of Psychiatry of the Albert Einstein College of Medicine had a contractual arrangement with the New York State Department of Mental Hygiene that gave the department a role in the recruitment of some of the psychiatric staff. These staff members held faculty appointments in the department in which they conducted teaching and research activities, for which they received added compensation.

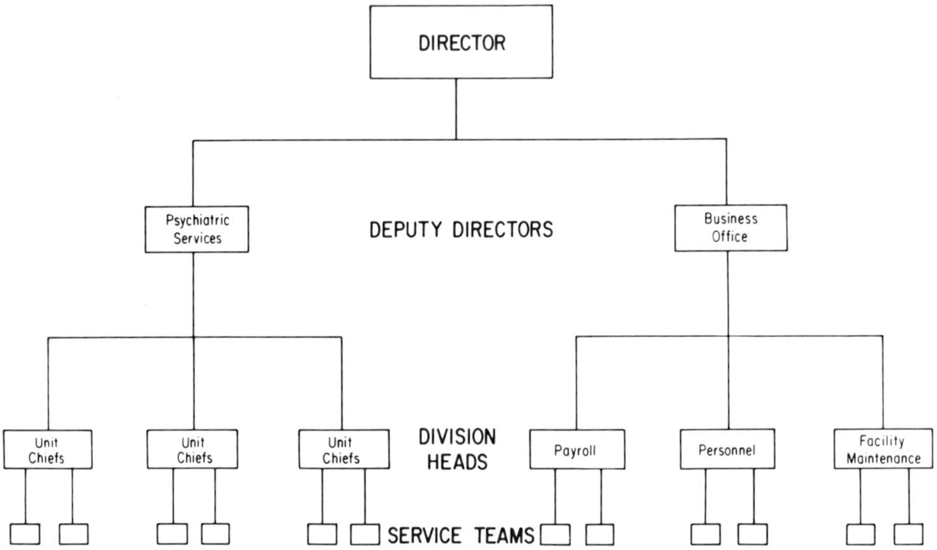

Figure 4-2. Model of a pyramid organizational structure.

public institutions. Many of the voluntary general hospitals have become large enterprises. For example, the operating budget of Montefiore Hospital and Medical Center, which has about 1800 inpatient beds and a staff of several thousand, is about $200 million. Unlike the situation in public hospitals, whose deficits are gururanteed by tax-levied public funds, private hospitals that cannot pay their bills are forced to close their doors, a not uncommon occurrence these days.

In response to this fiscal reality, reinforced recently by the prospective method used by third-party payers to determine hospital reimbursement rates, the business activities of voluntary hospitals have become increasingly standardized. The resultant formal structures for the administration of their business offices, although more complex than illustrated for state psychiatric hospitals, essentially are organized along hierarchical lines. Figure 4-3 illustrates the chain of command in a typical large private voluntary general hospital.

The boards of directors of voluntary general hospitals delegate to the directors of hospitals (medical centers) the power to establish defined administrative lines of authority for those activities for which the hospital has fiscal responsibility. These activities include the costs of providing room and board, nursing, laboratory and other ancillary services (the so-called hotel services), as well as the salaries of the interns and residents. In the larger complex private voluntary hospitals, these activities also include the costs of salaries for full-time physicians, i.e., the director of professional services, the chiefs of service, and ward chiefs (Fig. 4-3). These activities do not, however, include any salaries for the voluntary attending physicians, whose financial arrangements with their patients are independent of the hospital's business affairs.

The Administration of Professional Services

The general voluntary nonteaching hospital.—The autonomous role of the attending physician. The literature about the organization of professional services in recent years, particularly the literature about psychiatric services, has been

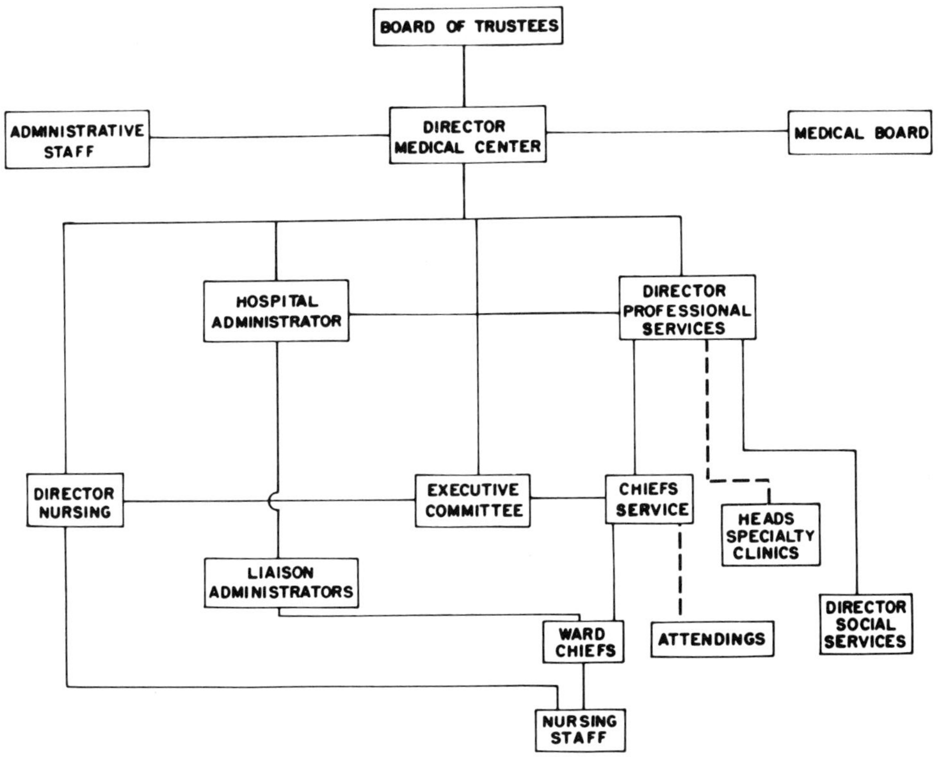

Figure 4-3. Administrative organization of a large voluntary medical center.

concerned primarily with state psychiatric hospitals or the psychiatric services in voluntary general hospitals in which many of the professionals hold full-time salaried positions. Their relationship to the administrative hierarchy of the institutions in which they function, however, is entirely different from that of voluntary attending physicians, who comprise the vast majority of physicians who provide medical services in hospitals.

Figure 4-4 has been constructed to illustrate the relationship of the voluntary attending physician to the administrative structures of a general voluntary nonteaching hospital. Figure 4-4 shows a broken line to the attending ward physicians and to the medical consultants to indicate their autonomy from the authority of the hospital's administration. The attending physicians, in fact, are not part of the formal organization of the hospital, although they are subject to the regulations contained in the bylaws of the medical board. Their voluntary use of the hospital's facilities for the treatment of their patients is the cardinal feature of a voluntary hospital. Where there is a surplus of beds in a community, the quality of the medical services and the financial solvency of the voluntary general hospital is dependent on the attending physicians' voluntary selective use of the hospital's facilities.

Figure 4-5 has been included to illustrate the similar autonomous role of the attending physician-psychiatrist in a general voluntary nonteaching hospital in which there is an "open" psychiatric service. (By "open," we refer to psychiatric inpatient services in which the admitting physician attends to the treatment of his patients.) Figure 4-5 also includes the presence of additional staff on psychiatric services, i.e., occupational therapists and psychiatric social workers.

—*The inverted pyramid structure.* Although it is tangential to this discussion, it

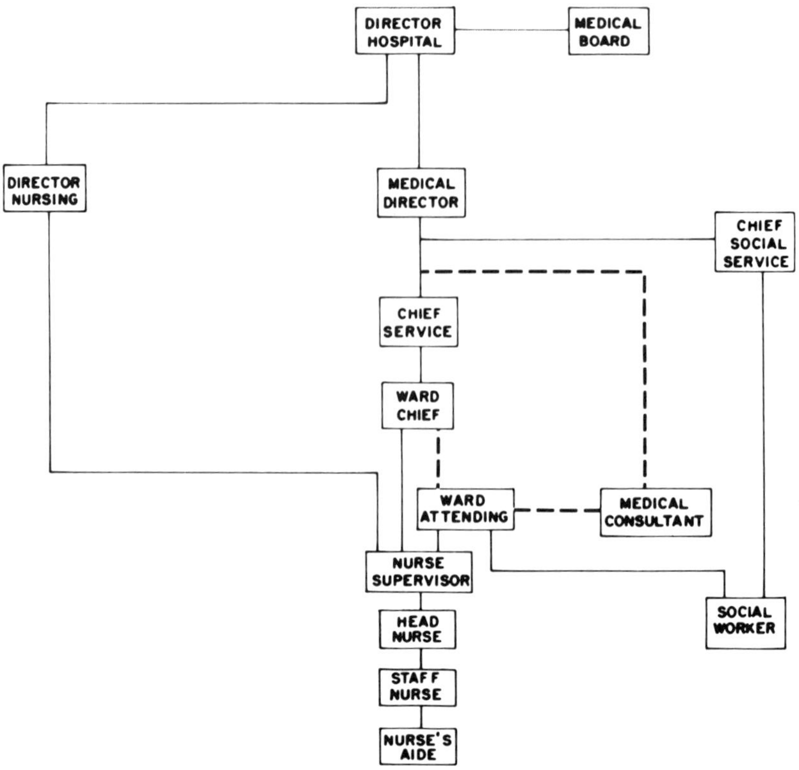

Figure 4-4. Professional organization of a typical medical ward in a general voluntary nonteaching hospital.

is of some importance to note the position of the staff nurse in the administrative structures illustrated in Figures 4-4 and 4-5. The nursing staff is by far the largest group of professionals under the administrative authority of the formal hospital hierarchy. (Other disciplines, in addition to the full-time salaried physicians, such as social workers, psychologists, and occupational therapists, also fall under the hospital's formal administrative structures, although their number is quite small by comparison to the nursing staff.) The position of the staff nurse is noted here in the context of the administrative structures. The position is subordinate to a number of professional superiors (the hospital's nursing hierarchy and the medical hierarchy, including the attending physicians and consultants), all of whom have authority over each staff nurse. This administrative structure, with multiple superiors, has been referred to as the "inverted pyramid" structure, in contrast to the "one person, one boss" of the typical pyramid structure. The position of the staff nurse, subordinate to a complex multiauthority administrative structure, is one of the major issues that underlies the problems of recruitment and retention of competent nursing staff.

The psychiatric service in a general voluntary teaching hospital The administration of psychiatric services in a general voluntary teaching hospital has a complex structure as a result of the presence of teaching faculty and psychiatric residents (and other students) and the presence of a range of supportive profes-

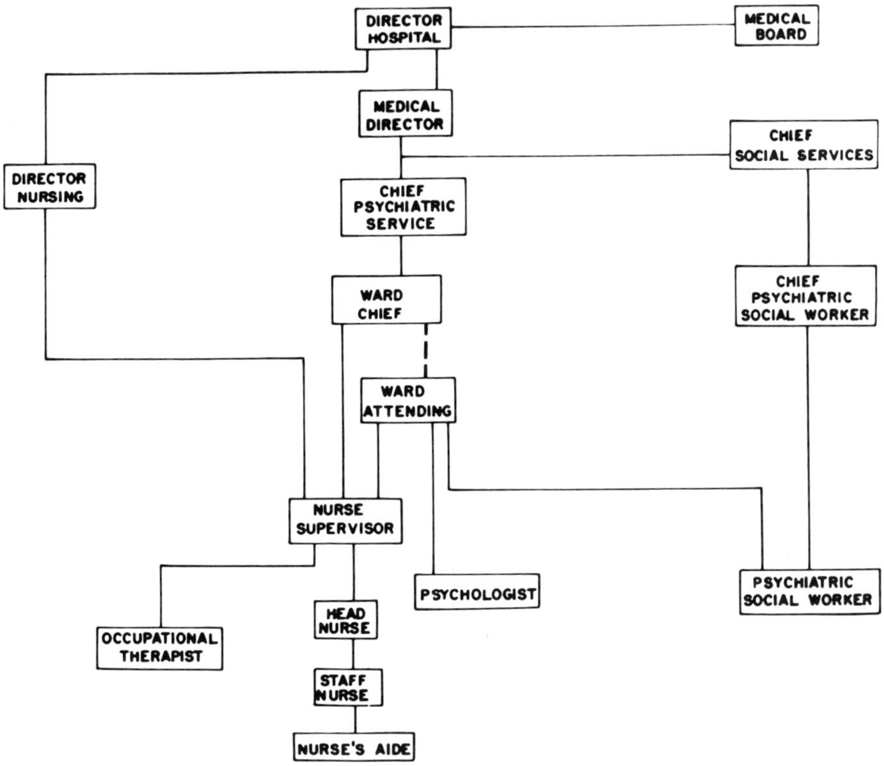

Figure 4-5. The professional organization of a typical psychiatric ward in a general voluntary nonteaching hospital.

sional staff (psychologists, occupational and recreational therapists, in addition to social work staff). This complex structure is illustrated in Figure 4-6.

The existence of multiple professional superiors, with authority over the "line" staff (residents, social workers, occupational/recreational therapists, as well as the nurses), represents a more complex example of the "inverted pyramid structure." The presence of a multiple-authority superstructure, which is typical of the structures on teaching psychiatric services, is particularly contrary to the objectives of an integrated program for the management of patient care. The nurses and other staff, who spend the most time with patients, have difficulty in communicating with one another and in obtaining coherent advice about patient care from psychiatrists and other senior professionals under such diffuse administrative structures. For this reason, there have been concerted efforts to develop models for the administrative structures of psychiatric services that would enable a multidisciplinary staff to function as an integrated and effective "team." The administrative structure illustrated in Figure 4-7 is an example of a model to facilitate the teamwork of an inpatient multidisciplinary team. This model is based on the concept of a matrix organization, described in Chapters 6 and 11.

It will be noted in Figure 4-7, as compared to Figure 4-6, that there is a reduction in the multiple professional positions with direct-line authority over the team members. For example, the clinical authority in Figure 4-6 of the director of the inpatient service and senior attendings, the chief psychologist, and chief social

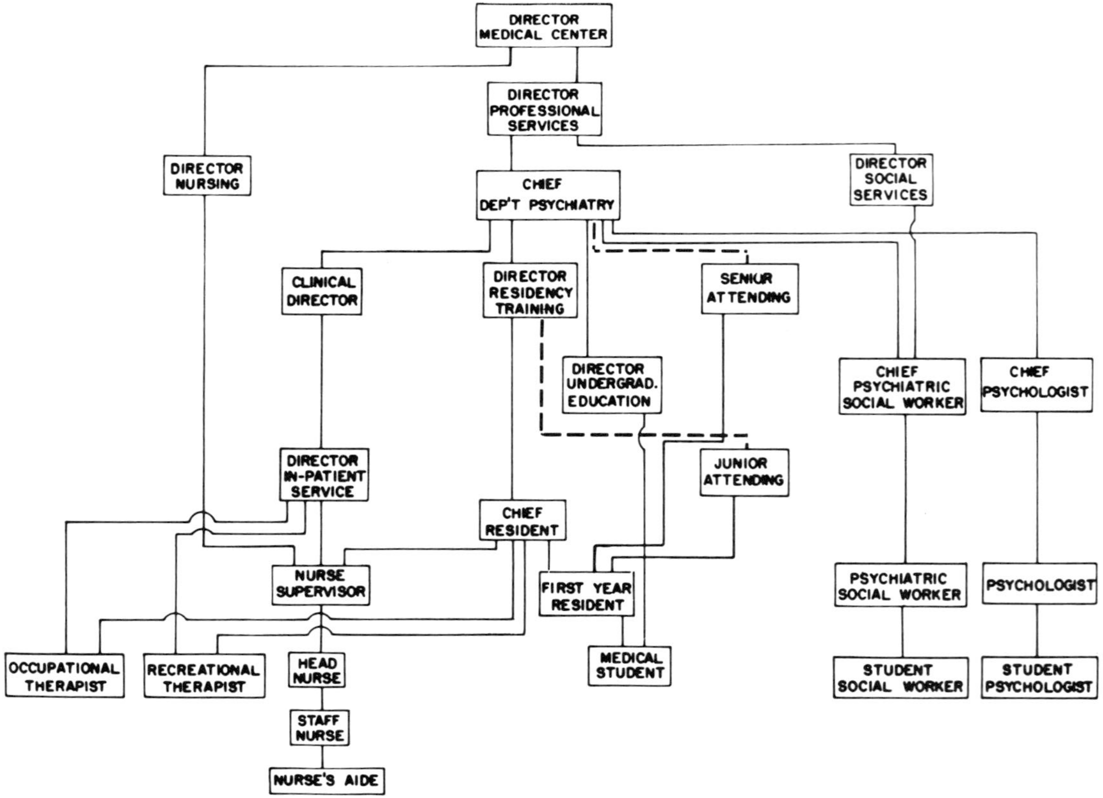

Figure 4-6. The professional organization of a psychiatric ward in a large general voluntary teaching center.

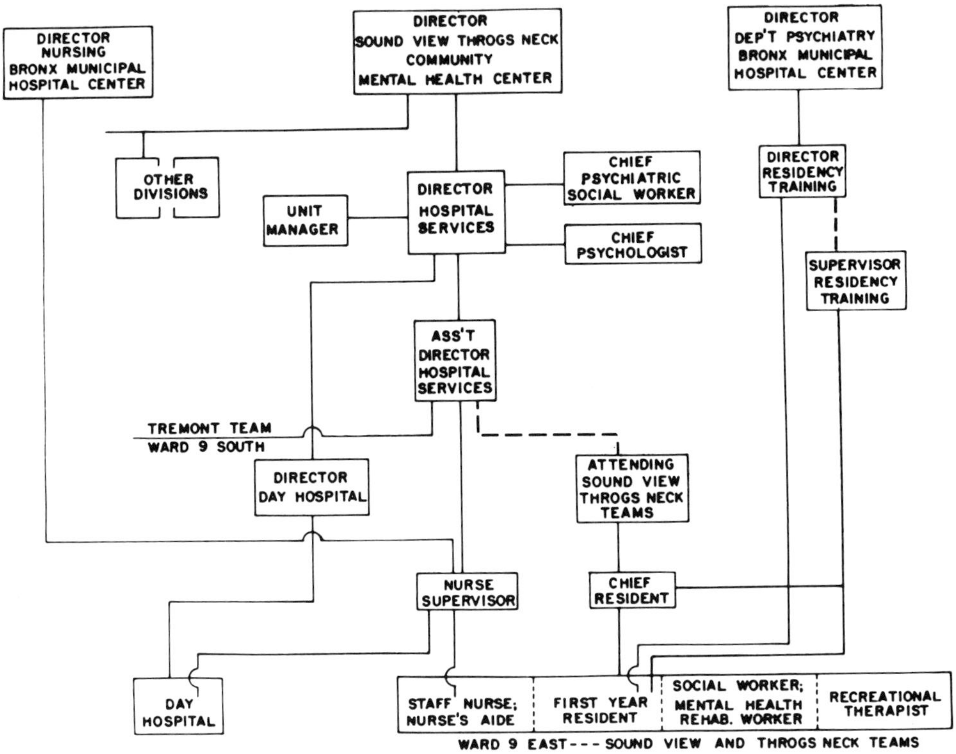

Figure 4-7. The professional organization of a psychiatric in-patient team in a general municipal teaching hospital (the Sound View Throgs Neck Community Mental Health Center model).

worker are in Figure 4-7 delegated to the position of the clinical team leader, as indicated by the position of the chief resident. There is a detailed discussion of the job description, performance standards, and criteria for evaluating the standards of the functions of the clinical team leader in Chapter 14.

Administrative structures of federally supported community mental health centers The formal structures for the administration of federally supported CMHCs embody the characteristics of the psychiatric institutions described above, according to the public or private (voluntary) status of their sponsoring institutions. There are, in addition, unique aspects of their formal structure as a result of the unusual nature of the federal public health laws (i.e., Public Law 88-164 and Public Law 94-63), under whose mandates the support for CMHC are authorized.

The unusual nature of these public health laws, particularly those of 1963 when the Federal Community Mental Health Act was passed, is that they delineated specific services and program structures that the health institutions, to which funds were granted, were mandated to provide. That is, previously, federal legislative bodies would decide which health categories would be supported and the amount of funds to be appropriated, but they did not dictate specific service requirements for each grant recipient. Figure 4-8 illustrates how these legislated requirements are reflected in the formal superordinate structures of a hypothetical federally supported CMHC.

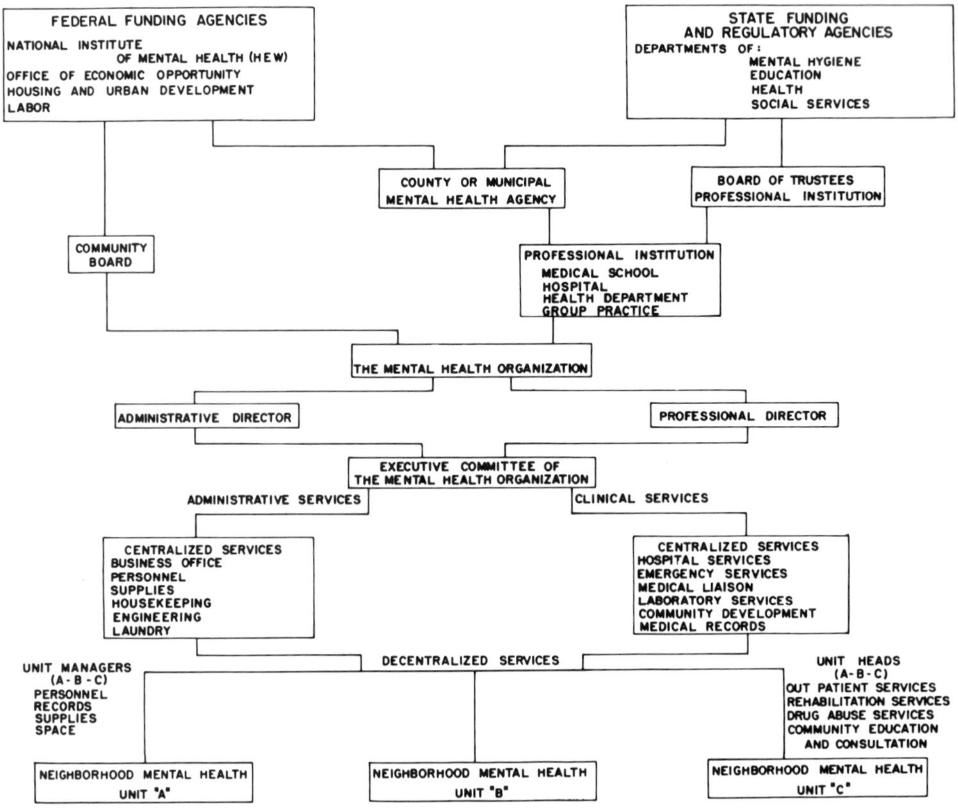

Figure 4-8. Hypothetical relationship of a community board to a decentralized mental health organization.

If the reader combines Figures 4-1 and 4-7 so that the federal agencies* are structurally superior to the New York City Health Services Administration, the result will represent the actual multiauthority superordinate relationships that existed for the Sound View Throgs Neck and Lincoln Hospital Community Mental Health Centers in 1970. One change in Figure 4-8, as the result of the regulations in Public Law 94-63, passed in 1975, is that federal grants awarded to governmental agencies were exempt from the mandates concerning community boards. That is, the New York City Department of Mental Health, as is the case in other municipalities, was the actual recipient of the grant, which it subcontracted to the Albert Einstein College of Medicine for the staffing of the Sound View Throgs Neck and Lincoln Community Mental Health Centers.

Figures 4-1 and 4-8 illustrate the complex formal administrative structures under which CMHCs operate. In Chapter 8, Ruiz and Tourlentes provide added details concerning the similarities and differences of the functions of CMHCs under public as compared to private sponsorship.

*Other federal agencies besides the National Institute of Mental Health are included in Figure 4-8 to indicate that some CMHCs received grant support for programs that were incorporated in their center. For example, Model Cities programs supported by HUD provided neighborhood health services and Office of Economic Opportunity (OEO)-sponsored specialized training programs.

Roger Peele, M.D.
John O. Lipkin, M.D.

5

Public Mental Hospitals

Although public mental hospitals have moved off the center stage in American psychiatry, they still provide invaluable services to one half million mentally ill patients annually. This chapter summarizes the public mental hospital's history, governance, organization, staffing, funding, programs, management-clinical interface, constraints, and future prospects. Veterans Administration (VA) hospitals will be considered separately.

HISTORY

The first public mental hospital opened in Virginia at Williamsburg in 1773, but only a small number were established over the next 70 years. In 1843, Dorothea Lynde Dix (1802–1887) began her lobbying, which resulted in the building of public mental hospitals in 15 or more states, in Canada, and in the District of Columbia. In 1844, the Association of Medical Superintendents of American Institutes for the Insane (later the American Psychiatric Association) was formed and provided professional impetus to the growth of the public mental hospital, which was intended to be of moderate size and emphasize moral treatment.[1] Over succeeding decades, this changed. Hospitals grew in size, the staff-to-patient ratios fell, and socioeconomic conditions and attitudes—"You can't treat the Irish"—produced impersonal, regimented institutions.[2] The humanistic optimism of moral therapy was replaced by a "scientific" focus on brain disease, pessimistic nihilism, and a Darwinistic attitude that the "unfit" needed a permanent protective asylum. By the 1880s, exposés and calls for reform were common, but public mental hospitals were not able to reverse the trends and problems over ensuing decades.

The seeds for change in American psychiatry were symbolized by five events in 1909. Freud visited Clark University; Healy established the first child guidance clinic in Chicago; the first psychopathic hospital was built in Ann Arbor; the National Mental Health Association was formed; and Adolf Meyer suggested that

Dr. Martin Giller and Mr. Robert Furano of the staff of Saint Elizabeths Hospital improved this text.

public mental hospitals move out into the communities to assist the mentally ill who lived there. Although there were exceptions, these five events symbolized 20th-century trends that bypassed state mental hospitals and coalesced a half century later in a call not to reform state hospitals but to abolish them. Mental illness was seen as prolonged and aggravated by public mental hospitals ("institutionalism"). In 1958, the president of the American Psychiatric Association, the organization that began as the Association of Medical Superintendents, called for the closing of public mental hospitals.[3] In the 1960s, this negativism toward public mental hospitals conjoined with community psychiatry's positive call for treatment of the mentally ill in their communities. Although some mental hospitals managed to ride the crest of community psychiatry through using Sivadon's unitization (see below), developed day treatment programs, established clinics, or provided consultation to community agencies, about half the public mental hospitals still provided only inpatient services.

The number of mentally ill in state and county psychiatric hospitals peaked in 1955 at 558,922; by the late 1970s, the number of inpatients had decreased to nearly 150,000. In addition, public mental hospitals reduced their average inpatient stays for adults to 2–3 weeks, and readmissions began to exceed new admissions by a ratio of two to one. Despite the huge reduction in beds, occupancy rates of about 90 percent have remained higher than in private psychiatric hospitals or in general hospital psychiatric wards.[4]

By 1977, there were about 300 public mental hospitals. Closings have taken place infrequently, and two decades after the call for their abolition, these 300 hospitals were receiving a total budget in excess of $3 billion annually.[4]

GOVERNANCE

Governmental Bodies

The policy-making authority for the governance of public mental hospitals rests with the legislative arm of government. The executive branch of the government and the bureaucratic structures it creates have the responsibility and authority to implement legislative policies. This statement contains many troubling features for public mental hospitals. The executive bureaucracy often imposes on hospitals a *modus operandi* that makes it difficult to provide optimum services for the patients.

Characteristically, executive structures are rarely constant and stable. Governors or mayors usually change every 4 years, and it takes time for them to get their political teams assembled and working as a group. As soon as the entire hierarchy is in place and working together to carry out major initiatives with the public mental hospitals, they may be on their way out. Mental health commissioners, for example, often serve only 2–3 years. With this inherent turnover, it is difficult for hospitals and their governance ever to see through a plan or policy to complete fruition. Psychiatric administrators can thus often "wait out" unsatisfactory initiatives, but this process is very frustrating when plans are in the patients' best interests.

In the legislative bodies, whether a city council or a state assembly, the patterns are similar. Within the legislature, there will be an oversight committee that focuses on health, social welfare, or some other broad category that includes public mental hospitals. Oversight or monitoring functions are often by a committee separate from the one that addresses the hospital's budget. Oversight tends to include actions like changes in commitment laws, investigations of hospitals, and so on. The roles of such committees may be dormant for extended periods; then something happens—too often a negative event such as a media exposé—and the committee suddenly becomes active. On the other hand, budget committees will address their function on a regular basis every year or every 2 years. Budget hearings can wander into any issue that may interest the legislators.[5]

Besides the legislative and executive arms of the government, the judiciary is another key dimension in the governance of public mental hospitals. Its power can control the quality and quantity of health services for involuntary and forensic patients. In addition to this regular influence, in the 1970s, a new form of sporadic but significant governance emerged: the class-action suit. This type of litigation may deal with conditions of treatment throughout public mental hospitals.

A few public mental hospitals have their own autonomous boards—elected or appointed—that either advise or make policy.[6] Some of these boards predate the concept of citizen participation of the 1960s. Many of them were vocal and vigorous in making mental health services more relevant to local needs. These boards can be an additional positive influence on other levels of governance and may lobby for the hospital.

Nongovernmental Influences on Governance

Traditionally, the media, unions, professional societies, and local or state mental health associations have had an influential role in the governance of public mental health hospitals.[5] Two major new forces were added in the 1970s: the Joint Commission on Accreditation of Hospitals (JCAH) and health insurance companies. While the JCAH has formally existed since the mid-1950s, it was not until 1968 that the psychiatric administrator realized its potential use. Medicare and Medicaid began that year and were tied to JCAH standards. In 1972, JCAH developed separate standards for free-standing private and public psychiatric hospitals, and the surveys became more meaningful.[7] Both because of fiscal aspects and the concern for adequate care that JCAH symbolized, psychiatric administrators were able to use the need for compliance with JCAH standards as a way of obtaining millions of dollars in additional resources. Some critics, however, felt that this gambit, while successful in getting the governing body to act, tended to focus the governance too much on the hospital's physical plant rather than on community services.

Health insurance, through its third-party payment policies, sometimes virtually dictates hospital practices. For instance, third parties forced a definition of "active therapy" on the institution and its patients. Critics believe striving for attainment of third-party standards has led to an excessive listing of activities that they claim is useless and wasteful for some patients.

The ability of directors of public mental hospitals to administer is affected by the constellation of the forces described. For any given institution, the specific constellation tends to be unique in its checks and balances. The psychiatric administrator must understand and interact effectively with all the direct and indirect elements that impact on his or her institution's governance.

Organization

The public mental hospital organization tends to have two major divisions: clinical and administrative. The definition of "clinical" and of "administrative" varies, making it difficult to generalize. As a rule, the number of clinical staff about doubles the administrative staff. The administrative organization usually includes various mixtures of the following: finance, budget, personnel, supplies, procurement, engineering, security, safety, housekeeping, and dietary. Some states or counties centralize personnel, budget, security, or other administrative functions at a high level so that the hospital's own administration is not responsible for those functions.

Organizing the administrative part of the hospital usually follows one of two patterns: (1) organizing by function or (2) organizing as a reflection of the clinical organization. "Organizing by function" means a table of organization with a budget unit, a personnel unit, and so on. Organizing to reflect the clinical structure means that a "generalist" in administration, budget, or personnel has responsibility for a specific clinical unit, such as performing the administrative tasks for Clinical Unit A or handling personnel tasks for the nursing department. There are few generally accepted rules about the organization of the administrative structure; however, superintendents of public mental hospitals should have direct and continuing access to the heads of their personnel and budget departments.

Organizing clinical responsibility is usually a combination of the following:[8]

1. Organizing around disciplines, e.g., a social work department
2. Organizing around a service or task ("functional"), e.g., day treatment unit, community consultation program, or family therapy service
3. Organizing around a building, e.g., Smith Pavilion Service
4. Organizing around the diagnosis or problems, e.g., acute ward, alcoholism program, or addiction service
5. Organizing around important characteristics of patients that exist in addition to their pathology, e.g., children's service, Hispanic unit, or mental health program for the deaf
6. Organizing around arbitrary criteria, e.g., a service takes all admissions on Monday, Wednesday, and Friday, and another service takes all admissions on Tuesday, Thursday, and weekends; or a program gets all of the odd-numbered admissions and another service gets all of the even-numbered admissions
7. Organizing around the community or population from which the patients come, e.g., community mental health centers (CMHCs), a psychiatric program for a naval base, or a university psychiatric clinic for students

Of course, there are combinations of the above such as an alcoholic day program for the Smith City area, which is defined by three of the above dimensions.

THE COMMUNITY PSYCHIATRY MOVEMENT

By the mid-1960s, with the community psychiatry movement, a community focus became the way to organize public mental hospitals. See point 7 in list above. Under geographical unitization, hospitals were reorganized with several major, relatively comprehensive subhospital programs that were expected to provide all of the services that hospital would have for a specific population.[9,10]

Unitization tended to replace an organization around professions. See point 1 in list above. In doing so, it "decentralized" the professional organizations and blurred/blended the professional roles. There was a ground swell of positive feelings about this trend because it increased the respect and power of those closer to the patients. Additionally, it coincided with the CMHC movement and allowed hospitals a sense of identity with new and modern goals. By about 1970, "deinstitutionalization" began to become a concern, and the concept of the need for the staff to "follow the patient into the community" was developed to reduce the abandonment of patients associated with deinstitutionalization. Theoretically, unitization allowed this to occur to a greater degree than other types of organization.

Not only did unitization become a popular internal way to organize hospitals, it also became a common method to define the whole hospital's responsibility. Most public mental hospitals by 1980 thus had their responsibilities defined in terms of a geographical region for which they were responsible.

Staffing

There is probably no major area of public mental hospital administration more unsettled than staffing. The quality of the staff needed to serve patients well and the quantity needed are not topics on which there is any consensus. In 1976, 297 state and county hospitals were staffed as described in Table 5-1.

In the 1960s, there developed an attitude that everyone could do anything for the patients. There also developed the interesting phenomenon that what each profession could contribute to therapeutic teams tended to represent the task that they did not want to do. Physicians did not want only to diagnose and prescribe, psychologists did not want only to be doing psychological tests, social workers did not want only to function as the persons who would relate to other agencies, and so on. Instead, most of the professions preferred to do individual, group, or family psychotherapy. Compounding these qualitative issues, continuing education, staff development, upward mobility, unions, racism, sexism, and concern about staff as well as patients becoming "institutionalized" all tended to keep staffing of the public mental hospitals unsettled.

Funding

By the late 1970s, public mental hospitals received more than $3 billion from state, county, or city revenues, an average of more than $10 million per hospital.

Psychiatric administrators usually are working on three budgets at any one time: (1) the current budget is being administered; (2) the next year's budget is being defended in the legislature and in other public settings; (3) the budget 2 years hence is under development.

Table 5-1.
Staff of 297 state and county hospitals in 1976.

	Total FTE* Staff	Percentage of Staff (%)	Average Staff For Each Hospital
Total	219,006	100	737
Psychiatrists	4,333	2	15
Other physicians	2,047	1	7
Psychologists	3,039	1	10
Social workers	5,949	3	20
Registered nurses	15,098	7	51
Other mental health professionals	10,551	5	36
Physical health professionals	5,580	3	19
LPN or equivalents	7,458	3	25
Other mental health workers, less than a BA	87,073	40	293
Administrative and other professionals (non health Staff)	3,686	2	12
All other (clerical, maintenance, etc.)	74,193	34	250

*FTE equals "full-time equivalents." For example, three social workers working two-thirds of an ordinary weekly tour of duty would represent two full-time equivalents.

Funding and budget development are closely tied to planning, and it is not uncommon to find that a hospital's only meaningful planning process is budget development.

Programs

Though the programs of public mental hospitals have a wide spectrum of activities that include virtually any psychiatric service imaginable, in comparison to other psychiatric services, public mental hospitals tend to have programs for psychiatric patients that are more severely ill, more chronically ill, or more dangerous. Despite the tendency, it is important to emphasize that a full gamut of programs can be found in some public mental hospitals. Day treatment, night hospitals, clinics, emergency services, foster homes, halfway houses, "quarterway" houses, cooperative apartments, nursing homes, consultation services, and public education programs can be found here and there as part of the public mental hospital's program. Yet half the state hospitals have only inpatient services.

Because of their relatively large populations, public mental hospitals have evolved specialized programs that would be difficult to visualize in smaller service systems, e.g., mental health programs for the deaf, mental health programs for the blind, or forensic programs.

In the 1960s, redefinitions of the mentally ill by the public, the profession, the legislatures, and the judiciary have prompted public mental hospital systems to assume responsibility for many patients who had previously entered the criminal system, especially alcoholics and drug addicts. In the District of Columbia, for example, the corrections department's alcoholic workhouse was turned over to the mental health administration, and the "prisoners" became "patients" overnight in exactly the same buildings. Also in the 1960s, nursing homes became more available to the mentally ill, and there was a reduction in potential nursing-home patients in public mental hospitals by the 1970s. The increases in alcoholics, drug addicts, and criminal patients and decreases in potential nursing-home patients led to a major change in the sex ratios in public mental hospitals. In 1965, there were more women than men, but 12 years later, there were 17 percent more men than women.[4]

As we enter the 1980s, a major programmatic goal, quite uneven in its achievement, is the integration of mental hospitals' efforts with other institutions. First, within psychiatric services, public mental hospitals have attempted to integrate their programs with general hospitals, university programs, and CMHC. Second and more broadly, public mental hospitals have attempted to integrate their programs with the social service, educational, and correctional systems. The ability of the psychiatric hospital's leadership to effectuate these programmatic integrations was a major factor in achieving a degree of freedom for the patients from their mental illnesses.[12–15]

Management and Its Clinical Interface

At the beginning of the 1970s, it was said that the mental health field suffered from data gluttony and information starvation.[16] A decade later, the typical public psychiatric hospital leader felt he or she was drowning from wave after wave of new information requirements in the name of accountability, efficiency, scientific management, "good" billing practices, and computer information processing technique requirements. Even so, the progress in meaningful information has been quite uneven.

Two main themes have dominated these requirements: the need for improved evaluation of psychiatric services and the need for improved processing of the information.

The need for improvements in evaluation of mental health services has taken many forms. The most important have been those in the rest of medicine: utilization review (UR), medical audits (MA), and professional standards review organizations (PSROs). UR and MA had their moments of success in producing useful studies; PSROs were more disappointing. For the public mental hospital, PSROs identified patients who should not be in the hospital, but too often there was no other option, so the only consequence was less money from Medicare reimbursement.

From management science came initiatives to objectivy the psychiatric administrators' decision-making process. "Cost-benefit analysis" and "management by objectives" became popular callings, but the criteria with which to define "benefit" or "objective" have proved a stumbling block for the public mental hospital. What is, for example, a satisfactory benefit or objective with a patient who has chronic paranoid schizophrenia? Critics of the emphasis on various evaluation techniques claimed that the new techniques that called for more rigorous accountability had not met rigorous tests themselves as to whether their use derived the benefits being claimed.[17,18] Many proposals met syllogistic tests of being reasonable but failed empirical tests of being useful.

While there were many problems with the new management techniques in the clinical area, more progress was attained in the business area. In the 1970s, the public mental hospital not connected with an IBM 360 felt anachronistic. Even so, the quantum jumps in information processing in many industries and in private psychiatric hospitals has yet to become characteristic of public mental hospitals. This is partially because new information systems follow the dollar and assist with billing. The inducements to follow the dollar have been less compelling in the public sector since vigorous billing often only adds money to local or state general coffers and does not add any funds directly to public mental hospitals. Automation of information about the three "m's"—money, manpower, and materials—has become sophisticated. Patient-related information systems have remained elementary. Missouri was one of the first states to develop an automated patient information system.[19] The staff at New York's Rockland State Hospital developed the Multi-State Information System (MSIS), which included a number of information systems to assist administrators in knowing more about their patients (see Chapter 22).

In summary, the goal of the management-clinical interface is to maximize benefits while minimizing costs. Great strides are anticipated in subgoals that are clearly measurable, but the management-clinical interface is going to continue to have strains and stresses in public mental hospitals because of difficulties in measuring benefits to patients.

The Constraints on Public Mental Hospitals

A whole book could be written about constraints on public mental hospitals—and Talbott has.[20] Space allows only a list of constraints, maybe one of the longest in this book; yet any experienced administrator could probably add more:[21]

1. The patients' illnesses are often those illnesses that are least responsive to today's treatment.
2. The patients' social and economic support system is often less substantial than that of patients in other systems.
3. The staff working with patients is relatively untrained.
4. The staff works within a bureaucracy that[21]:
    a. ultimately (at the top) has goals to meet political objectives, not to meet patients' needs;
    b. has a promotion system that pulls the best clinicians away from face-to-face contact with patients;
    c. has a regulatory system, built on mistrust, that is inflexible, restraining, and forces checkoffs for key decisions at hierarchical levels removed from the patients;
    d. has a personnel system that makes removal of incompetent staff quite difficult,
5. The public budget process is torpid, rigid, and stifles planning.

6. The state level makes key decisions that are too often founded on ignorance about the specific conditions and care of the patients.
7. The federal government and local government add regulatory requirements in addition to state regulatory webs.
8. Unions provide another restraint.
9. The courts in their adversarial and ponderous style restrain action. Legal advocates amplify this climate.
10. The legislature runs for office every 2 years and the governor every 4 years, and the mental health commissioner changes every 2 years. This provides an instability that virtually kills long-range planning.
11. The media tends to highlight the negative rather than the positive. It is not newsworthy, we are told, to headline "one thousand State Hospital patients did well yesterday." A single suicide or homicide is newsworthy. Hospitals can thus react to the media by stressing avoidance of the negative rather than achieving the positive.
12. While the accreditation process can point to many victories for improving the care of patients, accreditation bodies' frequent visits have made it difficult for marginal hospitals to plan beyond the next accreditation visit.
13. Overall funding, especially for inpatient services, tends to be inadequate.
14. The buildings of public mental hospitals are frequently not conducive to humane housing or effective treatment.
15. The location of public mental hospitals often compounds difficulties in staffing and in serving patients in their own communities.
16. The requirements of insurance companies generate paperwork and force clinicians to take wasteful actions.
17. General attitudes of prejudice against the mentally ill form the foundation for many of the troubles of public mental hospitals.
18. Another public attitude, a growing public attitude as of the early 1980s, is that "private" is good and "public" is bad.

Many patients' lives are saved or made less tragic by public mental hospitals despite the enormity of the restraints, which is a testimony to the potential of psychiatric treatment.

Future

Talbott suggested four options for public mental hospitals:[20]

1. Keep state hospitals as they are.
2. Drastically alter state hospitals.
3. Find new roles for state hospitals.
4. Close state hospitals.

While the last three options have been championed for a quarter of a century, it appears that no major redirections are likely in the near future. Regional rehabilitation programs are likely to characterize nearly all public mental hospitals, and many of those institutions not in regional programs offer specialized or community services. As long as private patients have their psychiatric hospitals and those hospitals are not available to all, public patients will have their hospitals.

VETERANS ADMINISTRATION

History

In 1593, the Parliament of England enacted the "Acte for Relief of Souldiours" to provide assistance to soldiers disabled by their military service. From this beginning in English law, there has developed a tradition of benefits for disabled veterans. During the 19th century, Congress established a number of "national veterans' homes," some of which are still used by the VA. In 1921, the newly formed U.S. Veterans Bureau began to build hospitals. In 1923, Congress approved the principle that empty beds in veterans' hospitals would be used to treat veterans who needed care even though the disability did not derive from their military service. Finally, in 1930, the three separate elements of the government's veterans' programs, the Bureau of Pensions, the National Homes for Disabled Volunteer Soldiers, and the Veterans Bureau were merged to form the VA.

In 1946, the VA began a period of intense development that included closer relationships with medical schools, active hospital construction, and development of medical—including psychiatric—residencies. The VA improved standards for public mental hospitals, changed mental hospital architecture, stimulated research at each psychiatric hospital, and operated the largest training program for psychiatrists and clinical psychologists in the world. Dr. Daniel Blain, as director, and Dr. Harvey Tompkins, as his deputy director of psychiatry, neurology, and psychology services, put forward new policies supporting rapid turnover in hospital units with follow-up in outpatient programs, utilization of all professionals in a therapeutic milieu, and an insistence on an eclectic approach. In the fifties and sixties, the VA decreased its total number of psychiatric beds, particularly in large neuropsychiatric hospitals. As new general hospitals were built, acute psychiatric units were included, making psychiatric care part of the mainstream of VA care.

By 1975, the conversion of psychiatric hospitals to general hospitals was largely accomplished. The decrease in psychiatric beds reached a level of 29,000 beds, or 32 percent of all beds. Chronic patients were managed in some hospitals, but more and more were placed in nursing homes and community facilities. New programs for alcohol- and drug-dependence treatment increased, and outpatient programs continued to be used extensively.

Governance

The VA has always been a part of the executive branch of government. Congress legislates a broad range of critical items that control operations, including budget, personnel ceiling, facility construction and replacement, and eligibility criteria. In some years, public conflicts between the legislative and executive branches of government have influenced the activity of the VA. House and Senate veterans' affairs committees closely monitor VA activities and have significant interest in proposed changes in policy and planning.

Organization

The VA of the 1980s has two major divisions under the administrator of Veterans' Affairs: the Department of Veterans Benefits and the Department of Medicine and Surgery. The Department of Veterans Benefits provides educational benefits, pensions, and compensation for veterans and their dependents and survivors.

Under the Department of Medicine and Surgery, health care policy decisions are made in the VA central office in Washington, D.C. The chief medical director has final authority for policy and operating budget decisions within the Department of Medicine and Surgery. Psychiatric policy decisions are developed for the chief medical director by the Mental Health and Behavioral Sciences Service and endorsed or modified by the Office of the Assistant Chief Medical Director for Professional Services. Following this endorsement, extensive staff concurrence is required at many levels before policy changes can be implemented by the associate deputy chief medical director for operations.

Research and education are separate from professional services. There are assistant chief medical directors for research and for education. In this way, research priorities and policies are established by the administrator of veterans' affairs, the chief medical director, and the assistant chief medical director for research. Individual disciplines, such as psychiatry, do not have direct responsibility for research in their areas. Research proposals are reviewed by merit review boards using a peer-review model.

Educational policy has central importance in the Department of Medicine and Surgery because affiliations with medical schools, first recommended in the 1920s and given high priority in 1946, have been used by the VA to provide high-quality patient care.

The VA currently has affiliations with 107 medical schools. Medical students and residents provide a significant percentage of the system's direct hands-on care supervised by staff physicians. The affiliations with medical schools established through an affiliation agreement and a "dean's committee" mechanism provide that the medical school departments will be responsible for assuring that educational quality is maintained, while VA medical center management will provide quality patient care, facilities, and research opportunity. VA physicians are jointly recruited by the VA and the medical school.

The complex structure of central management is balanced in some respects by the relative autonomy of local facilities. Despite the degree of centralized management and occasions for difficulty created by the interaction of many factors in Washington, D.C., including the tension between the legislative and executive branches of government, the complex divisions of responsibility in the VA central office, and the inherent difficulties in formulating regulations that adequately guide over 200 facilities, each local facility functions as an autonomous unit.

Medical centers have a director, a chief of staff, and a group of service chiefs. The center director and his or her staff make policy and planning decisions, allocate budget and personnel, and negotiate many issues with the VA central office, affiliated medical schools, and so on. Most directors in the VA have worked in many hospitals and the central office before becoming directors. This range of experience seems to add balance at many facilities.

The chief of staff serves the hospital director as the senior professional representative and is responsible for maintaining the quality of patient care. The chief of staff is often the principal contact with the medical school around professional issues.

Medical centers are also influenced by the "dean's committee." Dean's committees often make demands on the medical centers or the VA central office to provide special support for particular programs or, in times of declining resources, to leave favored programs alone. Whenever there is a cooperative relationship between the dean's committee and the management at the VA medical center (including service chiefs), patient care, education, and research tend to improve. When, however, medical school political battles are played out through the VA medical center, these programs often suffer.

In the role of a psychiatric service chief, successful administration requires complex negotiations at many levels. Daily contact with separate services, including medicine, surgery, psychology, nursing, engineering, and so on, governs local accomplishment.

The chief of psychiatry is responsible for all psychiatric care but does not have control of other professionals assigned to psychiatric units. A matrix administrative model governs these relationships, placing clinical care issues under the chief of psychiatry but reserving professional autonomy to the parallel chiefs of other disciplines.

Full integration with affiliated departments of psychiatry has been useful to many VA psychiatric services. Sometimes there are frictions between VA psychiatric services and the affiliated medical school departments of psychiatry. The most consistent friction derives from the difference in purpose of medical schools and VA medical centers. The VA hires staff psychiatrists primarily to provide patient care and, secondarily, to supervise residents or students, do research, and publish papers. At times, it seems, medical schools hire and promote faculty to do research, publish papers, teach, and secondarily, to take care of patients.

The attitude of many departments of psychiatry about chronic psychiatric illness has also made integration difficult. For many years, some medical schools have believed that certain patients were not good "teaching cases."

In summary, the VA has a complex mixture of horizontal and vertical management structures that challenge VA psychiatric service chiefs by allowing significant autonomy and many powerful, influential forces to cope with while maintaining clinical patient care, teaching, and research.

Facilities

The VA provides psychiatric inpatient services for 187,000 veterans each year. There are 172 medical centers and 34 clinics. VA psychiatric services have an average occupancy rate of 88 percent, with 21,000 patients in the hospital on a typical day. The outpatient programs had 3 million patient visits in 1980. There are 128 psychiatric services primarily in general hospital settings.

The VA employs 1101 full-time and 791 part-time psychiatrists, 47 percent are board certified, and 37 percent are foreign medical graduates. In 1980–1981, the VA trained psychiatric residents in 82 programs with 525 psychiatric residency positions.

Constraints

Generally, the VA has received increasingly tighter budgets since 1976. Continuing competition for scarce resources between medical, surgical, and psychiatric services can be disruptive and result in a narrower range of psychiatric care.

The shortage of psychiatrists in the United States poses a long-term challenge to the VA and the rest of public psychiatry. If the shortage continues to grow, the VA will have difficulty recruiting psychiatrists unless VA salaries and affiliations remain attractive.

The varieties of rules and restraints posed by recent commitment laws and right-to-treatment court decisions can make operation of a national program more difficult. Prior to new commitment statutes, many states allowed transfers within the VA system when needed. At this time, VA facilities cannot transfer committed patients and thus cannot develop specialized programs to serve large geographical areas. In some states, transfer across county lines leads to a new commitment hearing under very restrictive rules. Even though only 14 percent of VA psychiatric patients are committed, these restrictions complicate treatment planning.

Future

The future of VA psychiatry cannot be easily predicted. In the absence of war, however, the VA will become the treatment facility for increasing numbers of elderly patients. By 1990, a majority of veterans will be over 65, and there will be an increased need for psychiatric geriatric care.

VA psychiatry has two unusual features that will affect its future. First, the VA has built its clinical care system heavily on resident staffing. To run some VA facilities with active affiliations without residents would require additions of many physicians. For this reason, medical school affiliations and resident training will probably survive budget cuts. If other training money is eliminated, many medical schools will draw closer to their VA affiliates. The second unique feature of VA psychiatry is its relationship with veterans' organizations. These groups effectively promote better patient care for veterans and are one of the few lobbies devoted even partially to psychiatric patients.

The VA's greatest strength, however, lies in its staff. The future of VA psychiatry will be shaped positively by its growing cadre of effective clinicians, talented teachers, and innovative researchers. These physicians have largely retained a healthy balance of patient care and academic activities and will contribute to a resurgence of psychiatry in general and public psychiatry in particular.

REFERENCES

1. Barton WE: Administration in Psychiatry. Springfield, Ill, Thomas, 1962
2. Rothman DJ: The Discovery of the Asylum Social Order and Disorder in the New Republic. Boston, Little, Brown, 1971
3. Solomon H: Presidential address 1958. Am J Psychiatry 115:1–9, 1958
4. Division of Biometry, National Institute of Mental Health. Statistical Note Series. Rockville, Md, NIMH, 1975
5. Greenblatt M: Psychopolitics. New York, Grune & Stratton, 1978
6. Greenblatt M: Administration of the state hospital, in Freedman DX, Dyryd JE (eds): American Handbook of Psychiatry (ed 2), vol 5. New York, Basic Books, 1975, p 593–606
7. Joint Commission on Accreditation of Hospitals: Accreditation Manual for Psychiatric Facilities 1972. Chicago, JCAH, 1972
8. Peele R: Organizing to improve services: The structuring of public mental health services. Med Ann 41:495–495, 1972
9. Babow I, Johnson AC: Measuring staff attitudes toward decentralization. Hosp Community Psychiatry 19:118–211, 1968

10. Osterweil J, Brown BS: Critical factors in the unitization of mental hospitals. Int J Psychiatry 7:226–228, 1969
11. Rosenstein MJ, Taube CA: Staffing of Mental Health Facilities, United States 1976. Rockville, Md, NIMH, 1978
12. Arafeh MK, Fumiatti EK, Gregory ME, et al: Linking hospital and community care for psychiatric patients. Am J Nurs 68:1050–1056, 1968
13. Beigel A, Hanson D, Howard D: Partnerships in mental health planning: local state and federal relationships. Hosp Community Psychiatry 23:215–217, 1972
14. Kraft AM: The state hospital: cornerstone of community service. Hosp Community Psychiatry 18:243–244, 1967
15. Leopold RL: The West Philadelphia Mental Health Consortium: administrative planning in a multihospital catchment area. Am J Psychiatry 124:69–76, 1967
16. Holder HD: Evaluation methods and dynamics in program planning, in Wuster RR (ed): Statistics in Mental Health Programs. Washington, DC, NIMH, 1970, pp 433–442
17. Mushkin SJ: Evaluations: use with caution. Evaluation 2:30–35, 1973
18. Peele R, Palmer RR: Standards and quality control: problems and pitfalls. Adm Mental Health 3:146–155, 1976
19. Uleet BA, Sletten IW, Ameiss A, et al: Realities and prospects for the use of computers in psychiatric hospital management. Psychiatr Ann 3:27–53, 1973
20. Talbott JA: The Death of the Asylum. New York, Grune & Stratton, 1978
21. Arce A: Mission impossible: effects of bureaucratic rigidity, in Talbott (ed): State Mental Hospitals: Problems and Potentials. New York, Human Sciences Press, 1980, pp 47–99

Arthur T. Meyerson, M.D.
Samuel Davis, M.S.

6

General Hospitals

HISTORICAL BACKGROUND

The earliest example of a general hospital admitting psychiatric patients was the hospital at Saint Maria della Pieta in Rome,[1] founded in the 15th century and "dedicated to the care of all sick people, including those who are mentally sick." In the United States, the Pennsylvania Hospital treated "their first group of mentally ill patients" . . . who "were admitted in the cellar" as of 1756.[1] While general hospitals played a role in the care of the mentally ill, during the last century this role has been divorced from the necessity to plan in terms of comprehensive community service needs or the natural history of psychiatric illness. This was a result of the development, in the 19th century, of large-scale public (largely state) systems that have in great measure cared for the mentally ill. This separation of the public health priorities from general hospital planning is parallel to the instance of tuberculosis, for which the state also developed an independent system of care. The common denominator would appear to be the chronic and disabling aspects of the illnesses as well as the feelings of fear engendered in the "healthy" population. With this reliance on state systems for the bulk of services, the general hospital tended to focus on what is now called liaison psychiatry. "The seeds of liaison psychiatry were sown somewhat haphazardly whenever a medical staff member showed interest in mental disorders, whenever a disturbed patient had a medical problem, or whenever a medical patient had an emotional problem."[2]

Following World War II, with the appreciation of the broad psychiatric needs of the population, many general hospitals began to develop inpatient units, often devoted to patients suffering from so-called psychosomatic ailments. Unlike the community mental health centers (CHMCs) established under federal legislation in the early sixties,[3] the general hospital had no particular agenda for the development of a full range of psychiatric services for the mentally ill. General hospitals

The authors wish to express gratitude to Marvin Stein, M.D., and Arthur Schwartz, M.D., for their invaluable input.

devoted themselves to liaison/consultation services, small inpatient and emergency services, and ambulatory psychotherapy clinics. For many years prior to governmental deinstitutionalization, the general hospital had de facto revolving-door policies for many of the patients they treated. In 1955, prior to the largest wave of deinstitutionalization, the general hospital was responsible for 265,934 inpatient-related patient care episodes, a 20.5 percent share of the total of such episodes in the United States. The remainder were accounted for by state, county, Veterans Administration, (VA) and federal institutions.[4] By 1977, the number of inpatient-related patient care episodes in general hospitals had increased to 571,725, doubling the 1955 figure and now representing well over one-third of inpatient care episodes in the United States.

With the onset of deinstitutionalization (see Chapter 4), the general hospital has taken an increasing role in the provision of care for the psychiatrically disturbed. In 1972, the general hospital had 23,308 of the total of 471,800 psychiatric beds in the United States.[6] By 1978, while inpatient beds of all types had gone down over 35 percent to 301,011, those in the general hospital had increased to 29,384 (an increase of more than 25 percent).[7]

During the past decade, the inpatient psychiatric services in general hospitals have shown a trend toward a decrease in length of hospital stay for each index episode. The average length of stay has dropped from 60 days to less than 30 days. At the same time that external forces have been placing constraints on the length of hospital stay, pressure on the budgetary needs of general hospitals has often been in the direction of maintaining a high rate of occupancy.

The occupancy of psychiatric inpatient beds is of importance to the management and budgetary needs of voluntary general hospitals. As an example, Mount Sinai, a large voluntary general teaching hospital in New York City, has maintained an occupancy rate of over 90 percent over the last 5 years, approaching 97 percent for 1980. In general, there are substantial differences in the actual costs of medical and surgical beds as compared to psychiatric inpatient beds. As pointed out by Mesnikoff,[8] "In some instances, this difference is an important source of income and subsidy for the general hospital." Furthermore, Blue Cross reimburses voluntary hospitals at a higher rate than city, state, or free-standing psychiatric hospitals, which serves as further incentive for voluntary hospitals, and "in effect, the full utilization of psychiatric beds provides an ongoing subsidy for all services in the hospital."[8] In order to meet budgetary requirements as length of stay decreases, increased numbers of psychiatric patients must be admitted to maintain the total yearly number of patient days and consequent income. There is no difficulty with this approach in an urban general hospital, particularly during an era of deinstitutionalization and revolving door from state institutions, provided the general hospital department receives adequate funding to maintain quality care at a high rate of occupancy. A comprehensive program of integrated services is required that will provide quality care for a changing patient population during a brief hospital stay while at the same time considering the budgetary requirements of the institution and the department. An integrated service system must include a large ambulatory program, with inevitable readmission rates of 10–30 percent, which provides good long-term care while also serving as a source of clinically necessary inpatient admissions.

THE 1980s AND BEYOND

Rationale

Deinstitutionalization of state institutions has presented the general hospital psychiatric unit with two new patient populations. The first is the chronically ill and formerly hospitalized patient whose mental and physical health needs must be met. The second is the person suffering from schizophrenia or a major affective disorder, who appears de novo in the community and whose acute care and subsequent long-term care must be provided. The latter patient, after one or two episodes, would formerly become part of the large public system of care but no longer does so. Furthermore, the general hospital has become the core service agency in the community.

A brief review of some recent studies concerned with the treatment of the major psychoses, primarily schizophrenia, may provide some guidelines around which a general hospital can plan its services. It is important, however, to bear in mind that the department of psychiatry in a general hospital has cared for patients—and will continue to do so—with a wide range of less severe disorders.

Schizophrenia characteristically follows a chronic course, including quiescent periods interrupted by exacerbations of florid psychiatric symptoms and disorganized behavior. The essential feature in the treatment of schizophrenic patients has become the use of antipsychotic medications.[9] These drugs have totally restructured the modern management of schizophrenia.

In 1968, in a study investigating the treatment of schizophrenia, May[10] reported that the proportion of schizophrenic patients released from the hospital after successful treatment ranged from 58 percent to 65 percent for those who received milieu therapy or psychotherapy alone as compared to 95 percent and 96 percent, respectively, for those patients given psychotherapy plus phenothiazines or phenothiazines alone.

The availability of neuroleptic medication has considerably shortened the length of hospital stay for acute psychiatric episodes. This trend toward shorter periods of inpatient care has found support from the research of Swartzburg and Schwartz,[11] Glick,[12] and Weisman, Feirstein, and Thomas.[13] Recently, Klein and his colleagues[14] compared the outcome of patients hospitalized at Hillside Hospital for a short period (less than 90 days) with a long-term group (no limitation on length of stay). On the basis of their findings, they concluded that "considered with other previous findings, and other relevant studies, there is still little justification for recommending long-term hospitalization for the majority of psychiatric patients." As a result, hospital psychiatry has changed from a long-term, essentially custodial function to brief hospitalization utilizing a combination of medical treatment with psychopharmacologic agents and psychological support based on crisis intervention principles and rehabilitative interventions. Modern psychiatric inpatient management of schizophrenia, therefore, can be conducted effectively in voluntary general hospitals.

In addition, Davis,[15] in a comprehensive review of maintenance drug studies, has shown that there is universal agreement among 24 controlled studies that significantly more patients relapse on placebo than on maintenance antipsychotic medication. It is necessary, however, for patients to comply and remain on medication. In addition, many chronic patients are discharged well enough to be outside the hospital but not well enough to be self-sufficient and require a social support system. Aftercare programs, especially day care treatment centers, provide a critical means of delivering the required comprehensive services of medication maintenance and various forms of psychotherapeutic support such as supportive resocialization and rehabilitation programs. Hogarty et al.[16] evaluated the effect of drugs and sociotherapy in the aftercare of schizophrenic patients. The results of the study revealed that patients discharged into the community and maintained on placebo have a 70 percent rehospitalization rate within 1 year. The rehospitalization rate of patients maintained on phenothiazines is significantly reduced. The greatest reduction in rehospitalization was in those patients who complied in taking medication and for whom medication was combined with a resocialization program concerned with facilitating their social relationships.

Early[17] has suggested two "ladders" toward stabilization in the community. One is the occupational and the other is residential for patients who require arrangements outside the family setting. At different stages of the illness, a patient may need to be in the hospital, in a supervised group living setting, in supervised single living quarters, in a halfway house, or in his or her own home. Transitional living arrangments following discharge from an inpatient service have been shown to have an effect on some aspects of the course of schizophrenic patients. Several studies have followed patients who have moved from halfway houses to independent living. Recidivism rates 6 months following departure from halfway houses were 40 percent[18] and at 18 months were 50 percent.[19] These relapse rates did not differ from base-rate data. Wilder et al.,[18] however, reported a full-time employment rate at a 6-month follow-up of 53 percent, which was significantly greater than the base rate. This finding is consistent with the studies of Mosher[20] and Singer and Grob,[21] which have shown that transitional living does not affect recidivism rates but does result in a better quality of life during nonhospitalization periods.

Equally critical is the role of vocational rehabilitation. A graded variety of activities is necessary, ranging from re-education in a workshop to independent work with a number of intermediate sheltered employment situations. Brown[22] has noted that while domestic and occupational rehabilitation interact, at any point in time, they may function independently, and a patient may be further along one dimension than the other. In the long-term comprehensive care of schizophrenic patients, a range of resocialization, rehabilitative services, and living arrangements is therefore required to enable a patient to move freely without the danger of large gaps in time or level of achievement.

It has been demonstrated that the onset of the psychotic state is often preceded by a major change in family life.[22] High expression of emotion by family members is associated with greater relapse rates and work impairment in schizophrenic patients living with relatives.[22] It is of note that long-term medication is especially effective in patients who return to live with highly emotional relatives.[21] Family treatment provides an important aspect in the management of schizophrenic patients. Family involvement in the treatment program helps in the recognition and possible prevention of a crisis and provides assistance in managing psychotic behavior. The inclusion of the family in the treatment process also allows its members to have some insight into situations that may precipitate disturbed behavior and to obtain guidance about how to live with a schizophrenic patient or to contemplate possible separation from the patient.

Psychotherapy with schizophrenic patients, as reported by Vaillant, Semrad, and Ewalt,[23] has a positive effect on post-hospital interpersonal relations and provides a means of social rehabilitation. Baldessarini[9] recently commented:

> The contributions of psychoanalytic psychiatry to the understanding of the experience of being schizophrenic or living with a schizophrenic patient have been important, but, as a general rule, prolonged and intensive psychotherapy aimed at accomplishing fundamental changes in the personality has not been demonstrated to be an effective primary mode of treatment for severe schizophrenia."

Feinsilver and Gunderson[24] have reviewed the literature of the last two decades of psychotherapy of schizophrenia. They selected five representative studies with the best design and concluded that these five studies "have neither proved psychotherapy ineffective, nor provided any strong evidence of its helpfulness."

On the other hand, as pointed out by Baldessarini,[9] "active supportive psychotherapy not only is humane, but has much to offer in helping schizophrenic patients and their families to cope with what represents a lifetime of at least partial and unremediable disability." In addition, there remains the possibility of defining subgroups of schizophrenic patients who respond to psychotherapy. There is the further possibility that specific psychotherapeutic techniques will be developed and matched to selected patients.

Davis[15] has noted that "there is substantial evidence that psychological therapies improve social adjustment. However, the antipsychotic effects of the neuroleptics . . . are independent of the effects of psychotherapy; psychotherapy in no sense substitutes for drug treatment." The findings at present indicate that drug and psychological therapies have different functions. This appears to be in keeping with the treatment and management of depression. Klerman et al.[25] and Paykel et al.[26] have shown that tricyclic drugs had a substantial prophylactic effect in preventing relapses of depressed patients. Psychotherapy was not effective in preventing depressive relapse but did improve social adjustment.

The above review strongly suggests that a model general hospital program must include the use of drugs and recognize that the psychological, economic, vocational, and social aspects of schizophrenia are important to its long-term treatment. It appears that the hospital treatment of the schizophrenic patient should concentrate on amelioration of psychotic symptoms and restitution to the premorbid state. In contrast, the goal of ambulatory treatment should be stabilization of the personality. It is during the stabilization phase that psychotherapy, social therapy, and rehabilitation are likely to be most helpful. The overall treatment strategy, therefore, should center around effective and meaningful integration of hospital care and aftercare. A number of reports[27–29] have emphasized the need for a comprehensive and coordinated psychiatric treatment program. Such a program prevents patients from slipping "between the interstices of piecemeal services, even when these are readily accessible and well publicized."[29] The aim of a comprehensive integrated service is not only to prevent relapse and unnecessary hospitalizations but also to promote maximum rehabilitation and resocialization.

The General Hospital Program for the Eighties

A general hospital psychiatric program in the 1980s must develop a comprehensive integrated delivery system, utilizing the current state of knowledge in the field concerning patient care, teaching, and research. It must serve a wide range of patients in terms of diagnostic category, severity of illness, and acute and chronic care. Programs should continue to provide treatment to the group of patients who do not require hospitalization and to the group who may need acute hospitalization but not long-term care. These two groups in the past comprised the majority of patients both admitted to general hospitals and attending psychiatric outpatient clinics. With the changing nature of the patient population and advances in the field, general hospitals should develop programs for the management and treatment of a more seriously disturbed and impaired patient population in both acute and chronic stages. It is an objective of modern general hospital departments of psychiatry to attempt to provide an alternative to long-term hospitalization and enhance avoidance of "the deinstitutionalization effect" and "revolving-door" approach for these severely disturbed patients.

The components of the system should include:

1. Acute care services
2. Inpatient services
3. Resocialization and rehabilitation services
4. Transitional living arrangements
5. Outpatient psychiatric services

The key to such an array of services is the integration of component parts. In the past, the operating divisions of most general hospital departments of psychiatry functioned with relative autonomy and with overt or covert protective boundaries. This enabled each component of the program to pursue a limited mission without major disruptions but also without an overview of the course of the patient's illness and overall management. Several guidelines to ensure coordination of services are discussed below. It must be kept in mind that these guidelines governing integration are of the utmost importance, whether the general hospital develops a service completely under its own umbrella or, through contracts and other arrangements, develops an array of allied but independent services.

ADMINISTRATION AND ORGANIZATION OF INTEGRATED PSYCHIATRIC SERVICES

Administrative Guidelines

Clinical Administration

The clinical director of the general hospital psychiatric program should have the overall responsibility and authority for the clinical services. Under this unified directorship, the leader of the inpatient service will have the responsibility and authority for the inpatient units. The directors or leaders of ambulatory care will have the responsibility and authority for the acute care service, the day treatment center, and the psychiatric outpatient clinics. The directors for the inpatient service and ambulatory care should share the administrative and clinical responsibilities for patient care, and both should report directly to the clinical director or chairman of the department of psychiatry. Major program policy must be made on the basis of participative joint decisions and not unilaterally.

Lines of Responsibility and Authority

Mental health workers from all participating disciplines, e.g., psychiatry, social work, medicine, psychology, occupational therapy, vocational rehabilitation, and so on, must be clinically responsible to the director of the program to which they are assigned while remaining identified with the professional department or division for purposes of accreditation, professional education, assignment, promotion, and so on.[30] The directors of the department of psychiatry's clinical services should meet on a regular basis with other responsible senior professionals, e.g., the director of psychiatric social services, the director of psychiatric nursing, and so on, to prevent fragmentation of disciplines and to ensure a coordinated and integrated delivery system. Clinical responsibility for all services within the department lies with the division directors, reporting to the directors of inpatient and ambulatory care, and ultimately to the clinical director or chairman. Job descriptions of all professional and paraprofessional workers in psychiatry programs in general hospitals should be arrived at jointly between the department of psychiatry and the other departments or divisions involved. All hiring, recommendations for promotion, job changes, and dismissals should be done collaboratively. This matrix system, as applied at the Mount Sinai Hospital, will be described later.

Shared Staffing

Continuity of care is essential and implicit to the proposed system. Shared staffing is exemplified by the interface between the inpatient and day treatment programs. Each inpatient unit should be assigned personnel from the day treatment program with responsibility to assess the patient's long-range needs for rehabilitative treatment of social role and vocational disability. After appropriate assessment, it should be the task of this staff to introduce the gradually improving patient to those aspects of day treatment (rehabilitation–resocialization program) appropriate to his or her needs. Fox and Potter[31] have shown that patients do better in unified programs of inpatient and aftercare staff than patients referred to an aftercare program from another inpatient facility.

Case Management

The National Institute of Mental Health (NIMH) has recommended introduction of the case management model in a delivery system for the mentally ill. This is predicated on the notion that many patients cannot integrate the array of needs and services that confront them with the disease, disability, and environmental treatment axes required in a unified comprehensive program. The responsibility of the case manager is to organize the appropriate complex of services and to eliminate barriers between components of the system so that as patients improve or relapse, the appropriate modalities are available. Each patient in need should be assigned to a case manager or primary therapist who fulfills the responsibility by advocating and ensuring integration on a clinical level. As patients improve, case management responsibility becomes an increasing part of the patient's own independent capacities and functioning, although many patients have the prototypical improvement and relapse course, which will require reinvolvement of the case manager.

Unitary Record System

A unitary record system, at least partially on a problem-oriented basis, should prove appropriate and will enhance the transition of the patient from one component of the system to another. Unitary records should reinforce the need for decisions about the treatment and management of the patient being made jointly by all staff involved. In modern general hospitals, computerized unitary records, employed by all components of the program, should be considered. Such records can include appropriate mental status schedules, problem-oriented treatment plan forms, progress notes, outcome measures, and so on (See Chapter 19).

Administration and Management Support

Although general hospitals have a central hospital administrative staff, the type of integrated psychiatric delivery system that we are describing requires a full-time administrator of psychiatric clinical services. This administrator should have specific expertise and experience in psychiatric delivery systems, with federal, state, and local regulations, and in funding. The administrator should be directly responsible to the clinical director and chairman of the department. His responsibility should be for all components of the proposed system, thereby further augmenting and ensuring coordination and integration. The administrator of these clinical services should meet on a regular basis with the directors of the inpatient and ambulatory care services. Funding of individual components may be through appropriate inpatient or ambulatory procedures within the hospital. One administrator for all of the major components of the proposed psychiatric delivery system will provide a rational and unified approach to management of the program as well as foster the integration of the care of the patients.

Organization

Organization and Professional Indentification

Employees of large, complex hospitals experience conflicts in their identification and in their reporting relationships. They may identify with their peers, their immediate superior, their supervisor's superior, their section, their department, and the objectives of the institution all at the same time! In addition, they may identify with other colleagues in their discipline through membership in a professional organization such as the American Psychological Association, the American Nurses Association, and so on. Identification with tasks or professional specialization is strengthened by traditional patterns of hospital organization in which the emphasis is on function rather than on programs. In a general hospital psychiatric department, clinical programs may include adult psychiatry, child psychiatry, inpatient and outpatient care, research, training, community service, and community education. Programs embody the principal purposes of an organization or the "why." Management represents the process or the "how." Resources can be seen to represent the "with what." A hospital does not exist for its social service, psychology, and nursing departments; rather, those departments exist to serve program objectives. They are by definition, resource departments.

Program–Resource Concept

It is possible to organize the hospital on the basis of a dual line of command—the program–resource concept.[32,33] Under this system of management, almost every hospital employee serves two designated "masters"—one for programmatic functions and one for resource functions. A pattern of general hospital organization is developed that clearly describes who reports to whom and for what. Certainly, professional employees in a hospital will respond to the influence of clinical supervisors as well as to functional departmental chiefs. The director of nursing of the institution is a resource department head. The chief psychiatric nurse is a member of that department. Dual command allows the hospital employee to have dual identification. Under the program–resource concept, the chief nurse is able to identify herself not only as a member of the department of psychiatry but also as a member of the nursing profession. Similarly, in a psychiatric unit of a general hospital, the social worker is able to identify both with her profession and with the interdisciplinary treatment team.

Resource departments face no loss of status by being organized under the program–resource concept. Rather, resource department heads are able to set objectives effectively in the areas of competence for which they are able to assume responsibility. The basic functions of a resource department head are to recruit and hire personnel, train them in the discipline of the department, assign them to assume program responsibilities, supervise their work within the discipline, evaluate and promote them within the discipline, and dismiss those whose performance is unsatisfactory. The resource department head also serves as a consultant in his or her discipline to the program director.

Management By Objectives

While resource department heads have the responsibility for setting objectives that relate to their own disciplines and to the resources for which they are responsible, program directors are also able to function effectively under a system of management by objectives. Each program director must develop a general statement of objectives for his or her program. The measure of performance is how well the individual achieves the stated objectives. If resources are committed to the program consistent with those objectives, the program director is obliged to carry out the objectives. If resources are not committed, the program objectives have to be reduced in scope and content. The program-resource concept thus establishes a clear basis for organizational accountability and for the development of measures of performance.

The program–resource concept makes possible accurate cost analysis and cost control by requiring program budgeting. The resources required to meet program objectives, manpower, money, material, and space should be budgeted to reflect the cost of each program at its inception and annually thereafter. Departmental budgets also should be prepared to reflect the allocation of resources on a functional basis.

At Mount Sinai Hospital, as an example, the psychiatric department chairman sets the broad programmatic objectives for the department. Program directors report to him, and his responsibility, based on the authority derived from his status, experience, and training, is to make decisions about priorities among competing requests for resources. The overall determination of program priorities is among his primary responsibilities.

Under this system, the general hospital administrator has two basic responsibilities: to answer to the governing board for the effective use of the hospital resources and to serve as a consultant to the chairman of the department and to the division directors about applying the management process to achieve the program's objectives. In this regard, the administrator helps to define programs, to determine the necessary resources, and to develop measures of how well the program goals have been achieved.

Under the program–resource concept, the principal organizational objectives are set forth as programs, and resources are identified as serving those programs, thus creating what has been termed "A Matrix Organization"[34] (see Chapter 11). By such devices, problems of employee identification are addressed, cost control and program budgeting are made possible, task specialization is realized, and most important, scarce health personnel have time to do the work for which they were trained.

COMPONENTS AND STAFFING OF INTEGRATED DELIVERY SYSTEMS

Acute Care Service

The primary goal of the acute care service is to offer immediate care to individuals who cannot cope with emergency situations without help. It may also screen admissions to the inpatient program and thus provide care ranging from crisis intervention to hospitalization.

Another major goal is to establish liaison with intramural and extramural referral sources and to develop new community relationships wherever appropriate. Acute service personnel also follow some patients who are undergoing care in other parts of the system and, where necessary, serve as case managers.

Staffing

The following staff is for approximately 3000 patient visits/year. *A full-time psychiatrist* should serve as the director. All professional personnel will be clinically responsible to the director. *A full-time Ph.D. psychologist* serves to carry out liaison functions. This responsibility requires knowledge and experience in the assessment of a patient's vocational and social disabilities as well as expertise in outcome variables and program evaluation unique to clinical psychology. Neuropsychological and other diagnostic assessment skills are also significant. *Three psychiatric social workers* conduct liaison with referring agencies. They also perform a triage function, conduct crisis treatment of patients and families, and carry out case management. *A psychiatric nurse clinician* is required to care for the more disturbed patients, participate in triage functions, and administrater and monitor psychotropic medication. Liaison with, and inservice training for, nursing personnel in the medical-surgical emergency room and other areas of the hospital are vital. At least three trained male medical-surgical emergency department staff should be available on every shift to deal with acutely disturbed and violent patients.

A full-time psychiatrist or psychiatric resident with experience in emergency work must be available from nine to five p.m. and an additional psychiatrist should be available at all other times. *A trained social worker* must also be available in the peak evening hours until nine p.m. The service should be within the general emergency service. An acute service requires access to a 24-hr observation unit. A single-bed quiet room, appropriately designed to meet the needs of acutely violent and suicidal patients, must be available.

The Psychiatric Outpatient Clinic

Goals and Functions

The psychiatric outpatient clinic will provide a full array of ambulatory treatment modalities required for personality stabilization, resolution of neurotic and characterological disorders, and the ambulatory medical components of treatment required by patients suffering with major functional illnesses. This requires integration with the inpatient and day treatment services as well as with the acute treatment service. Modalities of treatment subsumed under this latter function will include the full range of psychotherapeutic techniques as well as medication maintenance and ambulatory ECT.

The modalities required for the treatment of the nonpsychotic and appropriate psychotic ambulatory population include individual psychotherapy, group psychotherapy, family and couples psychotherapy, behavior modification, and approaches and treatment techniques utilized for the care of patients suffering with sexual dysfunctions.

Staffing

The following staff is for a clinic of approximately 20,000 visits/year. *A full-time psychiatrist* should serve as the director of the psychiatric outpatient clinic. The director will be responsible for integrating ambulatory care into the comprehensive integrated delivery system. *A full-time Ph.D. psychologist* will be required in order to provide adequate diagnostic services and linkages to the acute care service, the rehabilitation–resocialization program, and sheltered living settings.

Program evaluation and outcome monitoring are an essential function of the outpatient clinic psychologist. *Five full-time social workers* will be required to provide liaison and case management functions with respect to the community and other components of the psychiatric delivery system, e.g., the emergency room, inpatient units, and the rehabilitation–resocialization program. In addition, the social workers will provide couples therapy, family therapy, and group and individual psychotherapy.

Twenty psychiatric residents (half time) or 7–10 full-time physicians are required to carry out the medical aspects of care and to supervise the total planning and implementation of patient care.

Inpatient Service

Goals and Functions

The overall goals of the inpatient service will be to provide rapid evaluation and treatment of psychiatric patients during a brief hospital stay. This must include assessment of the need for ambulatory care and its implementation.

Staff

A full-time psychiatrist is required to function as a unit chief of a 20–25 bed unit.[36] This does not include the responsibility for training medical students and house staff or performing clinical research, which are all an integral part of many teaching general hospitals. Each unit at the Mount Sinai Hospital has one fourth postgraduate year resident (PGY-4) and three PGY-1 or PGY-2 residents at any one time. *A Ph.D. psychologist* (half time/unit) is assigned to deal with diagnostic problems and to assess functional capacity in terms of employment and social reintegration. *Two social workers* each see 10–12 patients who need to be followed in appropriate aftercare programs and living and work situations. Each patient's family and social network requires intervention as well. *The minimum nursing requirement* per unit is 10 nurses and an equal number of aides, at least half of whom should be male. In addition, each unit requires a supervising psychiatric nurse, who is responsible for supervision and in-service training, and four senior clinical nurses. *One social and vocational rehabilitation counselor* will be required to evaluate patients and to implement the aftercare program when the patients are clinically ready.

Rehabilitation and Resocialization Program and Supervised Residential Settings

Goals and Functions

One goal of a rehabilitation and resocialization program is to assess and treat social and vocational dysfunction while integrating this aspect of care with ongoing treatment of the disabling symptoms of mental illness. An additional goal is to develop transitional and long-term living arrangements.

A rehabilitation and resocialization program provides a series of work, social, and living experiences that afford patients the opportunity to function optimally in the community.

Staffing

The core staff listed is to serve the needs of approximately 100 chronically ill and disabled patients in a day rehabilitation program. A psychiatrist plus two other professionals is required for every 100 additional patients. *A full-time psychiatrist* serves as the medical director of the rehabilitation and resocialization program and provides expertise in the areas of rehabilitative psychiatry and psychopharmacology. The guidelines of the American Psychiatric Association and NIMH indicate that one full-time psychiatrist is required for every 100–150 patients. The psychiatrist assumes responsibility for all medical treatment given to patients.

A full-time director of the rehabilitation and resocialization program collaborates with the medical director of the program and assumes supervisory responsibility for rehabilitative occupational therapy, art therapy, and activities therapy workers in both the ambulatory and inpatient components. The director is responsible for the development of linkages with industry to provide contract work and transitional employment and assumes overall clinical responsibility for the transitional housing program.

A full-time psychologist is required for ongoing assessment of patient's functional capacities and abilities to adapt to different life settings, supervision of ongoing treatment and counseling services, and program outcome and efficacy evaluation.

A clinical coordinator of the day treatment program will assume day-to-day responsibility for the implementation of therapeutic programs designed to foster social and vocational adaptation for debilitated and isolated patients, including group treatment, graded work experiences, and skills necessary for social adaptation.

Two social workers are required to work with families and to provide liaison with community agencies in order to minimize revolving-door treatment at multiple facilities.

Four social and vocational rehabilitation counselors are required to implement appropriate programs for the patients.

A nurse–clinician is required to ensure that psychopharmacological treatment is appropriately monitored and administrated, and to ensure appropriate outreach and liaison to alternative living, acute care, and inpatient components. Many of the patients will require long-term parenteral medication.

SPECIAL ISSUES

Geropsychiatry

The general hospital psychiatric unit becomes a natural environment for the diagnosis and treatment of problems of the aging. At the Mount Sinai Hospital, for example, 25 percent of the psychiatric beds are currently occupied by geropsychiatric patients, often suffering from a combination of medical and psychiatric illnesses. This requires the introduction of geropsychiatric expertise and coordination between the department of medicine, the liaison psychiatry division, and the inpatient services.

Child Psychiatry

With the development of behavioral pediatrics and infant psychiatry, the general hospital has an increased community of need. It is striking how few general hospitals have child inpatient psychiatric units. In New York City, with its many general hospital psychiatric units, only one private institution has a child inpatient unit. The difficulty in staffing, the shortages of child psychiatrists, and the small volume of patients may account for this. The existence of a child psychiatry inpatient unit requires contractual arrangements with the local school board for continuing education of the hospitalized child.

Consultation/Liaison

The consultation/liaison service has been the mainstay of general hospital psychiatry, as noted above, for the past 80 years. The administrative structure of consultation psychiatry in a general hospital has been adequately described elsewhere.[37,38] The services are generally easy to develop and are funded through third-party payment. Liaison psychiatry, in contrast, represents a specific problem in that third-party payers do not support its development. For a specific description of structure, programs, and administration of liaison psychiatric services, the work of Strain and others is recommended.[39,40]

The Role of Attending Physicians

The majority of patients in general hospitals are hospitalized by physicians in each specialty, including psychiatry, with admitting privileges. The requirements for service in exchange for these admitting privileges as well as the minimal educational requirements (board eligibility, board certification, Continuing Medical Education (CME) credits, and so on) will vary from hospital to hospital. The administrative problems inherent in such a situation include questions of who controls final clinical decisions about private patients, conflicts over peer review and utilization review, and quality of care issues.

In some large voluntary general teaching hospitals such as Mount Sinai, the final decisions about the treatment and management of most inpatients are made by salaried staff psychiatrists or psychiatric residents under the authority delegated by the chairman of the department. The effects of this arrangement on the administrative structures of a teaching psychiatric service have been noted above and are also described in Chapter 7.

REFERENCES

1. Mora G: Historical and theoretical trends in psychiatry, in Kaplan HI, Freedman AM, Sadock BJ (eds): Comprehensive Textbook of Psychiatry/III. Baltimore, Williams & Wilkins, 1980, pp 4–98
2. Hackett TP: Beginnings: liaison psychiatry in a general hospital, in Hackett TP, Cassem NH (eds): Massachusetts General Hospital Handbook of General Hospital Psychiatry. Saint Louis, Mosby, 1978, pp 1–14
3. Davis S: Public policy and private psychiatric hospitals. J Nat Assoc Private Psychiatric Hospitals 1: 1969 pp 13–18
4. Witkin MJ National Institute of Mental Health: Trends in patient care episodes in mental health facilities, 1955–1977. Mental Health Statistical Note No. 154, September 1980. (1955 figures)
5. Witkin MJ National Institute of Mental Health: Trends in patient care episodes in mental health facilities, 1955–1977. Mental Health Statistical Note No. 154, September 1980. (1977 figures)
6. Taube CA National Institute of Mental Health: State and regional distribution of psychiatric beds in 1972. Mental Health Statistical Note No. 98, November 1973
7. Witkin MJ National Institute of Mental Health: State and regional distribution of psychiatric beds in 1978. Mental Health Statistical Note No. 155 (in press)
8. Mesnikoff AM: One person's barrier another person's fence. Presented at President's Commission on Mental Health, Technical Conference on Overcoming Systems' Barriers to Delivery of Mental Health Services. Arlie, Va, Arlie House, July 1977
9. Baldessarini RJ: Schizophrenia. N Engl J Med 297:988, 1977
10. May PRA: Treatment of Schizophrenia: A Comparative Study of Five Treatment Methods. New York, Science House, 1968

11. Swartzburg M, Schwartz A: A five-year study of brief hospitalization. Am J Psychiatry 133:922, 1976
12. Glick, ID, Hargreaves WA, Drues J, et al: Short versus long hospitalization: a prospective controlled study. Am J Psychiatry 133:509, 1976
13. Weisman G, Feirstein A, Thomas C: Three-day hospitalization—a model for intensive intervention. Arch Gen Psychiatry 21:620, 1969
14. Mattes, JA, Rosen B, Klein DF: Comparison of the clinical effectiveness of "short" versus "long" stay psychiatric hospitalization. II. Results of a 3-year posthospital follow-up. J Nerv Ment Dis 165:387, 1977
15. Davis JA: Overview: maintenance therapy in psychiatry. I. Schizophrenia. Am J Psychiatry 132:1237, 1975
16. Hogarty GE, Goldberg SC, and the Collaborative Study Group, Baltimore: The collaborative study group: drug and sociotherapy in the after care of schizophrenic patients, one year relapse rates. Arch Gen Psychiatry 28:54, 1973
17. Early DF: in Freem H (ed): Symposium on Psychiatric Hospital Care, London, 1964. London, Bailliere, Tindall and Cassell, 1965, p 165–187
18. Wilder J, Kessel M, Caulfield S: Follow-up of "high-expectations" halfway house. Am J Psychiatry 124:1085, 1968
19. Lamb HR, Goertzel V: Discharged mental patients—are they really in the community? Arch Gen Psychiatry 24:29, 1971
20. Mosher LR, Menn AZ: Dinosaur or Astronaut? One year follow-up data from the Soteria project, in Greenblatt M, Budson RD (eds): A Symposium of Community Care. Am J Psychiatry 133:916–921, 1976
21. Singer JE, Grob MC: Short-term versus long-term hospitalization in a private psychiatric facility: A follow-up study. Hosp Community Psychiatry 26:745, 1975
22. Brown GW, Birley JLT, Wing JK: Influence of family life on the course of schizophrenic disorders: A replication. Br J Psychiatry 121:241, 1972
23. Vaillant GE, Semrad EV, Ewalt JR: Current therapeutic results in schizophrenia. N Engl J Med 271:280, 1964
24. Feinsilver DB, Gunderson JG: Psychiatry for schizophrenics: is it indicated? in Gunderson JG, Mosher LR (eds): Psychotherapy of Schizophrenia. New York Jason Aronson, 1975 p 403
25. Klerman GL, DiMascia A, Weissman M, et al: Treatment of depression by drugs and psychotherapy. Am J Psychiatry 131:186, 1974
26. Paykel ES, DiMascia A, Haskell D, et al: Effects of maintenance amitriptyline and psychotherapy on symptoms of depression. Psychol Med 5:67, 1975
27. Lamb HR: Coordination: The key to rehabilitation. Hosp Community Psychiatry 22:46, 1971
28. Gruenberg EM: Community mental health services and the nature of psychoses. Lancet 721:721–724 1969
29. Barten HH: Developing a multiphasic rehabilitation program for psychotic patients in a community mental health clinic. Psychiatr Q 47:159, 1973
30. Davis S: Organizing a psychiatric hospital on the program-resource concept. Hosp Community Psychiatry 1970 21:33–36, 70
31. Fox RP, Potter DN: Using inpatient staff for after care of severely disturbed chronic patients. Hosp Community Psychiatry 24:482, 1973
32. Davis S, Carswell WD: The program-resource concept for hospitals: an alternative management strategy. Mt Sinai J Med NY 44: 174–182 1977
33. Davis S, Carswell WD: The program-resource concept: a management approach for an academic health center. Mt Sinai J Med NY 44: 624–632 1977
34. Neuhrouser D: The hospital as a matrix organization. Hosp Adm. 17:8–25, 1972
35. Hall RCW, Gardner ER, Stickney SK, et al: Physical illness manifesting as psychiatric disease. Arch Gen Psychiatry 37:989–995, 1980
36. Sabshin M: American psychiatric association comments and recommendations to notice of intent. Fed Reg 42:15433–15438, 1977
37. Lipowsky ZJ: Consultation psychiatry in the general hospital. Compr Psychiatry 12:461–465, 1971
38. Lipowsky ZJ: Consultation liaison psychiatry: an overview. Am J Psychiatry 131:623–630, 1974
39. Strain J, Grossman S: Psychological Care of the Medically Ill. A Primer in Liaison Psychiatry. New York, Appleton-Century-Crofts, 1975
40. Strain J: Psychological Interventions in Medical Practice. New York, Appleton-Century-Crofts, 1978

Robert W. Gibson, M.D.
Alan I. Levenson, M.D.

7

Private Psychiatric Hospitals

Utilizing the principle of "moral suasion," many outstanding private psychiatric hospitals were founded during the 1800s. Several of these hospitals still exist today: Brattleboro Retreat in Vermont; The Institute of Living, Hartford, Connecticut; the Westchester Division of New York Hospital, White Plains, New York; The Sheppard and Enoch Pratt Hospital, Towson, Maryland; Friends Hospital, Philadelphia, Pennsylvania; McLean Hospital, Boston, Massachusetts. All these early hospitals stressed the moral treatment of the mentally ill in contrast to the use of physical restraint, sometimes even physical abuse, that was prevalent when mentally disturbed patients were handled in almshouses and prisons.

Later, as psychiatry became an accepted specialty, psychodynamically oriented treatment was utilized in the hospital, psychotropic medications were developed, and the character of the private psychiatric hospital changed. Further impetus was given to the development of private psychiatric hospitals by the organization of the National Association of Private Psychiatric Hospitals (NAPPH) in 1933. NAPPH stressed quality patient care through educational programs and was instrumental in setting standards of excellence for its membership. Through the programs of the Joint Commission on Accreditation of Hospitals (JCAH) and other professional organizations, these standards were further elaborated under the Accreditation Program for Psychiatric Facilities. For more detailed information on the role of the private psychiatric hospital, the reader should refer to the paper entitled "Private Psychiatric Hospitals: Excellence Is Their Watchword."[1]

During the 1960s, the number of patients served by private psychiatric hospitals and the distribution between inpatient and outpatient services remained relatively stable.[2] The number of hospitals stayed at about 150; inpatients in residence at year end varied from about 10,200 to 11,000; annual admissions fluctuated from a low of about 87,000 in 1970 to a high of 92,000 in 1969. By 1979, however, the number of private psychiatric hospitals had increased to about 240, with a total of 21,700 beds.[3] The increase was greatest in the investor-owned hospitals; approximately two-thirds of all private psychiatric hospitals are currently operated by corporations, individuals, or partnerships on a for-profit basis, with the other third operated by not-for-profit groups. Particularly dramatic has been the growth in multihospital investor-owned chains, which now operate 88 hospitals.

GOVERNANCE

The governance of any private psychiatric hospital is based on its establishment as a legal entity. A public hospital operates under the auspices of a governmental agency, but a private hospital operates under the auspices of a nongovernmental sponsoring organization that determines the pattern for the hospital.

Typically, a private psychiatric hospital can be established as (1) an independent, not-for-profit corporation; (2) an independent proprietary (investor-owned) corporation; or (3) a subsidiary of a multihospital chain. The not-for-profit (or voluntary) psychiatric hospital is organized as a tax-exempt corporation and is operated by a community board whose members derive no personal gain from the hospital's operations. A proprietary hospital, on the other hand, is organized as a business venture that is designed to produce a profit for its owners; the subsidiary of the multihospital chain functions as one of a number of operating units that are owned by a single parent corporation. At the present time, most of the multi--institutional chains operating psychiatric hospitals are organized as investor-owned (for-profit) business firms, but not-for-profit chains operating multiple psychiatric facilities are increasing in numbers.

Whatever the nature of the corporate structure, the legal responsibility for the operation of the hospital is placed in the hands of a governing board. In the case of a not-for-profit hospital, the governing body is referred to as the board of trustees, and it is composed of community representatives who oversee the affairs of the hospital without compensation. The board of trustees is usually composed of about a dozen members who serve for a specified term of office and are responsible for electing their own successors.

In the case of the investor-owned hospital, the governing body is a board of directors, comparable to the board of directors of any business firm. The board of such hospitals is usually composed of a half-dozen members or even fewer; each member of the board holds a personal ownership interest in the hospital or represents someone who holds such an interest.

Finally, in the case of the hospital that is a subsidiary of a multihospital chain, the true governing board is generally the board of directors of the parent corporation; or if the hospital is owned jointly by the multihospital chain and local investors, the hospital's governing board may be composed of persons representing these two interested parties. A local hospital that is a wholly owned subsidiary of a multihospital chain often has a local community advisory board that can carry out some of the functions of a not-for-profit hospital's governing board. For more detailed information, the reader should refer to the paper entitled "The Growth of Investor-Owned Psychiatric Hospitals."[4]

As the body legally responsible for the operation of the hospital, the governing board performs many functions: establishing basic policies for the hospital; appointing the chief executive officer (who is responsible for the management of the hospital's operations); overseeing the financial affairs of the hospital through the approval of an annual budget and the review of periodic financial reports;

establishing the organized medical staff and appointing each medical staff member; and periodically reviewing the hospital and medical staff functions to assure the quality of care provided in the hospital. Most important, the governing board has the ultimate authority to commit the hospital's resources to new service programs and construction of new or expanded facilities.

ORGANIZATION

Personnel within the private psychiatric hospital must provide services within three functional areas: (1) nonmedical clinical services provided by hospital staff (hospital-based patient care services); (2) nonclinical support services; and (3) medical services provided by physicians. The organizaitonal plan for carrying out these three sets of functions varies according to corporate status, hospital size, established hospital patterns in the community, and the individual preferences of the hospital's governing board, administration, and medical staff.

Hospital-based patient care services (psychology, nursing, social work, activity therapy, and so forth) are generally under the supervision of the hospital's chief medical officer, who carries the title of medical director. Nonclinical support services are under the direction of the hospital's chief administrative officer, who is referred to as the administrator. Medical services, when provided by a closed staff of employed physicians, are usually supervised by the medical director. When medical services are provided by private practitioners as members of an open staff, supervisory functions are often carried jointly by the medical director and the active medical staff, having an elected president and various committees.

In most hospitals, a psychiatrist functioning in the role of the medical director is the chief executive officer, reporting directly to the governing board and having ultimate responsibility for the overall direction and management of the hospital. Under this arrangement, the administrator reports to the medical director and has delegated authority for the direction of such nonclinical departments as finance, personnel, housekeeping, diet, maintenance, security. Placing the ultimate authority with a medical director with clinical training and experience is favored, because every aspect of the hospital experience impacts on the therapeutic needs of the patient.

In some hospitals, the medical director and a nonmedical administrator report to the governing board as coequals. Under this model, the areas of responsibility of the medical director and the administrator are defined, but in practice such a balance can seldom be achieved solely by a detailed job description. Rather, it requires a collaborative relationship between the two individuals with an appreciation and mutual respect for the special competencies and training of both. Dual authority and responsibility provide a balance between the therapeutic needs of patients and the requirements of administration.

In some hospitals, the nonmedical administrator is the chief executive officer. JCAH standards and common sense dictate that even under this arrangement, the medical director must have ultimate authority over decisions about the treatment of patients. Realistically, however, when the nonmedical administrator is the chief executive officer, he has substantial influence over the allocation of therapeutic resources available for the care of patients. Admittedly, the professionally trained administrator may be better qualifed to cope with the administrative and regulatory complexity of the present health care system.

In practice, all three models have produced clinical programs of excellence. To a high degree, the outcome depends on the skill of specific individuals and their capacity to collaborate. The increasing demands for leadership in both clinical practice and management have led many hospitals to establish the position of chief executive officer as well as that of medical director, with both positions filled by psychiatrists. In this model, the chief executive officer is responsible for the overall direction and management of the institution, with special emphasis on defining the hospital's mission, maintaining external relations, and securing financial resources.

The medical director, under the guidance of the chief executive officer, is responsible for the clinical services of the hospital and the quality of patient care. Consistent with the overall mission and goal of the hospital, the medical director has authority to direct the clinical programs and departments, including the supervising, coordinating, planning, organizing, staffing, budgeting, and control of clinical resources.

Most private psychiatric hospitals provide their own nonclinical management functions. There is a trend (particularly among small hospitals) toward the purchase of management services because of the growing complexity of hospital administrative procedures and the increasing cost of administrative functions. Those hospitals that are subsidiaries of multihospital chains rely heavily on specialized staff at the corporate level. Few independent psychiatric hospitals can afford staff competent to cope with all the complex problems of reimbursement, cost reporting, and certificate-of-need planning. The ability to handle these matters in a cost-efficient way (largely through economies of scale) has been an important factor in the growth of the multihospital chains; and it is this same ability of hospital management firms that has made their services attractive to independent psychiatric hospitals, both not for profit and investor owned.

Some twenty years ago, most private psychiatric hospitals had a closed staff of psychiatrists who were employees of the institution. Psychiatric services, whether covered in the daily rate or itemized, were billed by the institution. Many hospitals offered an opportunity for psychiatrists from the community to treat patients within the hospital, but this was more the exception than the rule.

In the past decade, a major shift has occurred away from the closed staff organization toward an open staff organization. This is particularly true in the investor-owned hospitals, more than three-fourths of which operate with an open staff arrangement. In the open staff hospital, which is similar to the general hospital, psychiatrists in private practice admit patients, provide services in accordance with organizational rules of the medical staff and bill privately. In some instances, a small group of psychiatrists treat most of the hospital's patients and may be organized into a corporation established separate from the institution. Not-for-profit hospitals have also moved toward open staff organization with slightly more than half having such an arrangement. Some hospitals have a small cadre of salaried psychiatrists with key responsibilities for clinical administration and rely on physicians from an attending staff to provide the bulk of the direct services to patients.

Psychiatrists in private practice find the open staff attractive because they can maintain the continuity of care of a patient needing hospitalization. In those areas having more than one private psychiatric hospital or having psychiatric units in general hospitals, the private practitioner has the freedom to select the hospital that he finds most acceptable to his mode of practice. Still another advantage occurs in those states having cost review commissions, because the private psychiatrist is exempt from regulations limiting charges that apply to employed hospital personnel.

Hospitals offering specialized services and accredited residency training programs tend to favor a closed staff because of the need for control over the assignment of patients and the organization of teaching services. Some private psychiatric hospitals with outstanding teaching programs, however, have an open staff. Even those hospitals with a closed staff usually allow some psychiatrists in the community to treat hospital patients and allow the physicians on the closed staff to engage in limited private practice.

As more hospitals have moved toward an open staff organization, the active medical staff has assumed a more prominent role. As the main source of patient referrals, the members of the medical staff assume greater influence over the governance of the hospital. The responsibility for overseeing the medical (physician-directed) aspects of the hospital's patient care program in the open staff hospital is often divided between the medical director and the elected president of the medical staff.

The medical director carries responsibility (and authority) for hospital-based patient care services provided by hospital employees. The president of the medical staff carries responsibility for overseeing the work of the medical staff; and it is the organized medical staff itself that oversees the work of the individual physicians, largely through a series of formalized peer-review mechanisms.

PROGRAMS AND SERVICES

There was a time when psychiatric hospitals were devoted almost exclusively to providing long-term care for chronically ill mental patients; this has changed dramatically. Private psychiatric hospitals now provide a wide range of services and serve patients of many different types. Long-term care is one of the services offered by today's private psychiatric hospitals; but, in addition, these facilities now offer short-term hospitalization and provide a variety of specialized diagnostic and treatment programs as well.

In 1979, 57 percent of the nation's nongovernmental psychiatric hospitals reported lengths of stay of under 30 days.[5] Moreover, on the basis of a 1980 survey of 175 private psychiatric hospitals, the NAPPH reported that only 20 of the association's 183 member hospitals now have average lengths of stay of 6 months or more.[6]

Approximately half of the NAPPH member hospitals in 1980 reported serving adults and adolescents, while one-quarter of the member hospitals served not only these two age groups but also children (up to the age of 12) as well. Sixteen percent of the hospitals reported having specialized treatment units for geriatric patients; half of the facilities reported specialized services for alcoholic patients and/or drug abusers.

To meet the needs of their diverse patient population, private psychiatric hospitals provide many different types of treatment services. Most hospitals have both open and closed units. The treatment modalities offered include not only individual and group therapy but also a wide range of other treatment approaches, such as activity therapy, occupational therapy, art therapy, and music therapy. To meet the standards of the JCAH, an individualized treatment plan that draws on all the hospital's therapeutic resources must be developed for each patient.

Unlike the general hospital psychiatric unit, which provides care for psychiatric patients as one small component of the hospital's total range of services, the private psychiatric hospital provides care for the mentally ill as its primary mission. Accordingly, the private psychiatric hospital can utilize all its resources and physical facilities to provide care uniquely tailored to the needs of the mentally ill. The private psychiatric hospital utilizes not only specially designed buildings but also has extensive indoor and outdoor activity and recreational facilities located on the hospital's own grounds.

Inpatient care continues to be the focal point of the services provided by the private psychiatric hospital. In addition, however, private hospitals offer hospitalization programs and in some cases halfway houses. These programs have been used both for transitional care of inpatients and as alternatives to inpatient care. Many private psychiatric hospitals have now established outpatient clinics, and some operate community mental health centers that provide the full range of federally mandated services to a designated geographical area.

As private psychiatric hospitals have developed community programs, much of the funding for these programs has come through contracts with state mental health agencies. While enabling private psychiatric hospitals to diversify their services, these contracts have also been enormously beneficial to the state mental health agencies. From a programmatic point of view, contract services provided by a private psychiatric hospital help considerably in the state agencies' efforts at deinstitutionalization. Moreover, from an administrative point of view, these contracts have allowed state agencies a degree of operational flexibility not found within the restrictions of governmental budgets and personnel systems. Given the advantages of these contractual arrangements between state mental health agencies and private psychiatric hospitals, it is not surprising that the range of services covered by them has been expanding.

Indeed, more and more private psychiatric hospitals are taking on contractual responsibility for services that traditionally have been provided by state agencies and state facilities. Private psychiatric hospitals have provided these services not only within their own facilities but also as specialized units of state hospitals and psychiatric units of prisons as independent contractors responsible to state agencies.

In addition to expanding the services provided to agencies in the public sector, private psychiatric hospitals have expanded their programs in private nonhospital settings. For example, many of the private psychiatric hospitals have developed consultation programs for industry. Through these programs, the hospital staff members provide clinical consultation for industrial medical departments and nonclinical consultation services for corporate management and supervisory personnel. Many private psychiatric hospitals have developed clinically oriented employee assistance programs, with services provided both on the job site and within the hospital. In most employee assistance programs, a business firm contracts with the hospital to provide both consultation and education services for supervisors and clinical services for employees at all levels. Services provided on a prepaid capitation basis typically include crisis intervention, evaluation, and short-term therapy.

STAFFING

Private psychiatric hospitals generally provide a higher ratio of staff to patients than do the psychiatric units of general hospitals and the state and county mental hospitals. According to Taube and Witkin,[7] in January 1974, the staff–patient ratio for all private mental hospitals was 204 full-time equivalents of staff for each 100 average resident patients, with patient care staff accounting for 124 of these full-time equivalents (66 professional/100 patients and 58 other). Not-for-profit private hospitals had a ratio of 238 total staff compared with 173 total staff/100 patients in investor-owned hospitals. Within the nonpublic general psychiatric hospital units, the total number of staff for each 100 patients was 130, with 115 patient-care staff (65 professional and 50 nonprofessional). In state and county mental hospitals, the total staff for each 100 patients was 88, with 57 patient-care staff (18 professional and 39 other).

These figures must be interpreted with some caution. For example, many not-for-profit psychiatric hospitals employ physicians, psychologists, social workers, and other professionals. In investor-owned hospitals, many of these professionals provide their services on a fee-for-services basis and thus would not be listed as employees. Furthermore, many investor-owned hospitals tend to have many of their nonclinical services provided on a contractual basis, thus further reducing the listed number of employees. To some extent, the same is true of the nonpublic general hospital psychiatric units. Other important factors are the patient population, severity of illness, treatment services offered, length of stay, and so forth.

In an effort to obtain more precise data, the NAPPH in 1980 conducted a survey of all private psychiatric hospitals.[8] A questionnaire was sent to all private psychiatric hospitals requesting information on staffing according to all major mental health disciplines, with a detailed breakdown identifying the level of professional training.

In addition, the hospitals were asked to provide data on staffing as they related to various major clinical programs (adult, child, adolescent, alcohol, geriatric, and mixed services). Usable responses from 69 hospitals showed a considerable variability in the data. This is not surprising considering the variety of hospital types: investor owned, not for profit; locally oriented, nationally oriented; open staff, closed staff; free standing, affiliated; short-term, long-term; and so forth.

To eliminate atypical hospitals from the sample, those showing "extreme" staffing patterns were dropped from the study. The largest number of hospitals indicated that they provided mixed services: adults, adolescents, substance abuse, and geriatric patients were all treated on the same patient units. For these mixed services, the mean staffing for each 100 patients was psychiatrists, 15; psychologists, 5; nursing, 88; social work, 9; activity therapy, 12. For specialized adolescent programs, the staffing for each 100 patients was nursing, 99; social work, 10; and because of the educational needs of patients, approximately 21 teachers for each 100 patients. On substance-abuse programs, the staffing for each 100 patients was psychiatrists, 20; nursing, only 71; and social work, 10. On geriatric units, the staffing for each 100 patients was psychiatrists, 20; nursing, up to 104; and activity staff, down to 8. These differences in staffing patterns clearly reflect the different needs of patients in the several types of programs.

FINANCING

All private psychiatric hospitals, whether investor owned or not for profit, must generate funds for the operation of the facility through the services provided. In contrast, the public hospital is funded through an annual appropriation from a governmental body. The annual budget of the public hospital is really a spending plan for the year. For the private psychiatric hospital, however, the budget is both a plan for expenditures and a projection of income. Not only must the hospital stay within the limits of its projected expenditures, it must meet its projections for income.

Because of the uncertaintly inherent in projecting the volume of services, the private psychiatric hospital is at financial risk every year. The governmental hospital operating within a fixed appropriation is relatively secure for a given year but in the long run is more vulnerable because of the uncertainties of the legislative and political process. On balance, the private psychiatric hospital with its opportunity to generate revenue from multiple sources has greater flexibility and opportunity for self-determination.

In addition to funds needed for operating expenditures, private psychiatric hospitals must generate revenues to meet capital needs, particularly new buildings, major modernization of existing facilities, equipment, and furnishings. Such investment capital for the private psychiatric hospital ordinarily comes from three major sources: internal generation of operating surpluses or profits, long-term debt, and expansion of equity (which in not-for-profit hospitals could take the form of charitable contributions).

Private psychiatric hospitals, both investor owned and not for profit, rely heavily on operating surpluses for their needed capital funds. Not-for-profit hospitals frequently are able to take advantage of tax-exempt hospital revenue bonds. Investor-owned hospitals can sometimes avail themselves of tax-exempt industrial revenue bonds, but these are often more restrictive. The larger hospital chains have greater access to capital funding. Mortgage notes and bonds are frequently utilized by these corporations to finance significant capital expenditures.

Because of their structure as investor-owned corporations, the multihospital chains are able to generate capital funds through the sale of stock; indeed, shares in the chains are traded actively on the nation's leading stock exchanges. In addition, given their equity (stock) capital base, these firms are in an excellent position to obtain additional financing from the banks and other commercial lending sources. Most not-for-profit private psychiatric hospitals engage in some fund raising, but except for a small number of the older and nationally known private psychiatric hospitals, such charitable contributions provide only a small fraction of their financing.

Some 20 years ago, most patients paid out of pocket an all-inclusive rate of some $20–$50 per day for private psychiatric hospital care. As the inflation of cost of all health care has increased about tenfold, it has become impossible for all but the wealthy to pay the total cost of care out of pocket. Fortunately, third-party payers, including the federal government, now provide increased coverage for inpatient psychiatric treatment, albeit generally less than they do for medical and surgical conditions.

In a study[9] of the total admissions to private psychiatric hospitals in 1975, the principal sources of payment were Blue Cross, 37 percent; commercial insurance, 30 percent; Medicare, 11 percent; other types of government payment, 10 percent; personal payment, only 6 percent. There is, of course, a high degree of variation from one private psychiatric hospital to another, depending on the location and types of patients typically treated. For example, a hospital located in an area where there is a high concentration of active-duty and retired military personnel may receive a substantial portion of its payments from the Civilian Health and Medical Program of the Uniformed Services (CHAMPUS) program. A hospital located in an area with a high concentration of federal employees will receive a higher proportion of payments from the Federal Employee Health Benefits Program. In any event, only a small percentage of payments are made by patients or families out of pocket in private psychiatric hospitals.

In recent years, private psychiatric hospitals have moved toward itemized billing of professional services. This was in part a response to third-party payers who demanded such itemized billing, but it also reflected the shift toward the open staff organization. A recent survey by the NAPPH showed that a few private psychiatric hospitals include the services of psychiatrists in the daily rate. In 85 percent of the responding investor-owned hospitals, psychiatrists bill privately; and even in 58 percent of the not-for-profit hospitals, the psychiatrists bill privately. Most hospitals still include in the daily rate the services provided by social workers, activity therapists, nurses, and educators, but there is a shift toward itemized billing even for these services.

During the 1960s and early 1970s, private psychiatric hospitals were able to take advantage of a number of grant programs, particularly in the area of education and research. These sources of funding were frequently limited to not-for-profit institutions, but many investor-owned hospitals established not-for-profit foundations that could receive such funding. Some private psychiatric hospitals have received state and county funds through grants or contracts to provide specific services. Federal grant programs have been cut substantially in recent years and probably will cease to be a significant source of funds. One source of funding that has continued to grow, however, is the payment by local boards of education for adolescent patients for educational programs within the hospitals.

The reimbursement restrictions imposed by health insurance carriers have made it difficult for private psychiatric hospitals to establish new and expanded services. For example, the development of partial hospitalization programs (both day hospitals and night hospitals) as a substitute for inpatient care and in some instances as a supplement to such care has been impeded because of the reluctance of insurance carriers to provide coverage for partial hospitalization programs even though the data prove these programs offer effective care at substantial savings.

Given their dependence on generating revenue and the problems that they face in obtaining funding, it is not surprising that private psychiatric hospitals today are making every effort to improve not only the quality of their services but also the cost effectiveness of their operations. Most private psychiatric hospitals (both not for profit and investor owned) have established active cost containment programs. In addition, to improve revenues, many hospitals have mounted active marketing campaigns through a variety of public information and public education activities designed to increase the hospitals' visibility and to expand their sources of referral.

CONSTRAINTS AND SPECIAL ISSUES

The proliferation of regulation and other forms of control affecting hospitals is staggering. There is regulation by governmental agencies at all levels, influence by voluntary agencies such as JCAH, management through the payment mechanism by third-party payers, and controls that are built into a wide range of health care legislation. Even beyond the regulatory efforts directed specifically toward health care, there is control from the Occupational Safety and Health Act, Equal Employment Opportunity Act, Pension Reform Act, and many others. President Reagan has expressed concern over the degree of regulation and has promised to stem the tide, if not to reverse it, but that will not be easy to do.

As government and third-party payers have come to play a more dominant role and as there has been increased demand for public accountability, the practice of psychiatry (and for that matter, the practice of all medicine) has come under such extensive public control that it assumes the characteristics of a public utility.

Despite disclaimers, the Medicare and Medicaid legislation in 1965 accelerated the move to regulate health care. The benefit package available to Medicare beneficiaries was designed to influence patterns of care through better benefits for psychiatric care in units of general hospitals than in private and public psychiatric hospitals; a requirement that psychiatric hospitals meet JCAH accreditation; and a lifetime limit for treatment in psychiatric hospitals that was not applied to general hospital psychiatric units.

Several pieces of legislation designed to control and presumably to make the health care system more cost effective have been enacted. For example, appropriations to assist health maintenance organizaitons were intended to stimulate organized systems of health care as opposed to individual private practice. Social security amendments mandating professional standards review organizations were designed to increase participation by physicians in utlization review activities. The National Health Planning and Resources Development Act established a vast network of local, state, and national citizen groups to plan, to coordinate, and to control health resources. Manpower legislation was designed to control that most important of all health resources—trained personnel.

A less apparent but enormously powerful force has been exerted by the various insurance carriers through claims review. In this process, the patient seeks help; a practitioner provides a service; a claim is submitted to a third-party payer; the claim is either paid, or it is not. This last step establishes a crucial feedback to the system. The standards and criteria used for denial influence the types of service provided and the administrative management of the hospitals.

There has been an increasing number of judicial decisions affecting psychiatric care: right-to-treatment cases, right-to-refuse-treatment cases, laws affecting involuntary commitment, the rights of minors. More recently, legislation has been passed in some states to control the use of medications. In most instances, these court decisions have been directed toward correcting some injustice or inequity. Unfortunately, the judicial system is not really designed to set standards and criteria for psychiatric care. Nevertheless, that is just what has been happening, and it appears to be increasing.

The National Health Planning and Resources Development Act set up state health coordinating councils (SHCC) in every state, and there are now over 200 health system agencies nationwide. Many states have established commissions to control the costs of health care. The Reagan administration has proposed the withdrawal of federal support for the system of health systems agencies (HSAs) and SHCCs, but it appears that some form of health planning will be retained under state auspices, and certainly the controls on cost will be retained.

Most of the regulatory efforts are well intentioned; unfortunately, however, the controls overlap, they are sometimes contradictory, they are constantly changing, and they add substantially to the cost of care. Preoccupation with these multiple requirements can distract mental health professionals from their main goal: providing high-quality treatment services appropriate to the patient's need. Many hospitals find it has become more important to document that regulatory requirements have been met than to provide services that will be really helpful to the patient. The hospital administrator must find ways to meet the mandatory regulatory requirements. At the same time, he must try to protect staff from the unnecessary and counterproductive paperwork that seems inherent in regulation.

THE FUTURE

Private hospitals should be expected to continue to provide inpatient care of high quality for children, adolescents, and adults. They will continue to expand outpatient and day treatment programs, particularly if third-party payers improve benefits. Alternatives to inpatient care, such as halfway houses and community services, will be developed under the auspices of private psychiatric hospitals. Private psychiatric hospitals have become more accessible and responsive to community needs through diagnostic, evaluation, emergency, and crisis intervention services.

With the cutbacks in governmental programs (federal, state, and county), there will be an increased need for private psychiatric hospitals to expand their services still further. The range of patients treated will be broadened by greater emphasis on alcoholism programs, active treatment for the elderly, programs for the drug abuser, and special education for the mentally disabled. Greater involvement is needed in preventive programs of (1) consultation to community agencies and industry; (2) public education, especially for those who influence others, such as executives, teachers, labor leaders, judges, and politicians; and (3) counseling, school guidance, and vocational rehabilitation. These programs are valuable in their own right but have an additional benefit in increasing the hospital's visibility and linkage to the community.

Private psychiatric hospitals can contribute to the training of mental health professionals, particularly through affiliations with academic centers. Many opportunities exist for research, particularly in the application and evaluation of newer therapeutic approaches. As many states seek to reduce their involvement in providing direct treatment services, private hospitals will have the opportunity to fill the gap on a contract basis. Although the per diem cost is likely to be greater under such arrangements, the overall cost will be less because of the elimination of the costly bureaucratic overhead. Similarly, contract arrangements with business and industry should be further explored.

Further growth is to be expected among the investor-owned psychiatric hospitals and particularly among the investor-owned multihospital chains. These investor-owned hospitals and chains have already demonstrated an impressive pattern of growth during the past decade. Their financial strength and economies of scale in providing complex management functions of the multihospital chains seem particularly suited for further growth and expansion in the years ahead. More and more hospitals that are now independent will become affiliated with the multihospital chains, in some instances through acquisition and in others through management contracts. Although there are now relatively few not-for-profit chains operating psychiatric hospitals, these may increase, and there will undoubtedly be an increase in collaboration among not-for-profit psychiatric hospitals through management networks.

Regulation with particular emphasis on cost containment will probably increase. Mental health services continue to be vulnerable to governmental and third-party payer economy moves. Private psychiatric hospitals through area-wide and national associations must continue as vigorous advocates and effective leaders in influencing the fiscal policies of government and private insurers. Above all, however, they must continue to strive for high-quality care. In addressing a recent annual meeting of NAPPH, Dr. Francis Braceland enunciated this clearly. "As to the future of the private psychiatric hospitals, it is bright, providing excellence is their watchword."[10]

REFERENCES

1. Gibson RW: Private psychiatric hospitals: excellence is their watchword. Am J Psychiatry 135(suppl):17–21, 1978
2. Bethel H: Trends in Total Additions and Resident Patients at End of Year in Private Mental Hospitals, 1968–1971. Statistical Note 99. Rockville, MD, National Institute of Mental Health, 1973
3. American Hospital Association: Hospital Statistics. Chicago, American Hospital Association, 1980
4. Levenson A: The growth of investor-owned psychiatric hospitals. Am J Psychiatry (in press)
5. Am Hospital Statistics, pp. 8–10
6. National Association of Private Psychiatric Hospitals: Directory of Member Hospitals 1980–1981. Washington, DC, National Association of Private Psychiatric Hospitals, 1980
7. Taube CA, Witkin MJ: Staff-Patient Ratios in Selected Inpatient Mental Health Facilities, January 1974. Statistical Note 129. Rockville, MD, National Institute of Mental Health, 1976

8. Gibson RW, Whitmarsh G: Summary of Staffing Pattern Survey, National Association of Private Psychiatric Hospitals, Fall 1980. Research Memo 512. Towson, The Sheppard and Enoch Pratt Hospital, May 1981
9. Regier DA: Expected Principal Payment Sources of Admissions to Private Psychiatric Hospitals in the United States. Memorandum 20. Rockville, MD, National Institute of Mental Health, 1977
10. Braceland FJ: Psychiatry in a world still more troubled. J Nat Assoc Private Psychiatric Hosp 3:5–12, 1971

Pedro Ruiz, M.D.
Thomas T. Tourlentes, M.D.

8

Community Mental Health Centers

HISTORICAL PERSPECTIVE

The latent concept of comprehensive community mental health centers (CMHCs) in this country finally emerged in the early 1960s when Congress passed Public Law 88-164 and the Community Mental Health Centers Act of 1963.[1] These pieces of legislation permitted, for the first time in history, the use of federal funds for construction, as well as staffing, of comprehensive community mental health programs. As initially defined, these programs were to receive seed funds for a period of 61 months for the development of services considered essential to the provision of comprehensive care, such as: (1) emergency services, (2) inpatient services, (3) partial hospitalization services, (4) outpatient services, and (5) prevention services. This act of Congress, in addition to its impact on the mental health care delivery system, has focused major attention and priority on the fields of social and community psychiatry.[2–5] It was the intention and goal of this legislation to assist local and state governments in establishing comprehensive community-based mental health programs in every possible geographical catchment (service) area in the nation, thus assuring provision of necessary mental health services to all sectors of the population, in particular to those not previously served, such as the poor, the socially disadvantaged, ethnic minorities, and other special groups considered to be at high risk of social extrusion. Furthermore, it was the intention of the law to ensure that state and local governments would maintain these newly created services for at least 20 years to prove their permanent worth. These new federal ventures have encouraged and facilitated initial development of one of the most ambitious mental health service delivery systems ever conceived.

More recently, the U.S. Congress has passed Public Law 94-63,[6] which reaffirms federal support and commitment to the CMHC concept and creates a series of new steps directed toward enhancement of previously approved legislation. This recent legislation made possible the development of new programs as well as creation of new fiscal opportunities within the CMHC model, of which the most relevant were the following:

1. Creation of conversion grants to allow service expansion when needed.
2. Redefinition of comprehensive services, increasing the number of essential services from the 5 previously enunciated to 12. Added were (a) special services for children, (b) alcoholism services, (c) services for drug abusers, (d) services for the elderly, (e) court screening services, (f) transitional services, and (g) follow-up care.
3. Prevention grants for the development of consultation and education services.
4. Financial distress grants for up to 3 years for centers facing financial difficulties, thus jeopardizing the maintenance of existing programs without additional federal assistance.

Continuity of federal support as well as broader public endorsement of CMHC concepts have been of such magnitude that by 1977 more than 730 federally funded CMHCs were operational, thus making comprehensive services available to a total of 97 million persons, or 47 percent of the total U.S. population.[7]

GOVERNANCE AND ORGANIZATIONAL FACTORS

While this new and bold approach in the mental health care delivery system in the United States offered a new and hopeful perspective, it also presented a new challenge to both the providers of services and consumers. To begin with, this new mental health center concept by its nature focused attention on the "public sector" due to the large and diverse populations that CMHCs were committed to serve. The legislation itself, particularly Public Law 94-63, also focused on the input that consumers should have in the planning, operating, and monitoring of these centers. This new legislative requirement not only emphasized the power of the consumers but also demanded greater flexibility on the part of providers of services.[8,9]

What in the beginning only appeared to be an interest on the part of consumers in service delivery aspects of these programs quickly evolved, in a period of a few years, into a major philosophical issue about genuine community control.[10] This was partially derived from the broad social movement that began in this country in the 1950s and that actively encouraged full citizen participation in all aspects of human services delivery, especially in the major urban areas of the country. While there has been much discussion and confusion regarding interpretation of these legislative mandates, Public Law 94-63 states with great specificity:

> The governing body of a community mental health center shall:
> (i) be composed, where practicable, of individuals who reside in the center's catchment area, and who, as a group, represent the residents of that area, taking into consideration their employment, age, sex, and place of residence, and other demographic characteristics of the area, and
> (ii) meet at least once a month, establish general policies for the center (including a schedule of hours during which services will be provided), approve the center's annual budget, and approve the selection of a director for the center.[11]

This emphasis on community input as well as the greater attention paid to the special interests and needs of ethnic minorities living in the United States not only represented a challenge in the governance and organization of these programs but also demanded a closer working partnership between providers and consumers of services, which, in addition to being new and unique in the mental health field, represented a most difficult situation for professional operation of these programs. As a result, some traditional providers of mental health services either withdrew from these programs or have not tried to move forward in developing additional services of this type. In other instances, community groups demanded input so fiercely that they put sheer survival of some programs at risk.[12] Though difficult to establish and maintain, however, consumer involvement in CMHC organization and governance has been seen by many as not only beneficial but necessary and essential to the continued well-being of these programs.[13–18] On occasion, the role of consumers in community-based programs has gone beyond issues related to governance and organization of these programs and has touched on other sensitive issues such as possible racism,[19] improving the quality of services,[20] and even preventing mental illness.[21]

PROGRAMMATIC AND SERVICE DELIVERY ASPECTS

The CMHC movement has, during the last two decades, laid down the basic ideas that have permitted the development of new service concepts and program models. These concepts and models have had a great impact on every component of the mental health care delivery system, not only those within the CMHC umbrella but those in virtually all parts of the mental health field. Some of these aspects need to be examined in detail, since they indicate current and future trends of the profession of psychiatry. To begin with, we should consider two major concepts ingrained in the basic philosophy of the Community Mental Health Centers Act. They are (1) "continuity of care" and (2) "comprehensiveness of services."

While continuity of care is difficult to implement and in some cases has been found not to be particularly effective,[22] it does represent a unique attempt to provide a systematic link between providers of essential services and individual patients in such a way that case records, manpower resources, and all facilities within the service network are put to work for the individualized benefit of all patients. This model of care may occasionally create demands and stresses on participating providers, particularly those in programs operating under a consortium-type organization or under autonomous sponsors. When effectively implemented, however, it certainly works well for most of the people served. Teamwork approaches present an advantage in achieving and maintaining continuity of care, particularly in those programs in which there is limited availability of professional staff.

In terms of comprehensiveness of services, the CMHC model offers for the first time the opportunity to eliminate traditional fragmentation of services within the mental health care delivery system. The implementation of this concept also is very challenging and demanding, particularly insofar as development of all 12 basic services required by Public Law 94-63 is concerned. The offering of a broad array of services within a single administrative umbrella represents not only an innovation but also a real necessity. There are, however, constraints on some providers who are incapable of developing certain basic programs, such as inpatient services, in competition with existing large institutions such as hospitals. Many centers manage to survive and prosper under these circumstances, both in urban and rural areas, provided there is adequate community support. In general, the twin concepts of "continuity of care" and "comprehensiveness of services" have not been perceived as absolutely essential during the initial development of CMHC but are regarded as mandatory features during subsequent developmental maturation and growth.[23]

Another relevant aspect, which has gained importance as a result of the CMHC movement, is the concept of "decentralization of services." This concept has grown out of the observation that CMHCs are generally more effective when services are located where the patients live, thus offering a firsthand perspective on the patients' realities and problems and their underlying psychological causes and consequences.[24,25] The decentralization model also grew out of consumer need for services to be available without delay as well as within easy reach.[26] This arrangement is particularly important for urban centers serving many patients from lower socioeconomic classes.

This community-focused approach also has suggested a fundamental shift in strategy for the handling of mental disorders. The view has been put forth that mental disorders are rooted in part within the social milieu in which patients live and that providers of services should therefore focus more on dealing with the role of the various social systems of which the community is composed than on individual treatment goals.[27]

Another aspect that, although present in the past, has gained new priority and perspective within the CMHC movement has to do with the cultural relevance of services. An intrinsic goal of the CMHC movement has been service availability to all regardless of the ability to pay. This, combined with outreach efforts emanating out of the decentralization model previously discussed, has resulted in centers reaching out to a new clientele, which by and large is not only poor but ethnically different. This new emphasis, particularly in urban areas, has required the creation of a new needs concept in which cultural relevancy becomes a major concern.[28,29] Traditional approaches to serving this new clientele are frequently perceived as irrelevant and therefore unacceptable. Some so-called pathological behavior is nothing more than an example of a culturally bound attempt to deal with stresses created by an unfamiliar or prejudicial environment.[30,31]

Another factor, which also has been perceived as playing a significant role in community programs, is family and group therapy.[32] Expanding demands for services, manpower shortages, culturally oriented needs, and increased utility of family and group therapies have all resulted in these treatment approaches being prominently requested in community-based programs, particularly in urban centers serving the poor and ethnically disadvantaged.

Finally, it should be noted that deinstitutionalization and the linkage aspects of community mental health have not only gained high visibility in the last decade but also have assumed additional importance in view of the massive relocation of the chronically ill outside state hospitals. Community linkage with state hospitals did not only evolve out of the mental health center movement but also was the result of the general public policy and concern about the chronically ill, which has become an increasingly major priority of the broader health field.[33,34] In either case, the CMHC movement has provided a unique model and organizational approach for state hospitals either to become full-fledged CMHCs or to participate more effectively as an integral part of the network of care expected of these programs.[35]

In this regard, one of the most advantageous benefits derived from the CMHC movement is the role the centers have played in decreasing the number of unnecessary state hospital admissions, thus not only diminishing the potential development of "chronicity" for these patients but also the social stigma associated with it by delivering more appropriate services in a less threatening setting, which is family oriented, more acceptable to patients, and presumably of higher quality.[36–38]

PREVENTION: SPECIAL CONSIDERATIONS

Among the many useful contributions of the CMHC model, incorporation of the public health concept of prevention is probably one of the most important. While prevention has been perceived within the framework of the Community Mental Health Centers Act as being synonymous with "primary prevention," it will be discussed here from a broader base, thus encompassing not only primary prevention but secondary and tertiary prevention aspects as well.

Primary Prevention

Primary prevention is the reduction in the incidence of mental illness and is one of the essential services required of all CMHCs receiving federal assistance through the Community Mental Health Centers Act. One no longer can comprehend fully the satisfactory provision of mental health services solely from a traditional point of view, but rather from a perspective that goes beyond the individual, to encompass his environment and every social factor that directly or indirectly influences his potential to stay healthy or become mentally ill. Mental health services must be understood not only in terms of traditional settings, such as clinics, hospitals, and individual offices, but also as extending to virtually every part of the community support system. In this context, CMHCs must attempt to increase opportunities for community development even if this means involvement in social action. Traditional ways of operating mental health services, such as frequent appointments, long-term individual psychotherapy, and emphasis on "working through," are not sufficient for achieving primary prevention results. One also must be aware and concerned with other key features of the community resident's life, such as employment, housing, education, recreation, sanitation, and the like.[39] It has been well established that individual psychological defenses are frequently influenced by the social organization surrounding the person.[40] In other words, we must look at both the individual and his environment in order to assess fully the state of his mental health. Such an approach is particularly relevant to the public sector because traditional therapeutic approaches based on "middle-class values" may lead to rejection and alienation and might even prove to be harmful to some patients.

The involvement of professionals in social action programs has been questioned because of their limited expertise in these particular areas. This kind of social involvement, however, is more traceable to the professional's personality than training.[41]

From the point of view of primary prevention, the model of mental health consultation[42] has been found to be quite helpful, considering the limited numbers of available mental health professionals and also, ideologically, recognizing that local citizens should be actively engaged in promoting services and programs. One must acknowledge, however, that little is really known about the effectiveness of these preventive efforts.

Enhancement of member leadership in all social systems becomes extremely important in these settings of low community cohesiveness with multiple social problems.[43] Many community welfare agencies can be perceived as part of the psychosocial care-giving system for prevention of mental disability, and as improving the general competence of the citizenry.[44] In discussing the best approaches for implementing primary prevention alternatives, one must underscore the several roles of neighborhood service centers, which are addressed to (1) increasing the competence of residents in coping with stress; (2) fostering a positive attitude toward helping others; (3) informing community residents of services available and how to use them; (4) supporing local community groups and organizations dedicated to the general improvement of neighborhood conditions; (5) stimulating social organizations of the neighborhoods to get involved in community affairs; (6) helping community residents get organized to tackle specific community issues; (7) developing linkages and liaisons between center staff and local agencies as well as other community groups in order to provide appropriate consultation when needed; and (8) assisting local agencies and groups in developing or improving their own services.[45]

Finally, one must consider the suitability of "medical model" approaches in the design of primary prevention programs, particularly when attempting to serve in the public sector. In view of the chronic and growing fiscal crisis affecting health and welfare services, one must re-evaluate strategies and priorities to best determine who should intervene, when to intervene, and how to intervene.

Secondary Prevention

Secondary prevention is the early diagnosis and treatment of manifest mental illness. While not a part of the original philosophy of the CMHC movement some special aspects of secondary prevention nevertheless have much relevancy. This is the result of the increasing emphasis on "primary health care," which has been encouraged more and more during the last decade. The greater interest in primary health care has been emphasized not only for solo or group medical practice and at teaching hospitals but also in neighborhood general health care centers as well.[46] Insofar as the provision of mental health-type diagnostic and treatment services are concerned, it has been repeatedly urged that these programs should be an integral part of the larger primary health care system.[47]

The inclusion of mental health programs as part of a neighborhood primary health care system offers several advantages in the provision of secondary prevention services: greater accessibility, earlier detection and intervention, crisis care, and reduction of chronicity. As far as outreach services are concerned, the neighborhood primary health care center model also offers definite advantages, particularly linkage for the effective and timely provision of the follow-up care.[48]

Neighborhood multiservice centers are becoming an increasingly acceptable method of delivering medical care, especially to underserved urban populations. They are a cost-effective way to offer crisis intervention, agency consultation, and family-oriented services.[49] Secondary prevention efforts along "medical model" lines are more easily designed and delivered through the existing institutional resource base.

Tertiary Prevention

Tertiary prevention is the provision of support services that minimize or shorten relapses and institutionalization. Appropriate care for the chronically ill has become the number-one national problem in the management of mental illness. In recent years, as a result of the indiscriminately pursued public policy of "deinstitutionalization," the treatment and maintenance of many such patients in the community has become very different qualitatively and quantitatively and has presented great challenges to the profession from a theoretical viewpoint. Community-based programs, particularly CMHCs, must play a greater role, providing active assistance with housing, employment, welfare benefits, medication, maintenance and socialization, or nothing less than the essential survival needs of many chronically ill individuals on a day-to-day basis.

Appropriate and timely intervention techniques are mandatory for the successful maintenance of many of these patients in the community. It has been demonstrated repeatedly that active patient assistance during the transitional period from institutional to community life through provision of suitable community-based mental health services has a positive impact on the relapse and hospital readmission rate of the chronically ill, particularly during the critical first 6 months following discharge.[50] These efforts to provide additional support services in the community as an alternative to long-term hospitalization have resulted, however, in some serious competition between inpatient services and community-based programs for the limited available dollar resources.[51]

Since there is no single medical or comprehensive social model that could be applied generally to the universal delivery of all mental health services, one should feel free to incorporate appropriate features of both the public health prevention model, including primary, secondary, and tertiary prevention strategies, as well as "balanced social services" approaches to the mental health delivery system of the country. This approach is likely to prove beneficial and viable not only from a mental health planning point of view but also economically.

STAFFING AND MANPOWER PERSPECTIVES

Analysis of staffing and manpower patterns within the CMHC movement is a very complex task because of the many factors that must be taken into consideration. To begin with, one must understand the relationship that exists between program philosophy and staffing patterns. In general, programs are staffed in accordance with the needs and goals of the services to be provided by a given system, whether they are medically or socially oriented.[52] This general postulate, although self-evident, must be applied with caution and only to CMHCs for the most part and is based on the fact that many emotionally distressed individuals are currently cared for within the general health care system rather than by CMHC programs.[53]

It also has been noted that all programs and services tend, by and large, to reflect the orientation and preferences of the providers offering such services.[54,55] In other words, programs under the sponsorship of a medical school may have an academic service delivery emphasis reflected in the professional staffing available to this provider, a program sponsored by a community hospital may tend to have a "private practice" character, and a program located in a disadvantaged neighborhood may be more socially oriented and rely more on the use of nonprofessional manpower resources.

The etiological determinants of the illness itself is another relevant factor in staffing. For instance, if one has a basic conviction that the main cause of mental illness is rooted in the social and economic system, the predominant type of manpower favored will be different from that selected if the etiological factors are tied to a particular biochemical process. This gets even more complicated when we consider the many different therapeutic approaches used in the treatment of the mentally ill. For instance, if psychotherapy is to be the treatment of choice, one might argue that this therapeutic method does not require medical knowledge and as a humanistic endeavor may be delivered by a variety of providers.[56]

In any case, there are a myriad of factors today that play significant roles in the evolving and shifting manpower and staffing patterns employed in various community mental health settings. A current concern has to do with the role of foreign medical graduates now and in the foreseeable future. Foreign medical graduates reportedly make up over 50 percent of the physicians who staff state and county institutions.[57] Under recent federal legislation (Health Professions Educational Assistance Act of 1976), however, the entry of foreign medical graduates into the United States is being greatly decreased, and this surely will have a significant impact on the future staffing patterns of these last-resort facilities.

Traditional Professions in CMHCs

Another factor to be considered in this connection is the role that the traditional professions will have in the service delivery and staffing of these programs. From 1960 to 1976, the number of psychiatrists in the United States for each 100,000 population only rose from 7.7 to 12.4, while psychologists increased from 10.3 to 19.5, social workers from 15.1 to 32.2, and nurses from 282 to 449.[58] These striking differences in professional ratios are playing a major role in terms of manpower availability, competition, and service mix.

All of the traditional disciplines, however, have been found wanting. For instance, involvement in social action programs is regarded as demeaning rather than enhancing by many professionals.[59] It also has been found that many professionals have difficulty in direct-service programs because they are asked to work in areas in which they have little familiarity or formal preparation.[60] From a more positive point of view, on the other hand, greater collaboration between professionals and local citizens has been beneficial in terms of better planning and distribution of manpower and coordination of services.[61] Professional "team" approaches also are considered an important asset by most programs.[62]

Nonprofessionals in CMHCs

The use of nonprofessionals in service delivery has played a prominent role in the history of the CMHC movement. This source of manpower has been considered an advantage for some community-based programs, especially in urban areas, since it offers unique insights about the neighborhood, its cultural characteristics, and their relationship to patient needs[63] in addition to performing many essential primary prevention tasks.[64] It also has been observed that utilization of familiar nonprofessional manpower in some CMHCs tends to increase service acceptance and utilization by local consumers.[65] Furthermore, as service demands increase, additional utilization of nonprofessional manpower takes place[66] even in the presence of a constant increase in traditional professional manpower.[67] One caveat, however, must be emphasized: utilization should not be equated with effectiveness in the absence of more scientific evaluation of this very important question.[68]

Psychiatrists in CMHCs

The presence of psychiatrists in CMHCs has been reported to be steadily declining.[69,70] This manpower decrease has been noted to be more predominant in CMHCs located in nonhospital settings, in urban slums, and in rural areas. This trend in terms of full-time positions is down from 6.8 in 1970 to 4.3 in 1977 and in terms of directors of centers is down from 55 percent in 1971 to 26 percent in 1976.[71] Informal "statistics" indicate that psychiatrists now provide less than 5 percent of reportable hours of CMHC professional service.

It also has been observed that many psychiatric administrators are, by and large, minimally prepared in traditional training programs for their challenging administrative responsibilities.[72] This trend toward less involvement of psychiatrists in CMHCs has continued and soon may become a crisis of major proportions. In this regard, the number of medical students evidencing interest in psychiatry reportedly also has been decreasing in recent years.[73] Such a shift in interest might result not only in a serious manpower shortage for CMHCs but also could shape the basic model of all services to be provided through these centers in the foreseeable future.

PRIVATE PROVIDER PARTICIPATION

The authors' emphasis thus far has been on the public contributions to the development of the community mental health movement in this country. The private sector also has been participating in various ways. The basic principles of the community mental health movement are not the sole domain of the public sector. It is advantageous for every provider, private as well as public, to be part of a comprehensive system that guarantees continuity. Private providers depend to a large degree on the public sector to make such a system possible through informal working arrangements or by means of legally mandated referrals. Economic pragmatism is the governing force.

Private providers obviously cannot survive without assurance of adequate reimbursement for their services. Consequently, it is necessary for private providers to work preferentially in those areas in which such assurances are forthcoming. This has been interpreted in some quarters as self-serving and exploitative of the public system and has led to mutual recriminations and polarized working relationships.[74,75] The unsubstantiated myths that "private is better" and "public is cheaper" have tended to keep these quarrels alive long beyond the time when there was any substance to these arguments.

Virtually everyone now knows that excessive reliance on long-term custodial care is not a cost-effective answer to the service needs of the vast majority of the mentally ill. It has led to massive and at times arbitrary emptying of state public institutions, with the result that many more people requiring special attention now reside in the community, where individual freedom and treatment rights are actively protected through determined advocacy and special legislation. Consequently, the proportional representation of individuals requiring active mental health services in the population has shifted and grown considerably. The elderly no longer represent the bulk of the deinstitutionalized active patient population. More than half of these patients are under the age of 40 now and have needs that tend to be quite different from those of the elderly.

Hospital-Sponsored Mental Health Centers

The change in patient mix has created new challenges and opportunities for all community providers, private as well as public. For example, interest in serving the mentally ill by general hospitals has increased dramatically, and more than 2000 now operate inpatient treatment units. Many also host alcoholism rehabilitation services. Virtually all others provide some limited crisis services. As a result, more than half of all acute inpatient care is now delivered through community hospitals. Much of this is made possible by improved health insurance coverage. For a substantial number of patients, however, these benefits are limited only to inpatient care. There is therefore considerable variation in pre- and posthospital arrangements for the delivery of other needed screening and follow-up services.

Some of these inpatients are the continuous responsibility of their attending psychiatrists, but others may come from, or be referred to, public providers for necessary outpatient services. These referral patterns may be based on reciprocal service agreements or may be informal, with heavier service obligations tending to fall on the public facility. In either instance, the general hospital's main responsibility and commitment is to furnish acute inpatient care, and then only to the extent that reimbursement for services delivered is assured.

Voluntary accreditation (Joint Commission of Accreditation of Hospitals) and mandatory standards (hospital licensure) will become more important if all hospital psychiatric services are to become part of an adequate continuum of care. This will make it increasingly difficult for some hospitals to restrict admissions to selected inpatients, and more of the revenue generated by profitable inpatient units will have to be used to support additional screening and outpatient and follow-up services. It will not be as easy to segregate inpatient economics from other programmatic considerations as separate public programs and funding sources shrink.

Some hospital-sponsored mental health centers have become largely self-sufficient through pooling of all revenue sources, including funds derived from inpatient psychiatric "profit centers." The Rock Island Franciscan Hospital is a good example. Multiple-source funding still must be used to meet all budgetary needs and programmatic commitments, but the amount of public subsidy generally is lower than in publically funded centers (less than 30 percent of a $6 million budget at Rock Island). In the hospital setting, of course, one can take full advantage of all available "medical model" health insurance coverage, which usually is not applicable when social welfare models are used to organize free-standing center services. Blue Cross, Medicare, and Medicaid programs, for example, pay only for services provided under traditional hospital/doctor auspices. This policy obviously has been designed to prevent proliferation of reimbursement claims for loosely defined social ills appearing in the vague guise of medical care. On the other hand, multidisciplinary teamwork is a recognized and reimbursable reality when it is supervised by responsible attending physicians functioning actively within the hospital-based center setting.[76,77] At Rock Island, for example, salaried and fee-for-service psychiatrists harmoniously provide team leadership that brings effective multidisciplinary services to over 6000 different patients annually.

Aggressive multiple-source funding through realistic individual fees, full insurance billing, and successful grant applications should make it possible for a hospital-based center to serve everyone in the same way without focusing on indivious distinctions between private and public patients and on who is paying for their care.

Everyone benefits from the commitment to an integrated one-class approach to the organization and delivery of hospital-based community mental health services in which unnecessary economic barriers no longer get in the way of quality clinical care. Patients are assured of appropriate attention, doctors are assured of adequate reimbursement, and hospitals are assured of a winning combination of self-supporting services. Private sector providers clearly gain from the programmatic economies of scale that a public partnership makes possible. The public sector also profits from the greater availability of highly trained and scarce professionals. Lastly, and most importantly, the patients of both benefit from greater access to a richer array of treatment resources, which generally are not available to either sector alone.

SOCIAL ACTION AND CASE-FINDING CONSIDERATIONS

Hospital-based CMHCs obviously must concentrate on well-defined clinical services that are usually reimbursable because third parties are reluctant, understandably, to assume potentially costly responsibility for peripheral social action activities. This does not, however, necessarily preclude private service providers from participating in and exerting influence in this important community sphere. Most hospital-based CMHCs enjoy a halo effect of respect and trust that can be used to cut across many socioeconomic and cultural barriers and effect change.

This is particularly true when hospital-based CMHC spokesmen enjoy favorable reputations as responsive and effective clinicians. Advice in broader social areas then carries more weight. Under these circumstances, community groups tend to become more interested in involving hospital-based CMHC people as consultants, advisers, and task force leaders. Occasionally, community groups are even willing to pay for the consultant time involved as a natural extension of the fee-for-service relationships established in clinical areas.

The measure of effectiveness of private providers is all too often the number of people they keep out of public facilities and programs. This "gate keeping" function tends to be emphasized at the expense of the equally important case-finding responsibility of effective community mental health programs. In the short run, of course, this misplaced "gate keeping" priority helps to control public costs by spreading the burden of care more widely. This approach, however, seems to overlook and conveniently discount the fact that community mental health services that are more available attract more people. That rising expectations of community residents are legitimate for the most part and certainly need to be recognized ultimately means that everyone will experience an expansion of service demands at all levels, and the question then becomes one of determining whether public facilities are being used appropriately, not if they are being used at all.

Rivalry and competition between public and private service providers is not inevitable or necessary, particularly in the majority of communities that historically have been underserved. A hospital-based and fully integrated community center is an effective case finder for all styles of practice and professional interests, and there is enough work to keep all providers, public and private, busy without duplicating effort or unnecessarily wasting dollars. Trying to do both jobs with the same dollars, however, is an obviously impossible goal that public funders are reluctant so far to admit or address in any significant way.

FUTURE OUTLOOK

To predict, or even envisage, the future outlook of the CMHCs movement is not an easy task. In any case, it seems self-evident that whatever happens to mental health centers in the next two or three decades will depend intrinsically on the overall future of the health care delivery system of this nation. It seems reasonable to assume that the CMHC model will survive in some form as one of the various prototypes for the delivery of health care in this country. Based on this premise, it behooves the authors to examine some of the key issues now facing the mental health care delivery system. In so doing, perhaps some of the more important future trends can be delineated.

Community Mental Health Centers and Academic Psychiatry

In spite of some of the confusion and concerns that have preoccupied the profession during the last decade regarding the place of psychiatry within CMHCs, we believe that centers will play a larger academic role for the profession. Several positive factors could be cited in this connection. Most medical schools (87 percent) in this country are currently utilizing, in one way or another, the center setting for academic purposes.[78] In addition, federal financial support for psychiatric education programs has decreased, thus making medical schools more dependent on public service programs for their academic survival.[79] Furthermore, medical schools in general are now being subjected to more consumer accountability. The role of psychiatrists in CMHC settings and the philosophy of this service model will undoubtedly play an influential part in these changes.

The Psychiatrist's Role in Community Mental Health Centers

We have previously noted the steady decline of psychiatric representation on CMHC staffs around the country, a situation that must be regarded with great concern since the future of the whole profession may be at stake. Such a decline will undoubtedly have a marked impact on what happens to the centers as key providers of mental health services. The problem has been blamed on the expedient deprofessionalization that has increasingly characterized the CMHCs, along with their seeming lack of clear purpose, funding uncertainties, and conflicts over authority, service delivery, and control.[80] The problem is now further compounded by the recent decline in medical student interest in psychiatry[81] and the general medical perception of psychiatry as having low professional status.[82–84] As the profession as a whole becomes better defined in terms of its social responsibilities, however, many of these problems will begin to disappear, and the influence of psychiatry over mental health center programs will definitely increase.

Service Delivery Model in Community Mental Health Centers

Needless to say, the community mental health movement as a whole has been confronted by a most difficult challenge insofar as prevailing models of service delivery is concerned. This crisis is not only complex but is still present and growing. Some authors[85,86] blame the community mental health movement itself for these difficulties, while others[87] refer to the general lack of substantive service evaluation efforts; still others[88] focus their criticisms on the largely unfulfilled real programmatic mission of many centers. It also has been suggested that CMHCs have not tried to define their boundaries and by attempting to be all things to all people have gotten overinvolved in areas in which mental health professionals have no real expertise,[89] not to mention the grandiose and wishful thinking of the 1960s that psychiatry, as a discipline, could provide solutions for most of the social problems facing mankind.[90] Despite most of these problems, it remains a hopeful fact that CMHCs and outpatient clinics deliver over 50 percent of all reportable mental health care in the United States today.[91]

Most of the efforts so far made to understand and resolve the problems facing CMHCs, although valid, have been rather limited and narrow in scope and, by and large, have failed to encompass the broader role of society and its impact on the mental health care delivery system and the profession. If one were to include these factors in assessing the current and future role of centers, it would be important to look at another layer of several problems.

National Health Insurance

As consumers demand and get more comprehensive health care, a clearer delineation will be made of what mental health services are to be offered and who is to provide these services. In this connection, one could predict that with the fiscal conservatism now prevailing in the country, CMHCs will gradually become limited outposts for hospital-based services, with emphasis on medically prescribed approaches. These efforts, however, will be focused primarily on cost-containment goals; therefore, disciplines other than that of psychiatrists probably will play a larger role, particularly in terms of psychological and socially oriented services. Services also will be more circumscribed in terms of eligibility, type of care, and duration.

Locus of Services

The diminishing role of the state hospital within the mental health care system seems inevitable, and the dominant locus of mental health care delivery will shift to community-based facilities. This will not, however, necessarily follow the decentralization model felt to be most appropriate in the past. As a result, as has already been mentioned,[92–94] emphasis on the chronically ill mental patient will increase, secondary and tertiary prevention services will grow in number, and primary prevention efforts will tend to diminish. Furthermore, fiscal constraints will force providers to organize more "consortium" models as well as move to the regionalization of certain type of programs such as forensic services, children's services, and geriatric services. A major emphasis on avoiding hospitalization will grow. This again will be based mainly on cost containment and other fiscal constraints. It should be remembered, however, that shortening the periods of hospitalization tends to lead to higher readmission rates. The mean length of stay also tends to be somewhat higher for comparable admissions in the private sector than in the public sector.[95]

Role of Psychiatrists

As the changing role of the profession begins to be better understood in the field, particularly as far as returning to mainstream medicine is concerned,[96,97] psychiatrists will begin to feel less threatened, and their current identity crisis will start to subside. In this new role, more psychiatrists will begin to re-examine their functions and responsibilities within the CMHC movement. These centers also will change their scope of services, and the profession then will find a more meaningful permanent role within these programs. This process undoubtedly will demand training curriculum revisions to assure more competence in social and community psychiatry as well as better evaluation and research strategies to avoid the mistakes of the past. Continuing manpower shortages, however, will force psychiatrists to assume more and more the role of consultants and managers of team care. The public and the private sectors will start to converge toward a single system of health care, which will offer not only a more equitable solution to the many problems now confronting the health care system but also a better qualitative approach to the treatment of the mentally ill.

REFERENCES

1. Morrison LJ: Barriers to self-sufficiency for mental health centers. Hosp Community Psychiatry 28:185–191, 1977
2. Wachpress M: Goals and functions of the community mental health center. Am J Psychiatry 129:187–190, 1972
3. Feldman S: Community mental health centers: a decade later. J Ment Health 3:19–34, 1974
4. Peck HB, Kaplan SR: A mental health program for the urban multiservice center, in Shore M (ed): Mental Health and the Community. New York, Behavioral Publications, 1969, pp 123–142
5. Beigel A, Levenson A (eds): The Community Mental Health Center: Strategies and Programs. New York, Basic Books, 1972
6. Sharfstein SS: Will community mental health survive in the 1980's?, Am J Psychiatry 135:1363–1365, 1978
7. Sharfstein SS: Community mental health centers: returning to basics. Am J Psychiatry 136:1077–1079, 1979
8. Ruiz P: Consumer participation in mental health programs. Hosp Community Psychiatry 24:38–40, 1973
9. Shaw R, Eagle C: Programmed failure: the Lincoln Hospital story. Community Ment Health J 7:255–263, 1971
10. Bolman WM: Community control of the community mental health center: I. Introduction. Am J Psychiatry 129:173–180, 1972
11. National Institute of Mental Health: Citizen Participation in Community Mental Health Centers. Washington, DC, US Government Printing Office: 260-943/1122, P.v., 1978
12. Ruiz P, Behrens M: Community control in mental health: how far can it go? Psychiat Q 47:317–324, 1973
13. Ahmed BM, Stein DD: Children's mental health services: a case study of a successful grant proposal. Hosp Community Psychiatry 25:591–595, 1974
14. Levine RA: Consumer participation in planning and evaluation of mental health services. Social Work 15:41–46, 1970
15. Mogulof MB: Advocates for themselves: citizen participation in federally supported community organizations. Community Ment Health J 10:66–76, 1974
16. Ozarin L, Feldman S, Spaner FE: Experience with Community Mental Health Centers. Am J Psychiatry 127:88–92, 1973
17. Rabiner CJ: On community advisory boards. World J Psychosynthesis 3:32–34, 1971
18. Williams CE, French N, Becker R: Neighborhood organization: prevention and psychiatry. Am J Orthopsychiatry 41:243–244, 1971
19. Cornely PB: Community participation and control: a possible answer to racism in health. Milbank Mem Fund Q 49:347–362, 1970
20. Smith MB, Hubbs N: The community and the community mental health center. Am Psychol 21:499–509, 1966
21. Johnson TJ, Boutwell CR, Hinkle AL: Community mental health center evaluation: a survey of mental health problems and professional services. Evaluation 2:18–19, 1975
22. Kline J, King M: Treatment dropouts from a community mental health center. Community Ment Health J 9:354–360, 1973
23. Austin MA: Developmental view of the comprehensive community mental health concept. Community Ment Health J 5:156–163, 1969
24. Fishman JR, McCormick J: Mental health without walls: program for the ghetto. Curr Psychiatr Ther 9:245–256, 1969
25. Fishman JR, McCormick J: Mental health without walls: community mental health in the ghetto. Am J Psychiatry 126:1461–1467, 1970
26. Kluger JM: The uninsulated case load in a neighborhood mental health center. Am J Psychiatry 126:1430–1436, 1970
27. Dorken H: A dimensional strategy for community-focused mental health services, in Rosenblum G (ed): Issues in Community Psychiatry and Preventive Mental Health. New York, Behavioral Publications, 1971, pp 75–87
28. Brooks CM: New mental health perspectives in the black community. Soc Casework 55:489–496, 1974
29. Ruiz P, Langrod J: The role of folk healers in community mental health services. Community Ment Health J 12:392–398, 1976
30. Griffith EH, Ruiz P: Cultural factors in the training of psychiatric residents in a Hispanic urban community. Psychiatr Q 49:29–37, 1977
31. Griffith EH, English T, Mayfield V: Possession, prayer, and testimony: therapeutic aspects of the Wednesday night meeting in a black church. Psychiatry 43:120–128, 1980
32. Sands RM, Young AK: The retooling of a child guidance center: changes and change-

over for the tasks of the seventies. Am J Orthopsychiatry 43:65–71, 1973

33. Talbott JA: Toward a public policy on the chronic mentally ill patient. Am J Orthopsychiatry 50:43–53, 1980
34. Williams DH, Bellis EC, Wellington SW: Deinstitutionalization and social policy: historical perspectives and present dilemmas. Am J Orthopsychiatry 50:54–64, 1980
35. Osterweil J, Brown BS: Critical factors in the unitization of mental hospitals. Int J Psychiatry 7:226–228, 1969
36. Dyck G: The effect of a community mental health center upon state hospital utilization. Am J Psychiatry 131:453–456, 1974
37. Ruiz P, Saiger G: Partial hospitalization within an urban slum. Am J Psychiatry 129:89–92, 1972
38. Ruiz P: Avoiding hospitalization for the urban poor: problems and prospects, in Lamb HR (ed): New Directions for Mental Health Services. San Francisco, Jossey-Bass, 1979, pp 65–72
39. Peck HB, Kaplan SR, Roman M: Prevention, treatment and social action: a strategy of intervention in a disadvantaged urban area. Am J Orthopsychiatry 36:57–69, 1966
40. Erikson EH: Identity and the life cycle. Psychol Issues 1: 1959.
41. Goodstein LD: Organizational development as a model for a community consultation. Hosp Community Psychiatry 23:165–168, 1972
42. Scheidlinger S, Strueing EL, Rabkin JG: Evaluation of a mental health consultation service in a ghetto area. Am J Psychother 24:485–493, 1970
43. Scheidlinger S, Sarcka A: A mental health Consultation-education program with group agencies in a disadvantaged community. Community Ment Health J 5:164–171, 1969
44. Rae-Grant QAF, Gladwin T, Bower E: Mental health, social competency, and the war on poverty. Am J Orthopsychiatry 36:652–664, 1966
45. Hallowitz E: The role of a neighborhood service center in community mental health. Am J Orthopsychiatry 38:705–714, 1968
46. Macht LB: Neighborhood health centers: perspectives on opportunity for comprehensive ambulatory health care. N Engl J Med 292:591–592, 1975
47. American Public Health Association resolution on mental health as an essential part of comprehensive health care programs. Am J Public Health 66:189–190, 1976
48. Borus JF: Neighborhood health centers as providers of primary mental health care. N Eng J Med 295:140–145, 1976
49. Scharfstein SS: Neighborhood psychiatry: new community approach. Community Ment Health J 10:77–83, 1974
50. Bene-Kociemba A, Cotton PG, Frank A: Predictors of community tenure of discharged state hospital patients. Am J Psychiatry 136:1556–1561, 1979
51. Osberg JW: Unifying state hospital and community mental health systems through area programs. Hosp Community Psychiatry 23:105–108, 1972
52. Du Mas FM: Medical, nonmedical, or antimedical models for mental health centers? Am J Psychiatry 131:875–878, 1974
53. Report to the President from the President's Commission on Mental Health, vol. 1, Washington, DC, 1978.
54. Agel J: the Radical Therapist. New York, Ballantine, 1971
55. Neugeboren B: Psychiatric Clinics: A Typology of Service Patterns. Metuchen, NJ, Scarecrow Press, 1970
56. Talbott JA: Radical psychiatry: an examination of the issues. Am J Psychiatry 131:121–128, 1974
57. Jenkins JJ, Witkin MJ: Foreign Medical Graduates Employed in State and County Mental Hospitals. Mental Health Statistical Note 131. Rockville, MD, National Institute of Mental Health, 1976
58. Langsley DG, Robinowitz CB: Psychiatric manpower: An overview. Hosp Community Psychiatry 30:749–755, 1979
59. Bolman WM: Community control of the community mental health center: II. Case examples. Am J Psychiatry 129:181–186, 1972
60. Baldwin BA: Alternative services, professional practice, and community mental health. Am J Orthopsychiatry 45:734–743, 1975
61. Kolb LC: Community mental health centers. Int J Psychiatry 9:283–293, 1970
62. Cowen DL: Denver's mental health program. JAMA 215:260–273, 1971
63. Herbert GK, Chevalier MC, Meyers CL: Factors contributing to the successful use of indigenous mental health workers. Hosp Community Psychiatry 25:308–310, 1974
64. Peck HB: A candid appraisal of a community mental health center as a public agency: a case history. Am J Public Health 59:459–469, 1969
65. Riessman CK: The supply-demand dilema in community mental health centers. Am J Orthopsychiatry 40:858–869, 1970

66. Rusk TN: Future changes in mental health care. Hosp Community Psychiatry 23:7–9, 1972
67. Felton GS, Wallace HF, Gallo CL: Training mental health workers to better meet patient needs. Hosp Community Psychiatry 25:299–302, 1974
68. Karlsruher AE: The nonprofessional as a psychotherapeutic agent. Am J Community Psychology 2:61–77, 1974
69. Sabshin M: Politics and the stalled revolution. Psychiatr Ann 7:98–102, 1977
70. Sharfstein SS, Wolfe JC: The community mental health centers program: expectations and realities. Hosp Community Psychiatry 29:46–49, 1978
71. Beigel A, Sharfstein SS, Wolfe JC: Toward increased psychiatric presence in community mental health centers. Hosp Community Psychiatry 30:763–767, 1979
72. Greenblatt M: Psychopolitics. Am J Psychiatry 131:1197–1203, 1974
73. Nielsen AC: The magnitude of declining psychiatric career choice. J Med Ed 54:632–637, 1979
74. Tourlentes TT: Audio-cassette Lecture: Complete Merger of Private and Center Practice Systems into a Unified Whole. University of Wisconsin Extension Health Services Unit, Continuing Education in Mental Health, 1973.
75. Tourlentes TT: Integration of Private Fee and Salaried Professional Practice in a Community Mental Health Center System Proceedings, Vth World Congress of Social Psychiatry, Athens, 1974
76. Tourlentes TT: Psychiatric administration: a unique mental health responsibility. Psychiat Opinion 15: 15:154–158, 1978
77. Tourlentes TT: Psychiatric administration and medical responsibility. Administration in Mental Health 9(2):154–158, 1981
78. Faulkner LR, Eaton JS: Administrative Relationships Between Community Mental Health Centers and Academic Psychiatric Departments, Am J Psychiatry 136:1040–1044, 1979
79. Eaton JS, Goldstein LS: Psychiatry in crisis. Am J Psychiatry 134:642–645, 1977
80. Fink PJ, Weinstein SP: Whatever happened to psychiatry? The deprofessionalization of community mental health centers. Am J Psychiatry 136:406–409, 1979
81. Nielsen AC: Choosing psychiatry: The importance of psychiatric education in medical school. Am J Psychiatry 137:428–431, 1980
82. Eagle PF, Marcos LR: Factors in medical students' choice of psychiatry. Am J Psychiatry 137:423–427, 1980
83. Zimet CN, Held ML: The development of views of specialties during four years of medical school. J Med Educ 50:157–166, 1975
84. Matteson MT, Smith SV: Selection of medical specialties: preferences versus choices. J Med Educ 52:548–554, 1977
85. Kubie LS: Pitfalls of community psychiatry. Arch Gen Psychiatry 18:257–266, 1968
86. Ketty SS: From rationalization to reason. Am J Psychiatry 131:957–963, 1974
87. Zusman J: Program evaluation and quality control in mental health services, in Bellak L, Barten HH (eds): Progress in Community Mental Health, vol. 3. New York, Brunnel & Mazel, 1975, pp 233–264
88. Zusman J, Lamb HR: In Defense of Community Mental Health, Am J Psychiatry 134:887–890, 1977
89. Borus JF: Issues critical to the survival of community mental health. Am J Psychiatry 135:1029–1035, 1978
90. Eaton JS, Daniels RS, Pardes, H: Psychiatric Education: State of the Art, 1976. Am J Psychiatry 134:2–6, 1977
91. Witkin MJ: Trends in Patient Care Episodes in Mental Health Facilities, Mental Health Statistical Note No. 154, DHHS Publication No. (ADM) 80-158, Rockville, MD, National Institute of Mental Health, 1980.
92. Kirk SA, Therrien ME: Community mental health myths and the fate of former hospitalized patients. Psychiatry 38:209–217, 1975
93. Robbins E, Robbins L: Charge to the community: some early effects of a state hospital system's change of policy. Am J Psychiatry 131:641–645, 1974
94. Lamb HR: Community Survival for Long Term Patients. San Francisco, Jossey-Bass, 1976
95. McNeill DN, Stevenson J, Longabaugh RH: Short-term inpatient care and readmission rates: the community mental health center approach versus the private approach. Hosp Community Psychiatry 31:751–755, 1980
96. Hackett TP: The psychiatrist: in the mainstream or on the banks of medicine? Am J Psychiatry 135:432–434, 1977
97. Engel GL: The need for a new medical model: a challenge for biomedicine. Science 196:129–136, 1977

PART III

Organizational and Administrative Theory

Alan M. Kraft, M.D.

9

Behavioral and Organizational Theories

Organizations consist of groups of people who consciously join to accomplish a stated purpose. Organizations are large or small, simple or complex, formal or informal. Yet their major elements are people and purpose. In the case of mental health service organizations, the purpose is service to the mentally ill; the work of the organization is prevention, care, treatment, and rehabilitation.

The more formal an organization and the larger it is, the more likely is it to have explicitly stated rules and regulations, procedures, and policies defining the goals and behavior of its members. In organizations made up of more than a few people, a certain amount of impersonality usually develops in the organization in its dealings with its staff and its public. The organization becomes a separate entity and is so viewed and dealt with. An organization is thus seen as a dynamic form that is managed, that may change, that acts and is acted upon. It is an organism or a system, a living thing quite independent of the people who make it up. As evidence of its independence of the people in it, it usually survives the tenure of the individuals who work in it.

The primary purpose of an organization is to deliver a service or to create a product that is sufficiently valued by its public that it receives in return the material rewards that, in turn, enable it to purchase the services of its employees, buy the materials it needs and in the case of a profit-making organization, return a financial gain to its owners or investors. The people in the organization are engaged in work that contributes directly or indirectly to the ultimate delivery of the service or product.

Though organizations were probably created in very early societies, they have grown in complexity in the last two centuries. It was not until recent decades that a great deal of attention was given to understanding them and the way they work. It became important to understand organizations when business and government grew in size and complexity and when, as a result, business and governmental organizations became critically important economic and political entities.

There is not a single coherent theory of organizational dynamics. There are, however, a number of important and useful conceptual frameworks.

Max Weber (1864–1920), a sociologist whose work is seminal, created the term *bureaucracy* and a theory of formal organizations. He was interested in the systematic division of tasks and authority and thus in organizational structure.

He recognized that there were different kinds of authority in an organization. He defined authority as the probability that a specific command will be obeyed.

Legitimate authority derives from the need to obey the rules of an organization. The individual with authority is granted power by the organization; in return, compliance is required by the organization. The order given and the order complied with are not personal in nature but flow from organizational structure. Legitimate authority is rational and legal. It is assigned in a rational manner to accomplish rational goals, and it has defined limits.

Weber also identifies two other kinds of authority, which are nonlegal and nonrational. These do not derive from the formal organizational relationship of two persons but rather from personal characteristics (charismatic authority) or from relationships existing outside the organization (traditional authority). *Charismatic* authority rests on the emotional and personal devotion of the follower to the leader. Its driving force lies in the personal characteristics of the leader that have special appeal to the follower. It is independent of the respective formal organizational roles of the persons involved. A charismatic leader may be or may not hold an office in the organization.

Traditional authority rests on the belief in the sacredness of the social order. Obedience in this case occurs because of the belief system that derives historically from the feudal system of lord and master and also from the family system of patient and child.

Weber's concept of bureaucracy is of a rational and legal system in which officeholders hold their positions because of competency for their tasks, not because of attractive personal qualities or because of age or wealth. As he described the bureaucratic organization, it has none of the prerogative connotation now associated with the term *bureaucracy*. It is a rational, competency-based organization, a meritocracy, resting on a logical hierarchical line of command. Rules, regulations, and policies regarding conduct are specified. Unlike an organization in which the owner is the manager, in bureaucracies, there is a separation of ownership from managership, as in contemporary large corporations, government, and most mental health organizations.

What is missing from Weber's theory is a consideration of the nonrational aspects of behavior that we have come to recognize and respect. Weber considered all the actors on the organizational stage to be motivated entirely by a rational consideration of the goals and rules of the organization.

Building on his work, others have given greater consideration to the nonrational but nonetheless significant motivations that influence behavior.[2–8]

Chester Bernard focused on motivation.[2] He defined organizations as systems of consciously coordinated personal activities or forces of one or more persons. A key concept is *cooperation,* which brings Bernard to address those psychological forces that mold and direct behaviors, i.e., motivation.

The concern of Bernard and other authors is the interface between the individual and the organization. This leads to a consideration of the central issue of personal motivation. The Bernard–Simon theory simply states:

1. An organization is a system of interrelated social behaviors of a number of persons who may be called *participants.*

2. Each participant receives from the organization inducements, in return for which he makes contributions.
3. Each participant will continue participation in an organization only so long as the inducements are as great or greater (according to his values) than the contribution he is asked to make.
4. The organization functions as a result of the contributions and, in turn, produces the necessary inducements.
5. The organization is solvent only so long as the contributions are sufficient to provide inducements adequate to draw forth these contributions. Inducements include wage and various other rewards, both material and psychological.

Levinson distinguishes role from social position.[7] *Social position* in an organization is an element of organizational anatomy. It defines the structural relationships between the people in an organization. *Role* is more complex. It has three different possible meanings. The term is used to describe the expected behaviors of people who occupy social positions. Role may define the person's expectations of how to fulfill the social position. Role is also defined as the actions of an individual in a social position. With regard to role, there may be greater or lesser congruency for an individual between organizatonal expectations and personal beliefs, values, goals, and interests.

Weber did not consider this congruency or lack of it. He was concerned only with the structure of the organization. If it is assumed that there is a high degree of congruency between organizational demands and personal needs, then one need not address the complexities of motivation.

Levinson sees role definition as an aspect of ego function, an expression of a person's ability to resolve conflicting demands, to utilize opportunities and to create new ones, and to find a balance between stability and change. As a consequence, the issue of a "fit" between the individual and the social position becomes a crucial one. It is not simply a matter of fitting skills to positions, but rather, in addition, a matter of considering the congruence between personality and position.

SYSTEMS THEORY

No proper discourse on organizational theory may exclude references to general systems theory.[9–10] Organizations are conceived as open systems that react directly with their environment. Open systems exchange information and goods and services across their boundaries with the external environment. Administrators manage this exchange across the boundary between the organization (or unit of an organization) and external world.

Systems have input functions that deal with the taking in of information, material, and services. In a hospital, the *input* functions are accomplished by various subsystems such as the admitting unit, which admits patients to the hospital, the personnel office, which recruits and processes new employees, and the purchasing–receiving unit, which procures food and other required goods and services.

Organizational systems also have *"throughput,"* or processing units. In a hospital, these would be the various units that accomplish the treatment process.

The *output* function is accomplished by the subsystems, which discharge patients, as well as create and distribute the various other products of the hospital. For example, another exportable product might be scientific research reports.

The various subsystems of the organization develop their own functions and manage transactions across their boundaries.

An important perspective that derives from this way of thinking about organizations is the awareness of the subsystems of which an organization is a part. For example, a hospital may be viewed as a subsystem of the health care system, a subsystem of the educational system, or a subsystem of the social control system.

The concept of *feedback* is a key one in systems theory. Every system and subsystem is dependent for survival on its ability to adjust its behavior based on the information it receives from its environment. Much of the complex work of organizations is concerned with selecting, processing, and interpreting information. Consequently, much of the work of the administrator is concerned with making judgments about information that has been received and with making decisions about the subsequent adjustments and changes in behavior that may be made by the organization.

APPLIED THEORY

The thinking and practice of managers and administrators have evolved as a result of the impact of these aforementioned theoretical considerations. During the first part of the 20th century, the most influential managerial theorist was Frederick W. Taylor.[11] An engineer who pioneered in conducting time and motion studies, he became the person most identified with "scientific management." Taylor's ideas were prevelant in the early industrial organizations. He proposed that the basic objective of management was to provide maximum prosperity for both the employer and employee. Taylor believed in the congruence of needs of organizations and the individual workers. Money was the only motivator. *Efficiency* was the measure of work by unit of time. Industrial engineers were "efficiency experts" who increased output of workers and machines. Individuals in industrial organizations were interchangeable and could be regulated, directed, and managed by scientific manipulation of the mechanisms of production. There was no concern or attention given to individual needs, wishes, or expectations.

Elton Mayo is generally credited with providing the basis for a very different perspective of the relationship of the individual and the organization. A university professor interested in the behavior of workers, he was studying the efforts of a group of "efficiency experts" who were observing the effects that changes in lighting had on workers at the Hawthorne plant of Western Electric. The Taylor-style efficiency engineers expected better lighting conditions to result in increased output. But Mayo found that things were not so simple. Paradoxically, the work output increased in some cases when the light level was reduced. He found that the factors that influenced the rise or fall in productivity were the relationships between the workers, their willingness to cooperate, and their motivations.[12] As the workers formed working groups and developed a sense of cohesion, their work output increased. He pointed to the personal futility of isolated solitary work that many industrial workers experienced. He stressed the significance to the worker as well as to the organization of cooperation for a sense of personal gratification on the part of the worker.

In this and his later work, Mayo brought attention to the powerful impact a group that is significant to its members may have on their behaviors. His writing resulted in a change in managerial behavior as well as a change in focus of studies of organizational behavior. Enlightened managers henceforth changed their focus from the output of individual workers and the manipulation of physical environment. More attention was given to the personal needs of workers and to the work groups they formed.

Douglas McGregor[13] had an enormous influence on the thinking of administrators. He defined management as a discipline or profession that had its own body of knowledge and practice. He indicated that adminstrators often make one of two quite different and contrasting assumptions about the nature of man and his relationship to work. He stated that each assumption would lead to different conclusions and actions.

With the first assumption,—he called it *Theory X*—the working person is inherently hostile to work and will avoid it if at all possible. The way to get work "out" of the workers, therefore, is to be threatening, coercive, and controlling. The average worker avoids work and responsibility and wants only security, to be controlled and told what to do.

When Theory X characterizes a manager's assumptions of behavior, it leads to very "soft" or very "hard" control and direction, with the expectation that being nice or firm will shame or force workers to work. Soft management McGreger says, leads to indolence. "Hard" management leads to hostility, antagonism, and militancy. Neither increases output.

The second set of assumptions, which he called *Theory Y,* state that work is a natural human activity that people may enjoy. Workers may direct themselves toward achieving work objectives and be gratified by their achievments. Important gratifications are internal, i.e., self-esteem. People will seek, not avoid, responsibility under proper conditions. People are capable of high degrees of interest, enthusiasm, creativity, and involvement in their work. The managerial consequences of Theory Y are more optimistic and humanistic. With these assumptions, workers are treated as individuals. They are neither coerced nor coddled. They are given opportunities to commit themselves to their work. Greater attention is given to the needs, wishes, and goals of workers rather than to coercion and control. Control is understood to be internal, within the properly motivated individual rather than within the manager. The task of the manager lies in the integration of the worker's needs with organizational goals.*

The implication of McGregor's work is that managers should encourage the participation of workers in the decision-making processes of the organization. Their level of participation is proportional to the level of commitment toward the goals of the organization. McGregor cautions, however, that just as it demeans the participative process if meaningless decisions are shared by management, it is

---

*For an excellent description of McGregor's work and the human relations school, the reader is referred to Rush.[14]

also not advisable to share all management decisions. He does not propose management by consensus. Instead, the decisions to be shared must be selected and appropriate to the experience and knowledge of the persons.

The work of Abraham Maslow,[15] an academic psychologist, has had significant influence on corporate managers. His contribution lies in his work on the basic nature of social motivation. He has defined a "hierarchy of needs"[16] for which individuals seek gratification. The lower order, or more basic the need, the more essential it is, and until and unless it is satisfied, the individual cannot be motivated by the next higher level of need. The very nature of motivation is that it is internally generated. People cannot be motivated by others. Persons seek gratification of their needs, and it is this need seeking that we know as motivated behavior. These needs, starting at the most basic level are as follows:

1. *Physiological needs* are the very basic bodily needs for shelter, food, warmth, water, sleep, and so on.
2. *Safety needs* are related to actual and perceived safety from physical and emotional danger.
3. *The need for belongingness and love* is a social need to be loved, valued, and accepted by others, to be part of a valued group. It implies both the need to give and to receive love.
4. *The need for esteem* is the need for self-respect, to value ones self and to be appreciated by others.
5. *The need for self-actualization* is the highest level of need, concerned with acquiring a sense that one is productively using one's abilities as fully as possible, exploiting all one's capabilities.

In organizational life, the significance of this schema is that workers are unlikely to be motivated by the higher order of needs unless and until the more fundamental needs are met. Adequate salaries, physical conditions of work, and safety are more fundamental and of greater primacy than self-esteem until they are satisfied. Once satisfied and continuing to be satisfied, the need becomes relatively less important as a motivating need. Self-esteem may then become a primary motivator. Self-actualization, the highest order of need, is the ultimate psychological growth need that drives people to realize their full human potential.

Maslow coined the word *eupsychian* to convey the idea of a society in which all members were self-actualizing. He believes that people have the capacity, if basic needs are met, to climb the motivational ladder and that upward movement is evidence of emotional maturity.

Another useful framework derives from the work of Frederick Herzberg.[15] His theory was developed as a result of a survey of work attitudes. He was able to differentiate two different kinds of motivating forces for working people. He called these *satisfiers* and *dissatisfiers*.

Satisfiers are factors that make people feel good about their work. These factors are related to job content and include the following:

1. Achievement: having a sense of accomplishment;
2. Recognition: being given credit for a job well done;
3. Work: having an interesting job that the person values, that he finds varied, that has opportunities for creativity, and that the person is challenged by;

4. Responsibility: having control of one's own job;
5. Advancement: having opportunities for upward movement;
6. Growth: having opportunities to learn new skills.

The presence of satisfiers adds to the motivation of persons at work. An interesting finding, however, was that the absence of these satisfiers resulted in less motivation but not in dissatisfaction.

Dissatisfaction results from the presence or absence of an entirely different set of factors, which include the following:

1. Company policy and administration
2. Competency of supervision
3. Physical working conditions
4. Salary
5. Status symbols
6. Job security

The presence of positive conditions for these factors did not lead to job satisfaction. If these conditions were negative, however, the result was job dissatisfaction.

The dissatisfiers rarely were significant factors in motivating individuals to greater investment in their work even when these conditions were positive. Herzberg called these factors "hygiene" factors because they represent basic needs for working conditions, but they do not lead to satisfaction. He called the satisfier factors "motivators" because they are important insofar as they touch on the personal needs of individuals that motivate them in their work. He advocates, therefore, that these two factors be treated in different ways. Basic needs must be met. Hygiene factors must be adequately addressed. But a very highly motivated, involved, creative staff can be best developed by attention to the satisfiers.

Motivators, Herzberg says,[17] should be introduced into the organizational system. He calls this process "job enrichment." Some of the factors entailed in job enrichment are the following:

1. Removing some controls while retaining accountability
2. Increasing the accountability of individuals for their own work
3. Giving a person a complete, natural unit of work
4. Granting additional authority to an employee in his activity
5. Introducing new and more difficult tasks

LEADERSHIP

The concept of leadership, clearly an important function in administration, is not easily defined and understood. For our purposes, we may consider this definition: leadership is the differential exertion of influence for the purpose of attaining organizational goals. Not all leaders are in positions of significant authority. Some leaders may influence people by means of their charismatic personal qualities in informal ways. Some managers are not leaders. These people have legitimate authority, as Weber defined it, but are not able to influence behavior except by demanding compliance. Ideally, the administrator or manager is also a leader.

Ideally, also, in an organization, persons with leadership ability are sprinkled throughout the organization and are able to influence behavior at various times and in situations in which they have the relevant knowledge and skill.

While it has been suggested by some that leaders are born and by others that leaders are merely in the right place at the right time, leadership is likely to be a more complex matter than either of these hypotheses imply. There is evidence that leadership skills may be learned and that leadership involves a complex interaction between leaders and followers.

In organizational terms, *power* is the ability to influence behavior. Whether or not an organization is effective or successful, the very process of organizational activity involves the exercise of power. In this sense, power is neither good or bad, though it may be used for good or bad purposes. Whenever one person influences the behavior of another, power is being exercised. What are the different kinds of power?

1. *Legitimate authority* (see previous discussion): this kind of power is derived from the organization's structure and the status or position of the individual in the organization. Subordinates generally obey orders given by supraordinates unless they are willing to accept appropriate penalties such as loss of job, pay, opportunities, and so on.
2. *Coercive power:* this kind of power relies on fear of punishment for its ability to influence.
3. *Rewards:* the promise of rewards may be used to influence behavior. People who are able to reward others have power.
4. *Charismatic power* (see previous discussion): Charisma is a personal characteristic that enables one person to influence the behavior of another. Charismatic power cannot be delegated, and it can exist without official "legitimate" authority.
5. *Expert or sapiential authority:* this power comes from the knowledge or skill a person has and may be independent of other powers. A physician often influences the behavior of others solely because of the knowledge he possesses. In an organization, the physician as consultant may influence behavior even though he is not the administrator or manager.

Successful leaders who are managers seem to have two special kinds of qualities. First, they have a *cognitive perspective* of the system that they manage. They understand the functions and structure of the organization and the nature of its environment. Second, effective leaders have *interpersonal skills.* They are articulate. They are able to reach people in affective terms. They can be convincing, yet are able to negotiate complex issues and arrive at compromises.

There are a variety of leadership styles. Many leaders develop their own individual style and vary that style little from issue to issue or person to person. As Blake and Mouton[18] suggest, however, it is not only possible but desirable for a manager to vary his *style of leadership,* depending on the type of decision being made, the skills of the group, and the environment in which he is operating.

Leaders must learn to balance the attention they give to instrumental functions and maintenance functions. *Instrumental* functions are those that are concerned with getting the job done. They are essentially task and production related. *Maintenance* functions are concerned with interpersonal relationships, morale, and the emotional supports that help sustain the staff in their task performance. Blake and Mouton have developed a "managerial grid" that they use in leadership workshops to elucidate the ways a leader balances emphasis on instrumental and maintenance functions.

Using a questionnaire device, a manager is able to locate his or her particular style along these two dimensions. Some examples are as follows:

1. High concern for people, low concern for production—"country club" management. The manager who gives thoughtful attention to the needs of people for satisfying relationships leads to a comfortable, friendly organizational atmosphere and work tempo.
2. High concern for production, low concern for people—authority, obedience. Efficiency in operation results from arranging conditions of work in such a way that human elements interfere to a minimum degree.
3. Modest concern for production, modest concern for people—organization man management. Adequate organizational performance is possible through balancing the necessity to get out the work along with maintaining the morale of people at a satisfying level.
4. High concern for people, high concern for production. Work accomplishment is from committed people; independence through a "common stake" in organizational purpose leads to relationships of trust and respect.

Another reported facet of leadership style is the way in which decisions are made and by whom. A continuum has been described[19] in which at one extreme decisions are made by the manager and simply announced and at the other extreme the manager permits subordinates to function within limits defined by the superior. It is suggested by Tannenbaum and Schmidt that *decision making* should be varied and that an effective leader should not utilize the same decision-making process in all situations. Decisions are best shared when:

1. Staff have high needs for independence.
2. Subordinates wish to assume responsibilities.
3. There is tolerance for ambiguity.
4. The staff understand and identify with the goals of the organization.

It is asserted that sharing decision-making functions raises staff morale, improves the quality of the decision, and develops teamwork.

Management by objectives (MBO) is a well-established and widely utilized method for increasing attention to task performance while also involving individuals in decision making. In this process, the supervisor and supervisee together discuss and describe the goals to be set for a specific time frame. The goals and specific outcomes are also defined by mutual agreement about what is to be expected in the way of work performance. At the end of the time period, the previous agreement is reviewed by worker and supervisor, and through discussion they rate the extent to which the objectives have been met. As a supervisory tool, MBO may be effective in raising morale and productivity. This same methodology (MBO) may be used for larger organizational units. Here each system administrator develops goals and objectives for the system and its various and subsystems.

MBO is a methodology that leads organizations to achievement of greater *accountability*. In the 1960s, when there was a relative richness of resources in the mental health system to an infusion of funds, there was a very large investment in training and in keeping good staff. Though *morale* is no less important an issue now than it was then, greater attention was given to it. Similarly, in the 1980s, there is a relative dearth of resources, and as a consequence, though task accountability is no more important than it ever was, far greater attention is given to it. Task accountability is at the height of emphasis when resources are limited. At the time of growth and innovation, morale factors receive greater attention.

In this chapter, some of the major elements of organizational theory have been described. In other chapter, the psychological, sociological, and political aspects of organizations will be addressed.

As theories of organizations developed, people were at first seen as extensions of machines and of organizations. Weber, a sociologist, described the structure of organizations he called bureaucracies in terms of hierarchical positions while ignoring all personal needs and other characteristics of the individuals in these positions. Taylor, an industrial engineer, considered the human part of the enterprise essentially a mechanical necessity. People were extensions of machines, and money was what fueled them.

During this century, the major development in organizational theory has been the discovery of the human being. Needs, wishes, and aspirations are linked to motivation, and motivation is an essential ingredient of effective work. Organizational effectiveness has come to be seen more as dependent on the system's ability to meet the personal needs of its staff while attaining its organizational goals.

Power, the ability to influence the behavior of others, is always a factor in organizational life. Leadership involves the skillful differential use of power.

The primary purpose of an organization is to produce goods or services. This involves the accomplishment of certain work or tasks by its employees. With the evolution of understanding of the relationship between organizations and the individuals who work in them, greater attention was given to the issue of individuals' personal needs and motivations.

The manager is faced with the need to maintain stability and achieve progress while balancing a variety of forces. The survival of the organization depends on its ability to produce services or goods that are sufficiently valued by the external environment to support the system. Survival also depends on the quality of staff and their productivity and morale, all of which are closely interrelated. Both the need for accountability of production and the need to support and maintain the quality of organizational life must be satisfied if the organization is to thrive.

REFERENCES

1. Weber M: Three types of legitimate rule. Preussioche Jahrbuecher 187:1–12, 1922
2. Bernard C: The Functions of the Executive. Cambridge, Mass, Harvard University Press, 1938
3. Selznick, P: Foundations of the theory of organizations. Am Sociol Rev 13:25–35, 1948
4. Parsons T: Suggestions for a sociologic approach to the theory of organization. Adm Sci Q 1:63–85, 1956
5. Merton RK: Bureaucratic Structures and Personality in Social Theory and Social Structure. Glencoe, Ill, Free Press, 1957
6. March J, Simon H: The Theory of Organizational Theory in Organizations. New York, Wiley, 1958

7. Levinson D: Role personality and social structures. J Abnorm Psychol, 58:179–180, 1958
8. Simon HA, Smithburg DW, Thomas VA: Public Administration. New York, Knopf, 1950
9. Von Bertalanffy L: General Systems Theory. New York, Braziller, 1968
10. Buckley W: Modern Systems Research for the Behavioral Scientist. Chicago, Aldine, 1968
11. Taylor FW: Scientific Management, New York, Harper & Row, 1911
12. Mayo V: The Human Problems of an Industrial Civilization. Cambridge, Mass., Harvard University Press, 1933
13. McGregor D: The Human Side of Enterprise. New York, McGraw-Hill, 1960
14. Rush HMF: Behaviorial Science: Concepts and Management Application. New York Conference Board, 1969
15. Maslow A: Eupsychian Management. Homewood, Ill, Irwin, 1965
16. Maslow A: Motivation and Personality. New York, Harper & Row, 1954
17. Herzberg F: One more time: how do you motivate employees. Harvard Business Review, Jan–Feb, 1968
18. Blake RR, Mouton JS: The New Managerial Grid. Houston, Gulf, 1978
19. Tannenbaum R, Schmidt W: How to choose a leadership pattern. Harvard Business Review, March–April, 1958

Judith R. Blau, Ph.D.

10

Sociological Theories

PROFESSIONS, ORGANIZATIONS, AND IDEOLOGIES: THE BEARING OF SOCIAL THEORY AND RESEARCH ON PRACTICES IN ADMINISTRATIVE PSYCHIATRY

At an earlier time when psychiatry was preoccupied with taxonomies of mental illness, sociology was developing taxonomies of its own. Many of these focus specifically on medicine and psychiatry, and others apply to them. A main form of taxonomy in the social sciences is the "ideal type," an analytical model that abstracts elements from empirical reality in order to accentuate the distinctive features underlying a particular process or structure. Relevant here are the ideal types dealing with the physician–patient relationship, the professional, the total institution, and the bureaucracy. Although these models do not provide genuine scientific explanations in that they are not subject to empirical testing and do not offer propositions concerning causality, they have yielded important insights and continue to influence, both positively and negatively, sociological research and theory. Indeed, it is difficult to trace the contributions of sociology in the fields of psychiatry and administration without reference to certain of these models.

Four Models

The *physician–patient relationship* was formulated by Parsons[1] as an ideal-type model. In certain respects, it is the psychiatrist–patient relation that defines the model best, and it provides an analogue for the role of the physician in any clinical setting. Parsons' view of the therapist's role—the legitimization of the sick person's deviance, social support, the temporary easement of family involvement, and the therapeutic denial of reciprocity that would perpetuate deviance—has sensitized physicians to the importance of interpersonal processes underlying therapy and recovery. At the same time, the model has served to reinforce the belief that therapy resides in the charismatic qualities of physicians as well as to legitimize the view that psychiatry is the sole agent of social control and treatment. A modification of the model must take into account that there currently exists a plurality of therapeutic roles and that the interpersonal relationship is but one of many therapeutic modes.

The ideal-type model of the *professional* derives largely from the attributes of physicians, although it is assumed that the model clarifies related attributes that characterize other professionals, notably lawyers, the clergy, and architects.[2–4] Professionals according to the model, have three core characteristics. First, they possess expert knowledge based on long training in a field that is scientifically grounded. Second, they act in the interests of the client, not in terms of their own self-interest. Third, they are oriented to a community of colleagues. It follows from these core characteristics that professional conduct is guided by ethical codes, lengthy professional socialization, and the opinions of peers. One implication derived from the model is that the tasks of professional review and regulations are, and ought to be, the responsibilities of professionals themselves. Another is that professional autonomy must be protected in the interest of quality service.

Criticisms of the model rest on considerations of the changes that have taken place in medicine itself within the past several decades as well as a re-evaluation of the underlying assumptions of the model. The typical physician implicit in the scheme is the solo practitioner. At the present time, however, the M.D. in a solo practice is in a marginal position, as health services are increasingly under the control of organizations, the state, and universities.[5] Moreover, medical and surgical physicians—and to some extent, psychiatrists—who work in bureaucratic settings, are specialists and deal less with people as patients and more with particular symptoms or treatments. Regulation by peers and the ethics that govern the professional—client relation are likely to become attenuated under such conditions.

The current conception of the professional rests less on assumptions about individual motivation and behavior and focuses more on the central interests of an entire profession in capturing a unique market and in securing the dependence of other occupational groups.[5,6] While not denying that individual professionals may be committed to the service ideal, the revised model fully recognizes that the integrity and advancement of an occupational group can only be achieved through the monopoly of a unique service, which partly depends on the exercise of power. A major contrast is that the older ideal type sought to explain individual behavior and attitudes, whereas the new model deals with the social structures of occupational life—professional associations, entire occupations, and specialties within a profession.

Two models of organizations—Goffman's[7] total institution and Weber's[8,9] bureaucracy—have guided research on hospitals and occupational roles within them. The *total institution,* according to Goffman, is the organization that serves the masses of inmates who live there and encompasses their total life and person. With its centralized authority, regimentation of activities, and severe restrictions on patients' physical mobility, the term *total institution* has become an epithet for any large custodial psychiatric hospital. While the model is indeed an indictment of custodial care, it also offers subtle insights into the effects of institutionalization, however humane or therapeutic the setting. For example, although the process of labeling behavior as deviant has chiefly been explained by social psychological theory,[10] Goffman views labeling as a function of institutional dynamics. Organizational needs for routinization are met by "stripping" patients of their personal possessions and their identities and then casting them with batches of others in roles that bear a stigma. The segmentation of the hospital personnel into staff and doctors may be a rational form of organization, but for inmates it creates an incompatible set of role demands; doctors evaluate behavior on the well-ill dimension, whereas other staff members are concerned with the good-bad dimension.[11] What may be perceived as a healthy adjustment by the psychiatrist may be manifest in what staff view as bad behavior. The description of the total institution may apply to few mental hospitals today, but all hospitals face the dilemma posed by Goffman, for it is the result of the need for bureaucratic routinization while also providing individualized care to patients.

Weber's ideal type of *bureaucracy* has been generally useful in organizational analysis, and it also has found specific application in the study of hospitals. For Weber, bureaucracy is the most rational and efficient means of carrying out complex tasks and coordinating work. The main defining attributes include the following: a complex division of labor evident in horizontal differentiation (such as programs and departments), vertical differentiation (levels), and distinct offices (specialties and occupations); clear lines of communication and supervision; formal rules and regulations; and a staff of administrators and clerks.

According to Weber, these attributes constitute the *sui generis* features of complex organizations, although in contemporary sociological research they have been translated into variable attributes of organizations in order to explain the interrelations among them. For example, it has been found in studies of many types of organizations, including hospitals, that large organizations tend to have relatively fewer administrative support staff compared with small organizations and in this sense are less "bureaucratic" than small organizations.[12]

It is necessary to incorporate into the model relevant other dimensions in explanations of organizational patterns in studies of health institutions. For one thing, hospitals have a sizable professional component, which Weber did not take into account, and for another, the activities and goals of hospitals influence, and are influenced by, a set of environments, including a community, other organizations, and a political environment. Furthermore, Weber's model deals primarily with government administration, but there are additional factors that are relevant in the study of people transforming organizations for which, again, the issue of rational organization versus individualized care poses a significant dilemma.

Work That Transforms People

It is important to point out the great difference between work that seeks significantly to *transform people* and other work. The contrast is that between jobs of the missionary, social worker, and school teacher, on the one hand, and those of the computer analyst, astronomer, and car mechanic, on the other. It is clearly a continuum, but work in mental health represents one extreme on it. The difference lies in part in the degree of direct responsibility to those whose transformation is being sought, but another important difference lies in the degree of uncertainty of the task and the capacity to standardize it.[13] Most knowledge of work that transforms people, though often derived from a scientific base, cannot be applied in a standardized fashion. Because work that aims to transform people involves much uncertainty and is not easily standardized, the implications for occupational roles and for organizations are profound.

Owing to the complex nature of the task—variable patients, difficulties of diagnosis, and the wide-ranging strategies of intervention—the performance of workers is difficult to evaluate, and standards for outcome are generally relative, not absolute. Moreover, because the task is uncertain, judging outcomes is difficult, and differences of opinion become easily translated into conflict. Politics, in the broad sense of the term, thus, plays an important role in occupational and organizational relations.[14] The factor of uncertainty coupled with the costliness of error help to account for the frequent reliance on an ideology for the justification of a particular approach. Finally, the importance of consultation and occupational autonomy and the fact that patient contact occurs at the very "bottom" of the organizational hierarchy make it likely that centralized control in mental health settings is achieved at the peril of staff morale and patient welfare.

Occupational Roles

The uncertainty that underlies clinical practice is multidimensional. As Fox[15] notes, there are two types of knowledge gaps in dealing with patients: one refers to those in scientific knowledge, and the other refers to gaps in personal knowledge. Distinguishing between these two creates, according to Fox, extraordinary role strain. Although Fox is dealing specifically with general medicine, one suspects that this problem is even more serious in fields of mental health. Davis[16] draws another distinction, that between substantive uncertainty involved in making the correct diagnosis and identifying the proper treatment and functional uncertaintly entailed by the problems of informing patients and managing their reactions. It is plausible that the division of activities in many psychiatric facilities between clinical and management staff provides a way of distributing these two sources of uncertainty.

Modern mental health facilities, however small, are typically staffed by persons with diverse occupational backgrounds, and the relations among them is a main source of ambiguity. In these facilities, there are varying conceptions of what each occupation is, of what it ought to be doing, and how it relates to other occupations.[17]

Wide variation exists among settings with respect to the *responsibilities and power* of different occupational groups. For example, in some, there is a marked division of responsibilities among different disciplines,[18] whereas in others there is considerable blurring of disciplinary boundaries.[19] Although a strict occupational division of labor can be defended on the grounds that there are differences in training and expertise, it is often argued that this creates a high degree of discontinuity in patient care.[20] One solution is to supplement a staff of specialists with a few generalists to maintain integrated care.[21]

There is some evidence that staffing and the occupational division of labor have changed since inception of the community mental health center (CMHC). Winslow[22] reports that psychiatrists are being utilized less now than at an earlier time, as their therapeutic and administrative functions are being assumed by other mental health professionals. A possible explanation for this is that drug therapy has routinized a certain area of work that was formerly within the clinical domain of psychiatrists, thereby increasing opportunities for other occupational groups.[23] Another study by Lorber and Satow,[24] however, provides evidence that in the psychoanalytically oriented CMHC, the substitution of psychiatrists by other occupational groups is less likely. They report that when individual therapy is the main form of treatment, psychiatrists take the "interesting cases" and assign chronic cases to social workers and paraprofessionals. Under these conditions, it is the nonpsychiatric staff who have the lowest morale and the highest rates of turnover.

Psychiatrist–Administrator

The institutionalization of medicine has largely undermined the charismatic authority of the physician, and at the same time, the line between the clinical authority and the administrative authority of the physician is relatively unclear.[25] The *role* of the psychiatric administrator is probably the least well defined of all medical specialties and undoubtedly the most variable. Much of the variability in the role can be accounted for by differences among clinics, private hospitals, and public hospitals.[26] Ambiguity of self-image is reported by Coser.[27] In her study of a psychoanalytically oriented hospital, administrative psychiatrists are more likely than other psychiatrists to report that they experience contradictions between the norms governing bureaucratic and clinical responsibilities. In a comparison with clinical psychiatrists, these administrative psychiatrists are found to have lower self-esteem and a weaker identification with the hospital, and both esteem and identification tend to decline over time.

Much of the sociological literature on psychiatric administration deals with the differences between appropriate styles of management for bureaucratic and clinical activities. For example, it has been suggested that administrative functions such as financial planning and accounting are best handled by means of *centralized* procedures and decision making, whereas the coordination and planning of clinical work ought to be *decentralized.*[28,29] In contrast, Wilensky[30] maintains that all aspects of administration in psychiatric settings be more or less decentralized, arguing that informal consultation and negotiation are most effective in dealing with diverse occupational groups.

One of the few intensive studies of the practice of psychiatric administration by several individuals rather than one is by Hodgson et al.[31] They view administration as based on a constellation of roles, and while that constellation can be composed of individuals with the same or different occupations, what they consider to be most important is that the individuals complement one another through different personalities and orientations.

These studies of psychiatric administration are mainly concerned with various aspects of intraorganizational management and coordination. As the result of recent legislation, however, the growing influence of consumer groups, and the lesser emphasis placed on comprehensive services, the psychiatric administrator must increasingly deal with external groups and agencies.[32] This is particularly the case in the public health sector because the service agency is a component of a multitiered structure. To illustrate the significance of such complexity, it appears that an increasing problem for administrators of local public service agencies is the incompatibility between the emphasis on quantity and efficiency by the central administration and the commitment to quality by staff members.[33]

In interorganizational negotiations in which administrators are increasingly involved, there are problems of communication, unequal resources, and power. Rogers and Molnar[34] distinguish between *role conflict,* which results when the administrator is faced with incompatible expectations, and *role ambiguity,* which occurs when the administrator has insufficient information or faces poorly defined expectations. They find that intraorganizational activities are the chief sources of role ambiguity, whereas interorganizational activities account for most role conflict. The boundary-spanning role of administrators is particularly susceptible to conflict because of the low control administrators have over other groups and the inconsistencies that accrue in this area.

Related topics include the structured relations among organizations and the systems approach to understanding interorganizational networks. A small number of empirical studies deal with these topics,[35–38] but the main focus of the discussion that follows is that of the internal characteristics of psychiatric facilities.

Organizations

The sociological perspective assumes that organizations and their characteristics—how large or small they are or how simply structured or how complex they are—exert constraints and create opportunities independently of the characteristics of the people who work in them. Perhaps in no other setting do characteristics of the organization exert more pronounced influences over staff and patients than in psychiatric settings owing to their relative degree of boundedness and the great importance attached to feelings and behavior.

In their classic studies, Caudill[39] and Stanton and Schwartz[40] draw attention to the effects of the *organization on patients.* Any reorganization in the hospital structure has reverberations—collective emotional disturbances—throughout the patient community. Coser's[41] analysis indicates that a decline in the social relational system of clinicians (decreased interaction, high turnover, and a decline in the frequency of meetings) results in an increase in the rate of patient suicides. In a replication of Coser's study in a large state hospital, the main effect on such patient incidents is found to be disorganization at the ward level rather than at higher clinical and administrative levels.[42]

Research carried out in large state hospitals during the 1950s and 1960s suggested that Goffman's total institution may not be an exaggerated model, after all, but a close approximation of reality. For example, Belknap's[43] study of a 2000-bed hospital indicates that custody is the only salient organizational objective; as he reports, patients who are "in continuous treatment" receive "no treatment." Part of the explanation is organizational: a three-way split between ward staff, administrators, and clinicians, according to Belknap, perpetuated communication problems and conflict. In a comparable facility, Dunham and Weinberg[44] report similar organizational problems accompanying inadequate patient care and treatment. As is generally known, such facilities as these have undergone tremendous changes as the result of deinstitutionalization, drug therapy, and a new emphasis on short-term care. The problems, it has been said, are transferred to the streets, and the resident institution is the "single room occupancy" hotel, not the hospital.

Most private and some public institutions differ in many respects from the custodial total institution. Because therapeutic approaches vary, as do organizational structures, the research questions for the private hospital focus primarily on the relations between ideology and organizational structure.

A consistent finding in studies of private hospitals is that there is a close correspondence between *organizational structure* and *therapeutic ideology*. For example, in a comparison of wards that emphasize either milieu, psychoanalytic, or drug therapy, Strauss et al.[45] report that the milieu ideology tends to promote a decentralized structure, whereas the other two types of wards are relatively centralized. Rubenstein and Lasswell[46] follow the transformation of a hospital from an emphasis on psychoanalytic techniques to milieu therapy and report that decentralization is accompanied by the blurring of occupational lines and the breakdown of traditional patterns of authority. Similar conclusions are reported in Greenblatt et al.[47] Perhaps the most optimistic account of the consequences of the link between a decentralized hospital structure and milieu therapy is provided by Rapoport.[48] Although according to Rapoport the ideology that "everything is treatment; all treatment is rehabilitation" results in high staff morale and wide sharing of responsibilities, Rubenstein and Lasswell detect some strain in the role relations of clinical and ward staff when such an ideology is adopted. In another study, King and Smith[49] find that when staff are oriented to milieu therapy, they are more likely to interact with patients, although the effectiveness of such an approach is more successful with the acutely ill than with the chronically ill. Moreover, Ellsworth et al.[50] suggest that this approach is effective in that it increases the independence and responsibility of patients, but does not reduce the length of time in treatment.

Of significance for any psychiatric facility is the clear evidence that clinical ideologies are not merely vague approaches to treatment but rather are deeply entrenched in the working lives of clinicians. Soskis[51] reports a close correspondence in a study of 335 psychiatrists between their views concerning etiology and their preferred treatment. Sharaf and Levinson[52] find a strong connection between the ideological commitments of psychiatric residents, their definitions of appropriate role relations with others, and their career aspirations.

Studies of therapeutic ideologies are helpful in understanding the treatment approach and organizational dynamics within a particular setting, or within a few, but they shed little light on how the formal characteristics of psychiatric facilities vary and how these characteristics are interrelated. Research questions that deal with this issue require large numbers of facilities for the purpose of comparison. It is Weber's model of bureaucracy that served to stimulate research on the formal organizational characteristics of psychiatric facilities, notably hospitals.

An early milestone in this research tradition is Heydebrand's[53] study of nearly 4000 hospitals, of which 313 are psychiatric. Results for the sample of psychiatric hospitals alone reveal that the variation in internal structure is largely a function of their size, whether they are teaching hospitals or not, and the complexity of their task structure (specifically, whether they have primarily custodial or treatment goals). The largest public custodial hospitals are bureaucratically coordinated by means of hierarchical control; small private facilities are coordinated through horizontal communication achieved by a balanced division of labor and a highly professionalized staff; and the large specialized Veteran's Administration hospitals are coordinated largely through administrative management. To put this another way, in simple structures, professionals can achieve coordination through collegial relations, but in larger, complex organizations, other forms of coordination are required. The form depends mainly on whether the task is routine or complex, that is, whether custodial or treatment goals predominate.

Because Heydebrand's study encompasses all types of hospitals, distinctive features of psychiatric hospitals are inevitably ignored. Other comparative studies of psychiatric facilities have been carried out in the past decade. Their main concerns are the nature and effects of bureaucratic control in organizations and the locus of authority.

How Much Bureaucracy?

There are three distinct views concerning the role of *bureaucratic control* in hospitals. Freidson[6] argues that peer regulation is insufficient and that hospitals need more formal mechanisms of bureaucratic control. Heydebrand, as we have seen, considers professionalization, administration, hierarchy, and the division of labor as constituting different forms of coordination, and which one is likely to be dominant in any given hospital depends on other organizational attributes. Mechanic[54] views growing bureaucratization in health settings with some concern and would grant institutions and their staff more freedom from bureaucratic constraints. There are clear problems of bureaucratic coordination *among* agencies and hospitals, but this is an issue different from bureaucratic coordination *within* organizations. It is the latter issue that most research has addressed.

In a study of 230 state hospitals, Smith and King[55] conclude that bureaucratic control through effective hierarchical supervision is related to staff morale and quality of care whereas bureaucratic coordination within and across departments has positive effects on organizational flexibility. In a study of halfway houses, Yancey and Segal[56] report similar findings. Bureaucratic characteristics such as administrative complexity increase staff members' expectations of patient functioning, which, in turn, is related to positive outcomes. Ullmann[57] reaches somewhat the same conclusion, reporting that large hospital size can impair patient treatment unless accompanied by unitization. To the extent that unitization helps to establish an intermediate level for the formalization of coordination and supervision, it represents a form of bureaucratic control.

Paradoxically, bureaucratic mechanisms for coordinating work tend to promote decentralization in organizations.[58] When formal procedures, committees, subunits, and rules are instituted, they tend to reduce the personal control of top administrators and increase the autonomy of staff. Many studies have found that decentralization of decision making is positively related to the autonomy of staff, open communications, staff morale, and the quality of care.[59,60] There is a main exception to the conclusion that decentralization increases effectiveness, however, and that involves areas that requires the adoption of innovative techniques. Empirical studies report that new innovations are more likely to be successfully adopted when decision making regarding the area of innovation is relatively centralized.[61–63] Fourcher's[64] conclusions in an observational study of a mental health center coincide with these empirical studies. He reports that a "loose reins" strategy works under most conditions because it recognizes the autonomy and special skills of professionals. But this strategy has shortcomings when a major innovation is sought for which centralized authority is most effective.

Bureaucracy and Quality of Care

When the subordinate's interests coincide with the superordinate's interests, authority can be described as conjoint. In most hierarchical authority relationships these interests do not coincide—*authority* is disjoint—and the subordinate has a significant residue of personal interest that is independent of the superordinate's.[65] Generally speaking, the authority relationships between any two highly trained professionals is conjoint. For example, although there are differences in authority between the attending and the resident psychiatrist, their interests are highly congruent.

Most authority relations in large, complex psychiatric organizations are not conjoint. Observed organizational pathology—high rates of turnover, low staff morale, and inferior patient care—largely stems from the predominance of disjoint authority relations over conjoint ones. The solution posed is a paradoxical one: the introduction of more bureaucratic forms of coordination.

One of the unique features of most psychiatric facilities is the high degree of occupational diversity. Studies reviewed indicate that when such diversity of expertness is ignored, for example, through a sharp split in responsibility and power, staff morale and the quality of care are jeopardized. It is consistent with theory and research on organizations that when staff members recognize the complementarity of interests and values and when differences among occupations are regarded as legitimate, the goals of the organization are better served.[66–70] The more heterogenous and complementary the values and role relations, therefore, the healthier the organization. The problem lies in maintaining this diversity and fully utilizing the distinctive expertise of each occupational group. It could be argued that full participatory democracy would best achieve this, but it is probably unrealistic to assume that psychiatric facilities, especially the largest and most complex ones, can be run democratically. An alternative solution is provided by a complex form of bureaucracy—the matrix organization.

In a *matrix organization,* people occupy multiple status positions and thus are linked with many others in a variety of capacities.[71] Multiple statuses may include one's main job as well as advisory positions, committee memberships, liaison roles, and team assignments. This maximizes the connections any given person has with others throughout the organization and helps to strengthen his or her commitment to organizational goals. Bureaucratic mechanisms of coordination become inseparable from the multiple lines of communication. Compliance with authority is no longer an issue because authority resides in the conglomerate of multiple statuses and penetrates the complex role relations that form communication networks.[72]

A person exercises power in that status in which he or she is expert, whereas in other capacities, that person is less knowledgeable and must seek advice from others. This helps to achieve organizational integration, an individual's feeling of worth, and, moreover, eliminates the problems associated with disjointed authority. It is inevitable that tolerance of others' opinions and values are increased owing to the complexity of the role relations built into the matrix. Furthermore, supervisors do less "checking up" on the work of subordinates because accountability and surveillance are built into the very fabric of the organization.

There is some empirical support that the introduction of the matrix structure into hospitals greatly enhances the quality of care. When nurses are given wider responsibilities and more contact with physcians, they have a more holistic understanding of patients' needs and are more attentive to patient care.[73] In a study of a private hospital, Gralnick[74] concludes that the level of patient care is highest when the complexity of the organizational structure is balanced with extensive communications and a balance of power among psychiatrists and other occupational groups. Greeley and Schoenherr[75] find that the autonomy of staff members is positively related to the level of human service, as reported by patients. These studies are not based on matrix organizations as such but on organizations that have certain elements associated with the matrix form. Positive outcomes suggest that the model deserves fuller consideration.

The matrix structure is being adopted in private enterprise, largely to offset the problems of worker morale. Its application in psychiatric settings where patients' welfare is also at stake, offers a creative challenge for administrators.

REFERENCES

1. Parsons T: Illness and the role of the physician. Am J Orthopsychiatry 21:454–460, 1951
2. Carr-Saunders AM, Wilson FA: The Professions. Oxford, Oxford University Press, 1933
3. Greenwood E: Attributes of a profession. Soc Work 2:44–55, 1957
4. Goode WJ: Community within a community: the professions. Am Sociol Rev 22:194–200, 1957
5. Larson MS: The Rise of Professionalism. Berkeley, University of California Press, 1977
6. Freidson E: Professional Dominance. New York, Atherton Press, 1970
7. Goffman E: Asylums. Chicago, Aldine, 1959, pp 1–124
8. Max Weber: Essays in Sociology, Gerth HH, Mills CW (eds) New York, Oxford University Press, 1946, pp 196–204
9. Max Weber: The Theory of Social and Economic Organization, Parsons T (ed): Glencoe, Ill, Free Press, 1947, pp 329–336
10. Lemert E: Social Pathology: A Systematic Approach to the Theory of Sociopathic Behavior. New York, McGraw-Hill, 1951
11. Goffman E: Asylums, pp 127–169
12. Blau PM: Independence and hierarchy in organizations. Soc Sci Res 1:1–24, 1972
13. Street D, Vinter RD, Perrow C: Organization for Treatment. New York, Free Press, 1966
14. Bucher R: Social process and power in a medical setting, in Zald MN (ed): Power in Organizations. Nashville, Vanderbilt University Press, 1970
15. Fox RC: Training for uncertainty, in Merton RK, Reader GG, Kendall PL et al (eds): The Student-Physician. Cambridge, Mass, Harvard University Press, 1957
16. Davis F: Uncertainty in medical prognoses. Am J Sociol 66:41–47, 1960
17. Hughes EC: Men and Their Work. Glencoe, Ill, Free Press, 1958, p 76
18. Simon AJ: Social structure of clinics and patient improvement. Adm Sci Q 4:197–206, 1959
19. Schulberg HC, Baker F: The Mental Hospital and Human Services. New York, Behavioral Publications, 1975
20. Henry J: On Sham, Vulnerability and Other Forms of Self-destruction. New York, Vintage, 1973, pp 1–16
21. Reichler RJ, Schopler E: Developmental therapy: a program model for providing individual services in the community, in Schopler E, Reichler RJ (eds): Psychopathology and Child Development. New York, Plenum Press, 1976
22. Winslow WW: The changing role of psychiatrists in community mental health centers. Am J Psychiatry 136:24–27, 1979
23. Crozier M: The Bureaucratic Phenomenon. Chicago, University of Chicago Press, 1964
24. Lorber J, Satow R: Creating a company of unequals: sources of occupational stratification in a ghetto community mental health center. Soc Work Occup 4:281–302, 1977
25. Wilson RN: The physician's changing role. Hum Org 18:177–183, 1959–1960.
26. Daniels AK: Advisory and coercive functions in psychiatry, in Albrect GL, Higgins

PC (eds): Health, Illness and Medicine. Chicago, Rand McNally, 1979
27. Coser RL: Training in Ambiguity. New York, Free Press, 1979
28. Perrow C: Analysis of goals in complex organizations. Am Sociol Rev 26:854–866, 1961
29. Gordon PJ: Top management triangle in voluntary hospitals. J Acad Management 4:205–214, 1961
30. Wilensky HL: Dynamics of professionalism: the case of hospital administration. Hosp Adm 7:6–24, 1962
31. Hodgson RC, Levinson DJ, Zaleznik A: The Executive Role Constellation. Cambridge, Harvard University Graduate School of Business Administration, 1965
32. O'Connor JT: The radically new medical care industry: implications for decision-making. J Appl Behav Sci 14:266–282, 1978
33. Wetten DA: Coping with incompatible expectations. Adm Sci Q 23:254–271, 1978
34. Rogers DL, Molnar D: Organizational antecedents of role conflict and ambiguity in top level administrators. Adm Sci Q 21:598–608, 1976
35. Ermann MD: The social control of organizations in the health care area. Health and Society 54:167–183, 1976
36. Alford RR: Health Care Politics. Chicago, University of Chicago Press, 1975
37. Pressman J, Wildarsky A: Implementation. Berkeley, University of California Press, 1973
38. Tichy NM: Diagnosis for complex health care delivery systems: a model and case study. J Appl Behav Sci 14:305–320, 1978
39. Caudill W: The Psychiatric Hospital as a Small Society. Cambridge, Mass, Harvard University Press, 1958
40. Stanton AH, Schwartz MS: The Mental Hospital. New York, Basic Books, 1954
41. Coser RL: Suicide and the relational system: A case study in a mental hospital. J Health Soc Behav 17:318–327, 1976
42. Berk BB: Staff stability and organizational effectiveness. Pacific Sociol Rev 20: 349–370, 1977
43. Belknap I: Human Problems of a State Mental Hospital. New York, McGraw-Hill, 1956
44. Dunham HW, Weinberg SK: The Culture of the State Mental Hospital. Detroit, Wayne State University Press, 1960
45. Strauss A, Schatzman L, Bucher R, et al: Psychiatric Ideologies and Institutions. New York, Free Press, 1964
46. Rubenstein R, Lasswell HD: The Sharing of Power in a Psychiatric Hospital. New Haven, Yale University Press, 1966, p 203–256
47. Greenblatt M, Levinson DJ, Williams RH (eds): The Patient and the Mental Hospital. Glencoe, Ill, Free Press, 1957
48. Rapoport RN: Community as Doctor. London, Tavistock, 1959
49. King JA, Smith CG: The effects of staff ideology and patient population characteristics on the treatment environment of the mental hospital. Soc Sci 51:161–169, 1976
50. Ellsworth R. Maroney R, Klett W, et al: Milieu characteristics of successful psychotic treatment programs. Am J Orthopsychiatry 31:427–441, 1971
51. Soskis DA: Aetiological models of schizophrenia: relationships to diagnosis and treatment. Br J Psychiatry 120:367–373, 1972
52. Sharaf MR, Levinson DJ: Patterns of ideology and role definition among psychiatric residents, in Greenblatt M, Levinson DJ, Williams RH (eds): The Patient and the Mental Hospital. Glencoe, Ill, Free Press, 1957
53. Heydebrand W: Hospital Bureaucracy: A Comparative Study of Organizations. New York, Dunellen, 1973
54. Mechanic D: The Growth of Bureaucratic Medicine. New York, Wiley, 1976, pp. 58–79
55. Smith CG, King JA: Mental Hospitals. Lexington, Mass, Heath, 1975
56. Yancey P, Segal B: Bureaucracy, size and staff expectations for client independence in halfway houses. J Health Soc Behav 18:376–390, 1977
57. Ullmann LP: Institution and Outcome. Oxford, Pergamon Press, 1967
58. Zey-Ferrell M: Dimensions of Organizations. Santa Monica, Calif, Goodyear, 1979, pp 157–164
59. Wessen AF: Hospital ideology and communication between ward personnel, in Jaco EG (ed): Patients, Physicians and Illness. Glencoe, Ill, Free Press, 1958
60. Seeman M, Evans JW: Stratification and hospital care. Am Sociol Rev 26:67–80; 193–204, 1961
61. Nathanson CA, Morlock LL: Control structure, values and innovation: A comparative study of hospitals. J Health Soc Behav 21:315–333, 1980
62. Flood AB, Scott WR: Professional power and professional effectiveness: the power of the surgical staff and the quality of surgical care in hospitals. J Health Soc Behav 19:240–254, 1978

63. Kaluzny AD, Veney JE, Gentry JT: Innovation of health services: a comparative study of hospitals and health departments. Health and Society 52:51–82, 1974
64. Fourcher LA: Compliance structures and change within mental health service organizations. Soc Work Occup 2:246–256, 1975
65. Coleman JS: Authority systems. Public Opinion Q 44:143–163, 1980
66. Kaplan SR: Teaching of community psychiatry in psychiatric residency training programs, in Lidz T, Edelson M (eds): Training Tomorrow's Psychiatrist. New Haven, Yale University Press, 1970
67. Turk H: Social cohesion through variant values: evidence from medical role relations. Am Sociol Rev 28:28–37, 1963
68. Hage J: Communication and Organizational Control. New York, Wiley, 1974
69. Coser RL: The complexity of roles as a seedbed of individual autonomy, in Coser L (ed): The Idea of Social Structure. New York, Harcourt Brace Jovanovich, 1975
70. Kriesburg L: Internal differentiation and the establishment of organizations, in Becker HS, Geer B, Riesman D, et al (eds): Institutions and the Person. Chicago, Aldine, 1968
71. Davis SM, Lawrence PR: Matrix. Reading, Mass, Addison-Wesley, 1977
72. Blau J: Paradoxical consequences of excess in structural complexity: a study of a state children's psychiatric hospital. Sociol, Health, Illn 2:277–292, 1980
73. Coser RL: Alienation and social structure: case analysis of a hospital, in Freidson E (ed): The Hospital in Modern Society. Glencoe, Ill, Free Press, 1963
74. Gralnick A: Humanizing the Psychiatric Hospital. New York, Jason Aronson, 1975
75. Greeley JR, Schoenherr RA: Organization effects on client satisfaction with humaneness of service. J Health Soc Behav 22:2–18, 1981

Herzl R. Spiro, M.D., Ph.D.

11

Psychodynamic Theories

Most psychiatric administrators are familiar with the essential ingredients of psychodynamic theory. In contrast to psychopolitics, administrative essentials, organizational theory, and sociologic theory, which comprise the remainder of this section, psychodynamic theory is part of a common language spoken by most psychiatrists.

For our purposes, we will consider psychodynamic theory as that set of constructs that concerns repression and the impact of the unconscious; the influence of development and life history on subsequent life events; the interplay of conflicting drives and forces in producing resultant symptoms, conditions, and adaptations; the sources of drive energy; the mechanisms of coping; and the dynamic unconscious influences that shape human behavior. This chapter deals with the application of this body of theory only as it applies to groups and organizations and thus to psychiatric administrative practice.

The administrator of a psychiatric organization is much more likely to have in-depth knowledge of group theory than the administrator of a business enterprise, an educational institution, or a governmental agency. On the other hand, psychiatric organizations do not seem to win frequent citation in organization management texts as models of stellar administrative practice. One might even conclude that in the predynamic era psychiatric administrators were more recognized as having particular hospital administrative expertise. (For instance, the first chief executive officer of the newly built Johns Hopkins Hospital in the late 19th century was a psychiatrist who had been superintendent of one of the insane asylums.) This writer shares the view of such diverse administrative theorists as Zaleznick,[1,2] Levinson,[3–6] and Field[7] that dynamic theory should enhance administrative practice. So why, in the era of dynamic psychiatry, have so many psychiatric facilities experienced major administrative problems? I believe that psychodynamic theory, like many meaningful theories, can be misused in a harmful manner just as it can be utililzed in an effective manner.

It is too easy a leap from "in-depth knowledge" of group theory to the false expectation that such knowledge automatically enhances effective organizational administrative practice. If a little knowledge is a dangerous thing, a great deal of knowledge almost exclusively derived from a totally separate universe of application becomes a disaster when torn from context or applied inappropriately.

Indeed, one's very familiarity with psychodynamic theory may breed unfortunate selective inattention or even contempt. Psychodynamic theory is usually only applied in individual or group psychotherapy after a careful case study and in-depth individual understanding. While the theory does shape therapeutic practice, true dynamic therapies demand restraint, meticulous understanding of each patient's uniqueness, and a carefully thought-through, structured set of role relationships and practices. Flip dynamic formulations based on a combination of metaphor and anecdote are hardly the stuff of serious psychiatry. The dangers of "wild analysis" were recognized by the earliest dynamic psychiatrists, including Freud himself.[8]

A psychiatric organization is not merely an aggregate of individuals. It certainly is not a series of therapy groups. Thorough data collection or structured role relationships of individual therapy or even of group therapy cannot be approached in work relationships and work organizations. Even the growing field of group psychodynamic theory must not be mistaken for a theory of organizations, though reliable insights have come forth from group work.

Fritz Redl, writing in 1942,[9] warned of the distinction between the study of "the emotional and instinctual relationships between persons who constitute groups" on the one hand and "the psychoanalytic study of the group or groups." Redl hoped for:

> . . . some blend between psychoanalytic and sociological insights . . . however, it is definitely felt that the time is not yet right. One cannot mix two things before one has them. Today there is a sociology of the group on one hand and a psychoanalytic psychology of the person on the other. These two do not blend.*

Redl's warning is far more applicable to organizational psychodynamic theory.

A REVIEW OF GROUP PSYCHODYNAMICS

The literature in group psychotherapy is a broad and expanding one. A very brief review of what readings contemporary psychiatric residents should cover and a summary of one epigenetic group developmental viewpoint will be presented.

Moore and Calder have summarized psychoanalytic contributions to understanding group process,[10] as has Ezriel with respect to British psychoanalysis.[11] Scheidlinger has contributed a series of seminal articles and collections that should be compulsory reading for the psychiatric administrator.[12–16]

Anthony bridges the gap to individual therapy.[17] Foulkes provides a broad systems framework and then collaborates with Anthony in summarizing an English-based psychoanalytic approach.[18,19] Slavson provides a classic volume based on U.S. concepts.[20] Semrad emphasizes egosyntonic and integrative aspects of group functioning of special interest to the psychiatric administrator.[21,22] Spanjard emphasizes emerging transference issues.[23] Broad summary work and collections by Jerome Frank,[24] Rosenbaum and Berger,[25] and Yalom[26] should be required reading. I have abbreviated these required resident reading lists for fear that some developing psychiatric administrators may not have had strong group training in dynamic theory during residency. Such group background reading is vital if one is to engage in critical examination of group theory applications to organizational development.

*From Redl F: Group Emotions and Leadership. Psychiatry 5:573–596, 1942. With permission.

An example: one could focus on developmental issues as groups and the organizations they constitute are founded, grow, and age. In a brilliant series of articles, Seymour Kaplan and his collaborators[27–37] utilize direct group observations, dream material, and systematic data collection to evolve a theory of group development that in our view has important implications for organizational evolution. Kaplan has postulated a theory of organizational psychogenesis that he discusses in Chapter 12. We believe that the epigenesis of organizations is a developing field and that each psychiatric administrator would benefit from awareness of what stage of development his organization may be approaching.

If the organization is closest to inception, one can expect a certain "looseness" of organization. One can anticipate that early undifferentiated group-as-a-unit phases will involve intense leader dependency. This stage is likely to change quickly into group-as-a-unit counterdependency, with a tendency to attack leadership. Individuals leading psychiatric organizations in which rapid change is occurring may go through these first two stages in the early phases of organization development. Subsequently, one may well encounter subgroup differentiation with power as a key issue. Absentee leadership, whatever the cause, may prove disastrous in these stages. This is followed by a late phase of development in which pairing, intimacy, and the phenomena of organizational aging are predominant. The leader-dependent early organization phase must be carefully distinguished from the highly differentiated subgroup "power" trip phase, or the director may find very traumatic consequences. Often the phase shifts are so subtle that even leadership well acquainted with epigenetic developmental theory as it applies to groups has difficulty applying the theory in organizations. At a minimum, the reader is urged to review carefully Kaplan and Razin's most recent piece on the dynamics of group cohesion (1981)[35] and the "parent" piece by Kaplan and Roman (1963)[37] as well as the application of these authors of group theory to organizational theory (1974).[31]

The author has approached this topic personally from three perspectives: as a practicing psychiatric administrator, as a psychoanalytic psychiatrist, and as a research worker with a degree in social psychology. It is my thesis that psychiatric organizations exhibit peculiarly difficult theoretical problems and that the familiarity of the psychiatric administrator with dynamic theory, in particular, may lead one beyond contempt to careless blunders based on loose extrapolations from dynamic theory.

Consequently, this brief overview of group literature will be followed by a section on "pitfalls" in hopes of warning the reader of possible dangers. From there, the chapter will proceed to a rather brief synopsis of central psychodynamic theories related to organizations. The third section will be an effort to apply the theories to psychiatric organizations with their particular unique attributes.

PITFALLS IN THE APPLICATION OF PSYCHODYNAMIC THEORY TO PSYCHIATRIC ADMINISTRATION

By bringing the pitfalls in application of psychodynamic theory into consciousness, the psychiatric administrator may avoid such pitfalls. The essense of psychodynamic theory involves bringing into consciousness unconscious material in such a way that ego structure can develop to channel the material in accord with reality principles and the goals and purposes that are important to the individual.

Regressive Phenomena

For much of this chapter, we will deal with the problems of individual regressive phenomena in psychiatric organizations. Some of these regressions relate to Oedipal struggles with parental figures transferred to individuals in positions of leadership and authority. Other regressions relate to basic oral dependency needs. Still others are related to anal compulsive power struggles. Staff of psychiatric institutions are no more immune to these phenomena than are the patients who come to see them in analysis or the individuals working in business enterprises. (See Zaleznick.[1,2]) The analysis of personality and role relations in management,[39] the power and political aspects of organizational life,[40] and the leadership patterns evolved by such politics[18] are well reviewed elsewhere.

The issues of power strivings,[41] organ inferiority,[42] acting out of Oedipal issues,[43] and specific acting out of executive role conflict,[44,45] are amply covered in other literature. They are hardly unique to psychiatric administration. The so-called pathos of power is ubiquitous.[46]

In this instance, though, there are specific regressive phenomena that occur as one has access to rather primitive unconscious material as a consequence of one's work. Oedipal and power issues come much closer to the surface. It is the awareness of the dangers of the regressive phenomena stirred up by readings of theory in the abstract that lead to the requirement of a personal analysis before one can be considered a trained psychoanalyst. Cognitive knowledge not only fails to produce mastery over difficult material in and of itself. It may actually contribute to regression and acting out of the very material under discussion. As one is constantly exposed to regressed patients and to one's own thoughts about materials that take origin in early life, one may uncover primitive aspects of organizational regression, fixation, and institutionalized acting out.

In psychoanalytic technique with individual patients, one overcomes this pitfall by structuring the role of the analyst and interdicting the acting out of the analyst's conflicts or personal regressive phenomena on the person of the patient. The psychiatric administrator lacks a similar code of structured rules. In fact, a certain institutionalized childish flaunting of anger and obsessive overcontrol may even be fostered in some organizations.

The Danger of "Loose Metaphor"

A principle of the scientific experiment is that data should be collected from a legitimate sample drawn from the appropriate universe of application if the constructs to be derived from the data are to have any validity. The constructs of psychodynamic theory have, by and large, been drawn from listening to individuals who come to see a therapist because of individual distress and who then interact with that therapist either in a one-to-one relationship or in a small group. The "demand characteristics" of the therapeutic situation involve relatively remote and neutral "Aesculapian" authority as well as meticulous applications of psychopathological principles. This means that individuals need to be labeled with a diagnosis based on generalized rules for making such diagnoses.

When these same principles are applied to work groups and to organizations, major difficulties may ensue. Metaphor and reality may become confused. When one speaks of a paranoid individual, one speaks of a specific pathological ego defense mechanism. It is entirely unclear what one means when one speaks of "a paranoid organization." One of the least effective division chiefs that the author has worked with was an individual who was fond of going about muttering, "This organization is psychotic." Needless to say, such generalized diagnosis was not very helpful when the division chief had to work with other division chiefs in specific problem solving. Repeatedly, the involved individual drew on an apparently endless store of psychopathological diagnoses used far more as epithets than descriptions. It was not clear whether the division chief expected everyone to go on phenothiazines or whether the communication was that the involved individual felt confused and uncertain about what he was to do. The very opposite of the purpose of psychopathological formulation resulted from this behavior. Psychopathological formulation is directed at precision of communication. Loose metaphors that lack a shared meaning in an organizational context lead to imprecise communication and a breakdown in problem-solving behaviors.

While a taxonomy of organizational pathology may prove highly useful in the future, one suspects that this taxonomy will need to remain far removed from medical diagnosis.

Poor Data Collection

It is not only that the metaphors may be imprecise in their meaning when they are drawn generally from medical and psychiatric nomenclature. It is also that the data collection may be of poor quality. In the consulting room, no psychiatrist would think of dropping labels on people without gathering sufficient data to know whether the label fits. Presumably, a physician–patient relationship is a prerequisite to making a diagnosis. Sophomore psychopathology game playing should not be confused with serious psychiatry. In order to apply psychodynamic theory to organizational situations, precise data need to be collected about the organization. For such data to be collected, there must be proper entry (e.g., the person collecting the data needs to be invited by the organization and needs to be given permission to gather information); there needs to be a thorough stage of data collection; and the data must be organized in a manner that involves knowledge of psychodynamic theory as it applies to organizations, not just individuals.

The confusion about data collection and the looseness of the metaphors lead to a corruption of language that, in turn, may ultimately result in inappropriate abandonment of psychodynamic theory as having no value in understanding organizations. For instance, a narcissistic character disorder is a serious treatment challenge to any clinician. The same term applied to an administrator often translates, "He insists on having his way and isn't letting me have my way." Obsessionalism may really mean, "He is being too demanding and too disciplined in what he insists on from me."

The psychiatric administrator should be far more (not far less) scrupulous about precise use of psychiatric language. The language must be based on precise application of the theory through proper data collection. One is rarely given license to collect psychiatric data concerning one's colleagues. If one seriously believes that a psychopathological state of serious proportions exists in one's colleagues, then perhaps the appropriate thing is to discuss referral to a neutral psychiatrist. Assuredly, the most inappropriate activity involves hurling about psychiatric terminology based on psychodynamic theory as a means of fighting rather than as a means of rendering care.

"Wild Interpretation"

Perhaps the most treacherous pitfall concerns the mental health professional who attends a few conferences on group behaviors and then proceeds to interpret the behavior of various individuals in the group without their invitation and without any real understanding of the involved individuals. Most persons who are deeply involved in the application of psychodynamic theory to individuals tend to be cautious about offering a putative, mutative interpretation outside the psychotherapeutic situation to a colleague in the corridor. For over 15 years of administration, the author has been impressed by the numbers of similarly well-trained mental health professionals who will take smatterings of ignorance concerning dynamic organizational theory and build extraordinarily complex (and equally useless) interpretations to be offered at staff meetings. Interpretation in psychiatry not only requires detailed data and detailed knowledge of the involved theory, but also a proper sense of timing. One interprets because one is in a therapeutic role and one anticipates that the interpretation will bring about change. Many of the groups that teach applications of psychodynamic theory through small group experience permit rapid interpretation based on brief exposures to the group. Students in such settings may find themselves modeling the behaviors of their teachers and interpreting what is occurring in a group rather than participating in the group's task and dealing with process issues in a constructive participant manner. The author defines wild interpretation as (1) interpretation made with insufficient data, or (2) with insufficient knowledge of the relevant applicable theory, or (3) in the absence of the proper sense of timing to produce change, or (4) with the absence of a social role in which generalized interpretive comments are role appropriate. A part of the uncomfortable state that occurs in psychiatric organizations is related to the tendency of staff to engage in "wild interpretation."

A strong recommendation to the psychiatric administrator is to be extremely parsimonious about interpretive behaviors in dealing with group phenomena. One needs to think through leadership roles to decide whether the discussion of the phenomena occurring in the group constitutes a generalized assault or truly constitutes an effort for both the leader and the group to understand what is occurring and to make changes. Is the social contract between the leader and the group constructed in such a way that interpretation is anticipated? Is the interpretation itself based on sufficient data? Is the interpretation likely to produce positive change, or is it merely a method of enhancing the power and authority of the leader? This psychiatric administrator has not found generalized group interpretations particularly useful as a leadership style. Psychiatric administrators may function most effectively by applying their knowledge of psychodynamic theory exclusively to themselves and to their own behaviors in groups. Perhaps the psychiatric administrator can model task-related activities and facilitation of interpersonal behaviors. In short, it would appear that the use of interpretation in dealing with psychiatric organizations is best confined to outside consultants who have gathered sufficient data (not whirlwind 1- or 2-day visits); know dynamic theory thoroughly; and have consciously selected interpretation rather than pure data feedback or structural intervention as the best way to help the organization accomplish its goals.

Inappropriate Emphasis

The body of psychodynamic theory involves many potential areas of emphasis. For instance, one can see the drive states that take origin in psychosexual conflict. Certainly some writers have been quite effective in applying these concepts. Others feel concern that many psychiatric administrators may unwittingly slip into McGregor Type X assumptions[47] in which the individual is seen as needing to be shaped by an authoritarian bureaucratic structure because the individual will be lazy, ineffectual, indolent, and otherwise fail in work tasks. Few organizations require McGregor Type Y management as much as psychiatric organizations. No psychiatric administrator can really know what goes on in each of the therapeutic encounters with patients. The real power of psychiatric organizations lies far at the periphery where the interaction with the patients and the outside environment occurs. The psychiatric administrator most usefully will see himself as being at the hub of a wheel where an intact and effective rim of contact with the environment is a necessity. The role is much more one of facilitation, coordination, and goal setting than manipulation of the actual encounters with the environment.

There is a broad area of psychodynamic theory that strongly supports the McGregor formulations. These are the Hartman formulations concerning the conflict-free areas of ego functioning.[48] If people can be seen as gaining their satisfactions from a sense of mastery over difficult tasks and as adult professional human beings who need respect rather than manipulation, the portion of dynamic theory that is the heart of modern ego psychoanalysis may help the psychiatric administrator. If the portion of dynamic theory that emphasizes the basic primitive drive states that influence behavior, seek out the conflicts people act out, emphasize regression, and so on; if, indeed, this is the primary body of theory to which the psychiatric administrator turns, justification may be found for an organizational structure that in the author's view will not work. Those subscribing to what the author sees as this pitfall might do well to include themselves with their colleagues for whom they are administratively responsible as they apply these conceptions to work behaviors (e.g., the administrator is lazy, indolent, and responds most to reward and punishment). The view that will be taken in this chapter is that the world of work ultimately needs to be related to Freud's formulations concerning effective ego development, Anna Freud's formulations concerning developmental lines, Grinker's concepts of mastery, Hartman's concepts of conflict-free areas of ego functioning, and so on. There is considerable discussion here of the more primitive regressive phenomena that at times dominate organizational life. These are emphasized as areas from which organization malfunction may evolve. Just as one needs to understand the destruction of tissues and the careful delineation of destroyed tissue in the treatment of burns, one also needs similar knowledge concerning dysfunction in organizations. On the other hand, the treatment of burns requires that new tissue grow in from healthy areas. Ultimately, the leadership of organizations similarly requires a knowledge of what makes individuals engage in healthy goal-oriented, task-oriented work activities.

CLASSIC PSYCHODYNAMIC THEORY IN ORGANIZATION ADMINISTRATION

Psychodynamic theory concerning organizations stems from Freud's general dynamic theories. Ellenberger's review of the origins of dynamic theory[49] and Rappaport's lucid systematic organization of Freud's meta-psychology[50] may help the reader review necessary background.

The theory draws on such early writers as LeBon,[51] McDougall,[52,53] Trotter,[54] and Cooley.[55] Early group and social psychology pioneers, including Pratt,[56] Trigent Burrow,[57] Paul Schilder,[58] George Herbert Mead,[59] and certainly Moreno,[60] heavily influenced emerging theory.

Psychodynamic theory of behavior in organizations begins with Freud. From the very outset, Freud emphasized such issues of organization context as becoming accustomed to the therapist or losing independence in relation to the therapist as the key resistance in the treatment of hysteria.[61] The basic theme of regression so crucial to the understanding of group and organizational behavior is introduced in *The Interpretation of Dreams.*[62] In the "Psychopathology of Everyday Life"[63] Freud draws examples from the military services to illustrate that all is to be remembered yet much is forgotten due to "extraorganizational motives." Freud's first full foray into the world of sociology comes in a short 1908 paper, "Civilized Sexual Morality and Modern Nervous Illness."[64] The antagonism between "organized" civilized life and instinctual life is considered as a cause for the neuroses. Rules of organizations such as schools are considered in mitigating the risk of suicide in a 1910 brief note.[65]

"Totem and Taboo" (1912)[66] contains Freud's hypothesis of the primal horde. Here he formulates the concept of the murder and ritual cannabalism of the primal father, with groups, organizations, and institutions taking origin from subsequent relationships among the murderous, mourning offspring. (See Eckstein[67] for applications in current groups and Slater[68] for a broad view of ritual "murder" and the fate of leaders.) Of particular concern is Freud's view of taboos about rulers (pp. 41–50), the dangerous magical power they possess, and the tendency to place such leaders in a position of torment, burden, and even bondage worse than the subjects. The elimination of the primal father by the rebellious sons and the reaction to these acts are seen as the cornerstone not only of organizational life but also as the basis of totemic art, totemic religion, and much of modern morality.

The boundary issues of organizations may well take origin from the exogamy drives meant to avoid further conflict among the primal sons. Freud returns to the parricide theme even in his last decade.[69] "Group Psychology and the Analysis of the Ego" (1921)[70] amplifies this theme, but other work comes first and needs review.

Freud also lays a foundation for object relations theory that has proved vital in understanding organizational development. As Kanzer emphasizes,[71] Freud's metapsychological theory of instincts and their vicissitudes defines instincts primarily in terms of the object world and the self.[72]

"On Narcissism" (1914)[73] presents a mirror image of object relations theory. Part three of this volume, entitled "Ego Ideal, Inheritor of Narcissism," sets the stage for group psychology and the analysis of the ego. The self-love directed at the actual ego in childhood becomes directed at a 1914 conception of the ego ideal in adulthood. The key role of the charismatic leader identified in LeBon's *Crowd*[51] is created because members of the crowd substitute the leader for the *then*-current concept of the ego ideal of "On Narcissism" and "Group Psychology and the Analysis of the Ego," which are essentially the same, although the concept of the superego and its relation to the ego ideal are formulated later.[73]

"Group Psychology and the Analysis of the Ego" is Freud's primary contribution to the psychology of organizations. Here Freud points out that in expressing instinctual impulses, the individual virtually always has someone else as a model, an object, an object, a helper, or an opponent. He reviews his concept of collective emotional life and the intensification of sentiment in group and organizations. Two artificial "groups" (which are really organizations) serve to illustrate: the church and the army. In each case, libidinal ties to leadership are formed. The ties include introjection, regressive introjection of the organization as part of the ego, and a sense of commonality with other group members bound to the same leader. A primary group is defined as a number of individuals who have put the same object in place of the ego ideal.

Freud's other formulations of organizational life provide insight into the organizational forces of negativism,[75,76] the inhibitions that make civilization possible,[77,78] and a global view of the nature of leadership and the binding of instincts so that groups of humans can coexist in ego-dominated reality-based relationships.[79,80]

Yet it is the earlier formulations of narcissism and the 1920's conception of the group that provide impetus to subsequent dynamic theory evolution. The effort to develop a concept of narcissism gave rise to Jacobson's conceptualization of the self in the object world,[81] to Balint's reformulation of primary narcissism,[82,83] as well as to the work of Bowlby[84] and Winnicut,[85] with their view of the vicissitudes of separation (with its administrative consequences). Ultimately, two related viewpoints emgerged in England: Fairbairn's formulation of object relations theory[86,87] and a body of theories that Wilfred Bion first developed [88,90] but are even more directly related to the work of Melanie Klein.[91,93]

TAVISTOCK PSYCHODYNAMIC ORGANIZATIONAL THEORY

Bion's concepts are related to small group task and regressive phenomena. A group of Kleinian analysts and social scientists at London's Tavistock Institute applied these theories over a period of decades. A. K. Rice, in particular, demonstrated the value of these theories in organizational life,[94,95] the demands of leadership,[96] and boundary monitoring.[97] Such writers as Trist and Sofer,[98–100] Jacque,[101] and Menzies[102] have applied what some refer to as "Tavistock Theory" to organizations ranging from factory life[94,103] to the university[104] and general hospital nursing services.[102] Rioch's lucid explications[105,106] should be utilized as essential to supplement this review, which is too brief to do the subject justice.

Bion's theories review group and organizational regression as a defense against internal objects and the part objects encountered in such social settings. Two levels produce these regressive phenomena: the neurotic family level noted by Freud and the more primitive paranoid-schizoid and depressive levels emphasized by Melanie Klein.[91]

The three "basic assumption behaviors" identified by Bion are the forms taken by such regressions. Bion's model is best experienced by a group attending a conference whose primary task is to understand behavior in groups as it happens. The presence of consultants who make group-centered interventions may foster regressions by their emulation of a psychoanalytically based stance of general abstinence. The absence of supportive interventions and the paradoxical nature of simultaneously acting and commenting on group behaviors[107] stimulates group regression. Nonetheless, the resultant behaviors are readily discernible in other settings, particularly in psychiatric organizations. The author has found application of these concepts of importance in formulations of prevention[108] as well as conceptualizations of psychiatric hospitals.[109,110]

Basic assumption dependency involves group behaviors to elicit positive, sustaining, gratifying, omnipotent, and omniscient behaviors from the leader. Basic assumption fight–flight involves threatening, competitive, vying, or fleeing behaviors either directed outside the group beyond an external boundary or across internal subgroup boundaries. Basic assumption pairing involves group discussions of a hopeful, future-oriented nature. There may be a Messianic quality, a sense that some special genious will soon arrive to serve the group. The group is marked by excited, high-energy interaction that may be sexually tinged. The tendency of charismatic leaders to reinforce their narcissistic needs by fusing leadership patterns with basic assumption regressive patterns has been described.[111,112]

More ego-integrative, reality-based behavior appears in groups and organizations when the tasks are clear and the members of an organization agree on those tasks. A. K. Rice, in particular, has explicated the nature of primary tasks as those tasks without which an organization would not exist and toward whose fulfillment the organization is structured. Industries whose putative primary task is profit making may, in reality, be organized to provide steady jobs for a group of employees. Some see similar trends in a few government hospitals whose task is supposed to be patient care. On the other hand, there may be occasional private health organizations whose real primary task is making money. Announced task and true primary task are not necessarily the same. Rice's study of a university setting best demonstrates this point.[104]

Moreover, the leadership task is so heavily weighted toward internal and external boundary maintenance that primary task may become a forgotten afterthought. How many excellent therapists go unrewarded because they come to the director's attention over boundary disputes rather than patient care? How many academic psychiatry leaders lose their posts because they fail to provide good undergraduate psychiatric curricula (their alleged primary task), and how many actually are blown away in a dispute over turf with some external chief or political rival? The administrator who thinks that task alone is sufficient and basic assumption behavior is to be ignored will not long remain a leader. Sabbaticals, national prominence with attendant absences from meetings, spells of illness, and other sources of absence are particularly potent prescriptions for group regression and leadership destruction.

OBJECT RELATIONS AND SELF-PSYCHOLOGY IN CURRENT ORGANIZATIONAL PSYCHODYNAMICS

The past decade has seen increasing convergence of Freud's 1920's formulations, ego psychoanalysis, object relations theory, and self-psychology. While Hartman and his colleagues developed an approach to ego analysis based on Freud's later formulations,[113,114] Erikson developed both a view of epigenesis[115–116] and psychohistory in relation to organizational constraints[117–118] that created foundations for a view of object relations and affect theory. (See Sandler and Sandler.[119]) Two contemporary additions to psychodynamic theory have resulted. Each requires careful study by the practitioner. One is Kohut's self-psychology,[120,121] a series of formulations that leads Kohut to a specific psychology of charisma, a group action, and of group creativity as it applies to Freud.[122] Of particular utility is Stone and Whitman's summary of self-psychology as it applies to group process.[123] George Pollock demonstrates the steps in the organizational mourning process requisite to creative organizational change,[124] a product of his original effective analysis of loss and grief plus the growing insight into positive creative processes.

Otto Kernberg has synthesized a contemporary view of object relations,[125,126] borderline states,[127] and narcissism[128–130] with his extensive knowledge of Bion's work and the Tavistock approach. He has written two classic articles on organizational regression issues found in psychiatric organizations.[131,132] No textbook chapter author has the right to attempt a summary of Kernberg's tight prose, which must be viewed as required reading for current "state of the art" concerning dynamic theory in psychiatric organizations, particularly the regressive forces in work groups and leaders.

PSYCHODYNAMIC ORGANIZATIONAL THEORY BASED ON FIELD THEORY, SOCIAL PSYCHOLOGY, AND COMMUNICATION THEORY

While these theories will primarily be covered in separate chapters, it is important to note the constant interchange between the American group dynamic school (especially the National Training Laboratory [NTL] at Bethel, Maine, founded by Kurt Lewin) and both the American and English psychoanalytic theorists. The author has found, through personal interviews, conclusive evidence of extensive exchanges both between the Tavistock group and NTL (dating back to 30 years ago) and between a series of American psychoanalytic theorists and NTL leaders. There is a dangerous tendency to dichotomize these fields and treat them as competitive rather than complementary. Lewin openly acknowledged his agreements with Freud even while maintaining his interest in the here-and-now social field.[133] Lewin's work on autocracy/democracy[134] and patterns of aggression in experimental social climates[135] remains of importance to the psychiatric administrator. The work of his colleague, Heider, is particularly central, and both balance theory and attribution theory deserve far more attention by psychiatrists than they currently receive.[136,137]

The problem has been that psychoanalytic-like silences by dynamically oriented administrators tend to produce regression and destructive organizational patterns. Bennis, Benne, and Chin[138] present far more effective change strategies grounded both in psychodynamics and modern social psychology. Argyris,[139–141] Bennis, and coworkers,[142–145] Blake and Mouton,[146] Lawrence and Lorch,[147] Likert,[148] Lippitt,[149] Shephard and Bennis,[150] Walton,[151] Eddy, et al.,[152] and Gelfand and Walker should not be viewed as being in conflict with psychodynamic approaches merely because their work is summarized in a different chapter of this text. Neither has this writer experienced difficulty integrating the body of modern social psychology and the systems theorists with classic analysis, although the connections are less obvious (and must be the subject for a future work). Particularly the Bales' groups,[154] the Mills' analysis of the sociology of these groups,[155] Cartwright and Zander's collection on group dynamics,[156] Etzioni's work on complex organizations,[157] and Breed's reformulation of these concepts[158] can be integrated with classic theory. Deutsch's cybernetic model[159] and both Parsons[160,161] and Merton[162,163] provide elaborated hypotheses that assuredly would have provoked Freud to extensive reformulation (given our knowledge of the impact far less profound theorists like LeBon had on Freud). The modern psychiatric administrator may be tempted to lump these extraordinary organizational dynamic theorists with Thibaut and Kelly's oversimplified learning-theory approach to groups.[164] This would be a grievous error. Finally, such key communication theorists as Ruesch, Bateson, and Watzlawik,[165–167] need integration into a comprehensive view of organizational psychodynamics.

SPECIAL DYNAMIC ISSUES IN PSYCHIATRIC HOSPITAL ADMINISTRATION—WHAT GOES WRONG

Regression as an Inherent Problem in Psychiatric Hospitals

With crisp primary tasks (patient care), leadership aware of the importance of fostering healthy ego function in staff, and a knowledge of social-science technology and its applications in preventing regressive behaviors, one might expect that such behaviors would be rarities in psychiatric organizations. The organizational and leadership regressive issues have been masterfully summarized in the two works by Otto Kernberg listed above.[131,132] Whence do these regressive issues take origin? Staff dealing with regressed individuals and regressed groups day in and day out cannot avoid being influenced by the nature of primitive issues that occupy most of their waking hours.

The leadership style of many psychiatric administrators is influenced by extensive experience with relatively "neutral" silent therapies or by group process experienced in which consultants model regression-promoting behaviors. The shift from behind-the-couch chair to the director's chair is a difficult shift.

Unconsciously, leaders may foster regression as though group therapy were the primary task. The leader may feel more comfortable managing regressed groups than leading task groups. One may play autocratic doctor when diplomatic leadership is required. One must avoid inappropriate overreliance on charisma in contrast to task leadership and boundary maintenance.

Poor Information Flow

Information flow in organizations is a major factor in organizational adaptation to change and application of innovation. George Field,[7] writing from the perspective of management consultation and professorship in business administration, describes processes by which organizations repress key information in a manner analogous to psychodynamic formulations concerning repression in individual psychology. Even with task clarity in profit-making organizations, information that upsets organizational homeostasis is consistently denied. (See Bennis, Benne, and Chin.[138]) Such repression is especially prominent in old hospital structures in which anxiety and threat may be much higher. Persons far removed from leadership roles tend to be particularly ignored. (See Whyte.[168]) This is a fact of particular concern in psychiatric facilities in which the most important data emerge from patient encounters far removed from executive offices. Habits of confidentiality, institutionalized distrust of funding agencies, or even distrust of nonmedical executives may cause severe disruption of vital information flow. Communication of problem-related information is negatively correlated with advancement in business organizations.[169] In hospital hierarchies, we have not often found great rewards produced for individuals offering information about impending accreditation issues.

Moreover, computer-based systems may further filter information flow to delete selectively affective concerns and reduce data to stylized irrelevancy. As a field trying to become a high-technology "scientific" field, psychiatry is particularly prone to the misuse of computer systems.

Field argues that nonprofit corporations, particularly universities, are far more (not less) subject to unconscious censoring of data to fit superego functions. The psychiatric organization appears most susceptible to such inattention. Service chiefs tend to tailor information to support staff increases but rarely provide accurate information on such subjects as failure to perform adequate examinations, abuse of restraints and medications, insensitivity, rudeness, or even cruelty by staff, and so on. When outside reporting sources bring such information to light, the organizational response is often to develop a siege mentality.

Psychiatric administrators who emphasize abuses within their own organization tend to be denied access to top posts or shunted aside. Furious intraorganizational fights may develop between internal critics pressing for institutional change and persons in authority fearful of accreditation loss, newspaper exposures, or other "dangerous" effects of "rocking the boat." We believe that the recurrent tendency of psychiatric hospitals to deteriorate to snake pits in various societies and in various ages is in large measure attributable to systematic denial and repression of uncomfortable information in psychiatric institutions.[109,110]

The psychiatric administrator who moves too rapidly in lifting such repression is in constant peril. (Any derepression will be interpreted as "too rapid change" by some members of medical hierarchies.) One can almost certainly anticipate gratuitous comments from individuals invested in the system that more information should have been gathered before any information was transmitted or any change was offered.

Moreover, the spread of technological innovation in a rapidly changing field is seriously impaired by such institutional repression. Morrison[170] cites the experience of a U.S. naval officer named Sims who attempted to gain acceptance of a new continuous-aim firing technique for U.S. naval vessels at a time when only 121 of 1500 shots fired at close range found their mark. Only the direct intervention of President Teddy Roosevelt enabled Sims to survive in the navy. Field provides multiple examples of persons fired or penalized as a consequence of presenting unpleasant data to individuals in authority and then refusing to disappear when they were politely ignored. Psychiatric organizations in particular have been slow to accept institutionalized external sources of data besides the rather distorted exposures that appear in newspapers. (See Breed, 1955[171] concerning problems of utilizing newspaper exposures as sources of data to produce change.)

One example studied by the author was the upheaval produced when a psychiatric director supported the presence of mental health association-selected, medical college-trained ombudsmen to help patients in a county psychiatric hospital. The potential consequences of systematic flow of patient dissatisfaction information to the director's desk was seen as disastrous by the service chiefs, and it required much of the director's energy to ward off attacks from threatened department heads over the next 5 years.

There is support for a view that some balance between institutional internal accountability systems and regular, thorough external evaluation by highly critical reviewers is a necessity merely to get relevant information to the directors.

Deutsch emphasizes a cybernetic feedback system in the political process as important in the theory of leadership.[159] Psychiatrists, of all people, should know better than to try to function without vital cognitive information.

Specifics

What, then, are the particular dynamic theoretical problems of the psychiatric facility?

1. The *patients* by the nature of their illness tend to be regressed and to uncover primitive unconscious processes in therapists.
2. The *process* involves intense attentivity to dynamic issues, which in turn may tend to be acted out in work groups. The work group involves high levels of interaction around charged issues.
3. The *staff* tends to select itself by the fascination of individuals with psychological process and at least occasionally as a consequence of personal experience with emotional dysfunction. A certain level of narcissism is a necessity in personnel who must render life-and-death decisions. That same narcissism may predispose the staff to overreliance on charismatic leadership rather than task leadership. A high level of obsessionalism is practically a prerequisite to passage of preclinical and professional course work. Such obsessionalism may blind the leader to broader issues.

4. The *nature of the art* involved unrealistic societal expectations not met by current technological innovation. The art is in a state of rapid flux requiring rapid change. A position strongly held by a leader one day may be proved incorrect by emerging research developments in a matter of a few years. There are always those political figures who will blame the leader rather than credit the advances in the state of the art.
5. The *milieu* involves stigma, "blame the victim" social fears, and intense political process. The psychiatrist–administrator is like a person walking a tightrope in a hurricane. While striving to keep one's balance, one must avoid even the most minor slips.

Needless to say, the dynamics of psychiatric administration are unlikely to draw hordes of volunteers. Yet for those who are willing to try, who understand that even brief "sprints" of success are socially important and worthwhile, and who are willing to keep learning as they experience some of the consequences of psychodynamic organizational theory, the work remains fascinating, satisfying, and at times even emotionally rewarding.

REFERENCES

1. Zaleznick A, Kets deVries M: Power and the Corporate Mind. New York, Houghton Mifflin, 1975
2. Zaleznick A: The Human Dilemma of Leadership. New York, Harper & Row, 1960
3. Levinson H: The Great Jackass Fallacy. Boston, Harvard University Press, 1973
4. Levinson H: The Exceptional Executive. Cambridge, Mass, Harvard University Press, 1968
5. Levinson H: Emotional Health: The World of Work. New York, Harper & Row, 1964
6. Levinson H: Organizational Diagnosis. Boston, Harvard University Press, 1972
7. Field GA: The unconscious organization. Psychoanal Rev 61:333–354, 1974
8. Freud S: Wild psychoanalysis (1910), in Strachey J (ed): Standard Edition of the Complete Psychological Works of Freud, vol. 11 London, Hogarth Press, 1910, 219–230
9. Redl F: Group emotions and leadership. Psychiatry 5:573–596, 1942
10. Moore BE, Calder, KJ: Psychoanalytic knowledge of group process. J Am Psychoanal Assoc 27:145–156, 1979
11. Ezriel HE: A psychoanalytic approach to group treatment. Br J Med Psychol 23:59–75, 1950
12. Scheidlinger S: Psychoanalysis and Group Behavior. New York, Norton, 1952
13. Scheidlinger S: Group process in group psychotherapy. Arch Psychother 14:104–120; 346–363, 1960
14. Scheidlinger S: The concept of regression in group psychotherapy. Int J Group Psychother 18:3–20, 1960
15. Scheidlinger S: Identification: The source of belonging and identity in small groups. Int J Group Psychother 14:291–306, 1964
16. Scheidlinger S: (ed): Psychoanalytic Group Dynamics. Basic Reading. New York, International University Press, 1980
17. Anthony EJ: The generic elements in dyadic and group psychotherapy. Int J Group Psychother 17:57–70, 1967
18. Foulkes SH: Therapeutic Group Analysis. New York, International Universities Press, 1965
19. Foulkes SH, Anthony EJ: Group Psychotherapy. The Psychoanalytic Approach. London, Penguin Books, 1957
20. Slavson SR: Analytic Group Psychotherapy. New York, Columbia University Press, 1950
21. Arsenian J, Semrad EV, Shapiro D: An analysis of integral function in groups. Int J Group Psychother 12:421–431, 1962
22. Semrad EV, et al: The field of group psychotherapy. Int J Group Psychother 13:452–475, 1963
23. Spanjard J: Transference neurosis and psychoanalytic group therapy. Int J Group Psychother 9:31–42, 1959

24. Frank JD: Persuasion and Healing. London, Oxford Press, 1961
25. Rosenbaum M, Berger MM: Group Psychotherapy and Group Function (rev ed). New York, Basic Books, 1975
26. Yalom I: The Theory and Practice of Group Therapy. New York, Basic Books, 1970
27. Kaplan SR: Therapy groups and training groups: Similarities and differences. Int J Group Psychother 17:473–504, 1967
28. Kaplan SR. Symposium: Dreams and the group setting. Int J Group Psychother 23:387–393, 1973
29. Kaplan SR: The "group dream." Int J Psychother 23:421–431, 1973
30. Kaplan SR: Reader's forum on Kohut. Int J Psychother 28:129–131, 1978
31. Kaplan SR: Characteristic phases of development in organizations, in Millman DS, Goldman GD (eds): Group Process Today. Evaluation and Perspectives. Springfield, Ill, Thomas, 1974
32. Kaplan SR, Ahmed B: Group strategies for disadvantaged populations. The role of the public mental health setting, in Seligman M (ed): Group Counselling and Group Psychotherapies. Springfield, Ill, Thomas, 1977
33. Kaplan SR, Razin A: The psychological substate of self help groups. J Operational Psychology 9:57–69, 1978
34. Kaplan SR: Nature of object relations in closed adult therapy groups (in preparation)
35. Kaplan SR, Razin A: Psychosocial dynamics of group cohesion, in Kellerman H (ed): Group Cohesion: Theoretical and Clinical Perspectives. New York, Grune and Stratton, 1981
36. Kaplan SR, Roman MS: Characteristic response in adult therapy groups to the introduction of a new member: a reflection of group process. Int J Group Psychotherapy 11:372–381, 1961
37. Kaplan JR, Roman M: Phases of development in an adult therapy group. Int J Group Psychother 13:10–26, 1963
38. Hodgson RC, Levinson DJ, Zaleznik A: The Executive Role Constellation: An Analysis of Personality and Role Relations in Management. Boston, Harvard University Press, 1965
39. Zaleznik A: Power and politics in organizational life. Harvard Business Review, May-June 1970, pp 47–60
40. Zaleznik A: Charismatic and consensus leaders. Bull Menninger Clin 38:222–238, 1974
41. Ansbacher H, Ansbacher R: The Individual Psychology of Alfred Adler. New York, Basic Books, 1956
42. Adler H: Superiority and the Social Interest (ed 3). Ansbacher H, Ansbacher R (eds): New York, Viking, 1973
43. Coleman D: Oedipus in the board room. Psychology Today 45:125, 1977.
44. Henry WE: The business executive: psychodynamics of a social role. Am J Sociol 54:286–291, 1949
45. Henry WE: The psychodynamics of the executive role, in Werner WC, Martin NH (eds): Industrial Man. New York, Harper & Row, 1959
46. Clark K: The pathos of power: a psychological perspective. Am Psychol 26:1047–1057, 1971
47. McGregor D: The Human Side of the Enterprise. New York, McGraw-Hill, 1960
48. Hartman H: Ego Psychology and the Problem of Adaptation. New York, International Universities Press, 1939
49. Ellenberger HF: The Discovery of the Unconscious: The History and Evolution of Dynamic Psychiatry. New York, International Universities Press, 1980
50. Rappaport D: The Structure of Psychoanalytic Theory: A Systematizing Attempt. Psychological Issues, Monograph 6. New York, International Universities Press, 1960
51. LeBon G: The Crowd: A Study of the Popular Mind. London, Fisher-Unwin, 1922
52. McDougall W: Social Psychology. New York, Norton, 1908
53. McDougall W: The Group Mind. New York, Putnam, 1920
54. Trotter W: Instincts of the Herd in Peace and War. London, Fisher-Unwin, 1916
55. Cooley CH: Human Nature and the Social Order. New York, Scribner, 1902
56. Pratt DH: The Cass method of treating consumption in the poor. JAMA 49:755–759, 1907
57. Burrow TL: The group method of analysis. Psychoanal Rev 14:268–280, 1924
58. Schilder P: Results and problems in group psychotherapy in severe neurosis. Ment Hyg 23:87–98, 1939
59. Mead GH: Mind, Self, and Society. Chicago, University of Chicago Press, 1934
60. Moreno JL: Psychodrama and group therapy. Sociometry 9:249–253, 1946
61. Freud S: Studies on Hysteria (1893–1895), chap 4 in Strachey J (ed): Complete Psychological Works, vol. 2. London, Hogarth Press, 1955, pp. 235–325

62. Freud S: The Interpretation of Dreams (1900), chap 7. The psychology of the dream process (B) Regression, in Strachey J (ed): Complete Psychological Works, vol. 5. London, Hogarth Press, 1953, pp 533–549
63. Freud S: The Psychopathology of Everyday Life (1901), chap 7: The forgetting of impressions and intentions, in Strachey J (ed): Complete Psychological Works, vol. 6. London, Hogarth Press, 1960, pp 151–161
64. Freud S: "Civilized" sexual ethics and modern nervous sickness (1908), in Strachey J (ed): Complete Psychological Works, vol. 9. London, Hogarth Press, 1959, pp 179–204
65. Freud S: Contributions to a discussion on suicide (1910) in Strachey J (ed): Complete Psychological Works, vol. 11 London, Hogarth Press, 1955, pp 231–232
66. Freud S: Totem and taboo (1913), in Strachey J (ed): Complete Psychological Works, vol. 13. London, Hogarth Press, 1955, pp 1–16
67. Eckstein R: The search and yearning for and the rebellion against the father—a group dilemma. Int J Group Psychother 28:435–444, 1978
68. Slater PE: Microcosm: Structural, Psychological and Religious Evolution in Groups. New York, Wiley, 1966
69. Freud S: Dostoevsky and parricide, in Strachey J (ed): Complete Psychological Works, vol. 21. London, Hogarth Press, 1958
70. Freud S: Group psychology and the analysis of the ego (1921), in Strachey J (ed): Complete Psychological Works, vol. 18. London, Hogarth Press, 1955, pp 67–143
71. Kanzer M: Object relations theory: An introduction. J Am Psychoanal Assoc. 27:313–325, 1979
72. Freud S: Instincts and their vicissitudes (1915), in Strachey J (ed): Complete Psychological Works, vol. 14. London, Hogarth Press, 1957, pp 117–170.
73. Freud S: On narcissism. An introduction. Part III. Ego-ideal, inheritor of narcissism (1914), in Strachey J (ed): Complete Psychological Works, vol. 14. London, Hogarth Press, 1957, pp 92–104
74. Freud S: The ego and the id. Part III: The ego and the superego (ego ideal) (1923), in Strachey J (ed): Complete Psychological Works, vol. 19. London, Hogarth Press, 1961, pp 28–39
75. Freud S: Beyond the pleasure principle (1920), in Strachey J (ed): Complete Psychological Works, vol. 18. London, Hogarth Press, 1955, pp 3–64
76. Freud S: Why war? (1933), in Strachey J (ed): Complete Psychological Works, vol. 22. London, Hogarth Press, 1964, pp 197–215
77. Freud S: Inhibitions, symptoms, and anxiety (1926), in Strachey J (ed): Complete Psychological Works, vol. 20. London, Hogarth Press, 1926, pp 77–174
78. Freud S: The future of an illusion. Civilization and its discontents (1927), in Strachey J (ed): Complete Psychological Works, vol. 21. London, Hogarth Press, 1958
79. Freud S: Moses and monotheism (1937), in Strachey J (ed): Complete Psychological Works, vol. 23. London, Hogarth Press, pp 3–140
80. Freud S: An outline of psychoanalysis (1939), in Strachey J (ed): Complete Psychological Works, vol. 23. London, Hogarth Press, pp 197–215
81. Jacobson E: The Self and the Object World. New York, International Universities Press, 1964.
82. Balint M: Primary narcissism and primary love. Psychoanal Q 29:6–45, 1960.
83. Balint M: Identification. Int J Psychoanal 24:97–107, 1943
84. Bowlby J. Separation anxiety: A critical review of the literature. J Child Psychol Psychiatry 1:251–169, 1962
85. Winnicott OW: Transitional objects and transitional phenomena. Int J Psychoanal 34:89–97, 1953
86. Fairbairn WRO: Synopis of an object relation theory of the personality. Int J Psychoanalysis 44:224, 1963
87. Fairbairn WRO: Psychoanalytic Studies of the Personality. London, Tavistock, 1952
88. Bion WR: Group dynamics: a review. Int J Psychoanalysis 33:235–247, 1951
89. Bion WR: Group dynamics—a review, in Klien M (ed): New Directions in Psychoanalysis. New York, Basic Books, 1955
90. Bion WR: Experiences in Groups. New York, Basic Books, 1961
91. Klein M: Contributions to Psychoanalysis 1921—1945. London, Hogarth Press, 1948
92. Klein M: Notes on some schizoid mechanisms (1946), in Riviere J (ed): Developments in Psychoanalysis. London, Hogarth Press, 1955, pp 292–320
93. Klein M: The importance of symbol formation in the development of the ego, in Klein M (ed): Contributions to Psychoanalysis 1921–1945. London, Hogarth Press, 1948

94. Rice AK: The Enterprise and Its Environment. London, Tavistock, 1963
95. Rice AK: Productivity and Social Organization. London, Tavistock, 1958
96. Rice AK: Learning for Leadership. London, Tavistock, 1965
97. Rice AK: Individual, group, and intergroup process. Hum Rel 22:565, 1969
98. Trist EL, et al: Organizational Choice. London, Tavistock, 1963
99. Sofer C: The Organization from Within. London, Tavistock, 1961
100. Trist EL, Sofer C: Exploration in Group Relations. Leicester, Leicester University Press, 1959
101. Jacques E: Work, Creativity and Social Justice. New York, International Universities Press, 1970 pp 113–129
102. Menzies IEP: A case study on the functioning of social systems as a defense against anxiety: A report on the study of the nursing service of a general hospital. Hum Rel 15:95–121, 1960
103. Jacques E: The Changing Culture of a Factory. London, Tavistock, 1951
104. Rice AK: The Modern University. London, Tavistock, 1970
105. Rioch MS: The work of Wilfred Bion on groups. Psychiatry 33:56–66, 1970
106. Rioch MJ: Group relations: rationale and technique, Internat. J Group Psychother 10:340–355, 1970
107. Spiro HR: The "old:new land" of group psychotherapy, in Masserman J (ed): Science and Psychoanalysis, vol. 18. New York, Grune & Statton, 1971
108. Spiro HR: Prevention in psychiatry, in Kaplan HI, Saddock BJ, Freedman AM (eds): Comprehensive Textbook of Psychiatry—III. Baltimore, Williams & Wilkins, 1981
109. Spiro HR: The psychiatric hospital. Asylum or snakepit? in Hall RCW (ed): Crisis in American Psychiatry. New York, Plenum, 1982
110. Spiro HR: The future of the state hospital. Hosp Community Psychiatry (in press)
111. Spiro HR: The nature of charismatic and task leadership in groups. Proceedings of the American Group Psychotherapy Association, February 1978. Int J Group Psychother (in press)
112. Volkan V: Narcissistic personality organization and "reparative" leadership. Int J Group Psychother 30:131–153, 1980
113. Hartman H: Psychoanalysis and developmental psychology, in Hartman H (ed): Essays on Ego Psychology. New York, International Universities Press, 1964
114. Schafer R: Regression in the service of the ego, in Lindzey G (ed): Assessment of Human Nature. New York, Reinhart, 1958, pp 119–148
115. Erikson EH: Childhood and Society (ed 2) New York, Norton, 1963
116. Erikson EH: Identity and the Life Cycle. New York, International Universities Press, 1959
117. Erikson EH: Ghandi's Truth or the Origins of Militant Nonviolence. New York, Norton, 1969
118. Erikson EH: Young Martin Luther: A Study in Psychoanalysis and History. New York, Norton, 1958
119. Sandler J, Sandler AM: On the development of object relationship and affects. Int J Psychoanal 59:285–296, 1978
120. Kohut H: Analysis of the Self. New York, International Universities Press, 1971
121. Kobut H: The Restoration of the Self. New York, International Universities Press, 1977
122. Kohut H: Creativeness, charisma, and group psychology. Psychol Issues 9:379–425, 1976
123. Stone WN, Whitman RM: Contributions to the psychology of the self by group process and group therapy. Int J Group Psychother 27:343—359, 1977
124. Pollock GH: The mourning process and the creative organizational change. J Am Psychoanal Assoc 25:3–34, 1977
125. Kernberg O: Structural derivatives of object relationships. Int J Psychoanalysis 47:236–253, 1966
126. Kernberg O: Object Relations Theory and Clinical Psychoanalysis. New York, Jason Aronson, 1976
127. Kernberg O: Borderline personality organization. J Am Psychoanal Assoc 15:641–685, 1967
128. Kernberg O: Factors in the psychoanalytic treatment of narcissistic personalities. J Am Psychoanal Assoc 18:51–85, 1970
129. Kernberg O: Further contributions to the treatment of narcissistic personalities. Int J Psychoanal 55:215–240, 1974
130. Kernberg O: Borderline Conditions and Pathologic Narcissism. New York, Jacob Aronson, 1975
131. Kernberg O: Leadership and organizational functioning: organizational regression. Int J Group Psychother 28:3–25, 1978
132. Kernberg O: Regression in organizational leadership. Psychiatry 42:24–39, 1979

133. Lewin K: Field Theory in Social Science. New York, Harper & Row, 1951
134. Lewin K, Lippitt, R: An experimental approach to the study of autocracy and democracy: a preliminary note. Sociometry 1:292–300, 1938
135. Lewin K, Lippitt R, White RK: Patterns of aggressive behavior in experimentally created social "climates." J Soc Psychol 10:271, 1939
136. Heider F: The Psychology of Interpersonal Relations. New York, Wiley, 1958
137. Heider F: Attitudes and cognitive organization. J Psychol 21:107–112, 1946
138. Bennis WG, Benne KD, Chin R (ed): The Planning of Change. New York, Holt, Rinehart, and Winston, 1969
139. Argyris C: Personality and Organization. New York, Harper & Row, 1957
140. Argyris C: Integrating the Individual and the Organization. New York, Wiley, 1964
141. Argyris C: Intervention Theory and Method: A Behavioral Science View. Reading, Mass, Addison Wesley, 1970
143. Bennis WG: Organizational Development: Its Nature, Origens and Prospects. Reading, Mass, Addison Wesley, 1969
144. Bennis WG, Shephard HA: A theory of group development. Hum Rel 9:415–457, 1956
145. Bennis WG, Slater, PE: The Temporary Society. New York, Harper & Row, 1968
146. Blake RP, Mouton, JS: Building a Dynamic Corporation through Grid Organization Development. Reading, Mass, Addison Wesley, 1969
147. Lawrence PR, Lorch, JW: Developing Organizations: Prognosis and Action. Reading, Mass, Addison Wesley, 1969
148. Likert R: New Patterns of Management. New York, McGraw-Hill, 1961
149. Lippitt GL: Implications of the Behavioral Sciences for Management. Washington, DC, Society for Personnel Adminstration, 1966
150. Shephard HA, Bennis WG: A theory of training by group methods. Hum Rel 9:403–414, 1956
151. Walton CC: Ethos and the Executive. Values in Managerial Decision Making. Englewood Cliffs, NJ, Prentice-Hall, 1969
152. Eddy WP, Burke WW, Dupre VA, et al (eds): Behavioral Science and the Manger's Role. Washington, DC, National Institute for Applied Behavioral Science, 1969
153. Gelfand AE, Walker C: A system theoretic approach to the management of complex organizations: Management by consensus level and its interaction with other management strategies. Behavioral Science 25:250–260, 1980
154. Bales RF: Interaction Process Analysis: A Method for the Study of Small Groups. Reading, Mass, Addison Wesley, 1950
155. Mills T: The Sociology of Small Groups. New York, Prentice-Hall, 1957
156. Cartwright D, Zander A: Group Dynamics. New York, Harper & Row, 1960.
157. Etzioni A: Complex Organizations: A Sociological Reader. New York, Holt, Rinehart, and Winston, 1961
158. Breed W: The Self Guiding Society. New York, Free Press, 1971
159. Deutsch KW: The Nerves of Government. Glencoe, Ill, Free Press, 1963.
160. Parsons T: The Social System. Glencoe, Ill, Free Press, 1951
161. Parsons T: Suggestions for a sociological approach to the theory of organizations. I and II. Adm Sci Q 1:63–85; 2:225–239, 1976
162. Merton RS: Bureaucratic structure and organization, in Merton RK, Grey AP, Hockey B, et al (eds): Reader in Bureaucracy. Glencoe, Ill, Free Press, 1952
163. Merton RK: Social Theory and Social Structure. New York, Free Press, 1968
164. Thibaut JW, Kelley HH: the Social Psychology of Groups. New York, Wiley, 1959
165. Ruesch J: Therapeutic Communication. New York, Norton, 1961
166. Ruesch J, Bateson O: Communication. The Social Matrix of Psychiatry. New York, Norton, 1951
167. Watzlawick P, Beavin JH, Hackson DP: Pragmatics of Human Communication. New York, Norton, 1967
168. Whyte FW: Human Relations in the Restaurant Industry. New York, McGraw-Hill, 1948
169. Read WH: Upward communication in industrial hierarchies. Hum Rel 15:3–15, 1962
170. Morrison EE: A case study of innovation, Bennis WG, Benne KD, Chin R (eds): The Planning of Change. New York, Holt, 1961, pp 592–605
171. Breed W: Social control in the newsroom: A functional analysis. Social Forces 33: 1955

Seymour R. Kaplan, M.D.

12

Phases of Development in Psychiatric Organizations

A hypothetical model of phases of development in psychiatric organizations will be presented in this chapter. The purpose of the model is to provide a basis for comparison of the similarities and differences in structures and interactions that occur over time in different psychiatric settings. The formulations that will be presented are extrapolations from theoretical constructs about characteristic small group processes and from practical experiences with a variety of psychiatric programs.

The author's interest in group processes stems from observations made during the late 1950s of the characteristic responses of therapy groups to the introduction of new members. The opportunity to make these observations came from the author's responsibility for the supervision of psychiatric residents at the Albert Einstein College of Medicine who were conducting a number of treatment groups. It was at that time also that the publications of Bion[1] and Foulkes[2] appeared in which they described their observations of characteristic group processes. Although neither delineated group developmental phases per se, Bion in particular based his construct of "basic assumption" group mentality on group events in which the members manifested phase-specific fantasies, attitudes, and behaviors.

The construct of phases of group development, in which sequences of phases are postulated, has since been used by a number of investigators. Apart from its inherent use, the author has found the construct to have heuristic value as a means of organizing material about the structure, processes, and interactions that he has observed in a variety of groups. These groups, composed of patients, staff, or students, numbered about 8–10 members in the instance of therapy groups; 12–15 members in the human relations or "T" groups; 30–50 members in therapeutic community meetings on a psychiatric ward or in a day hospital; and a similar number in staff development meetings. The groups varied in duration from 10–15 weekly sessions to monthly meetings convened over a period of years. There are a number of publications based on the observations of these group experiences.[3–13]

During the 1960s, the author participated in the development of the affiliated psychiatric programs of the Department of Psychiatry of the Albert Einstein

College of Medicine. The scope and diversity of these psychiatric programs were described in Chapter 4. Some of these programs, particularly the two community mental health centers (CMHCs) underwent the rapid expansion that was characteristic of federally supported services during that era. The changes in the structures and processes of these and other organizations described in the literature appeared to have similarities to that which I had observed in small groups. In the following section, a hypothetical model of the sequence of organizational changes, using the construct of developmental phases, will be presented. The first part of the discussion includes a description of the phases of the hypothetical organization and is followed by constructs of the symbolic role of the leader during each developmental phase. Publications describing aspects of the Einstein programs on which the following section is based are cited in references 14–23.

DESCRIPTION OF PHASES OF DEVELOPMENT

Phase I: the Beginning

At the beginning of phase I, when the organizational goals and purposes exist only on paper as general ideas and concepts, the professional membership will be identified by their prior career experiences. The task at hand is the initiation of the programmatic objectives so that hard work, commitment, and optimism are personality attributes valued by all the members. The sanction and assistance of the sponsoring institution will be necessary in the early stages of recruitment of staff and the arrangements for facilities.

In phase I, therefore, there will not be any complex intraorganizational issues with which to contend until such time as the characteristics unique to its structure and membership have emerged. This is not to say that there will not be any interpersonal difficulties among the members or any organizational problems, but these will reflect the relationship of the sponsoring institutions or the idiosyncratic nature of individual members.

Phase II: Accelerated Expansion

It is characteristic of a successful organization, after its initial recruitment and arrangements, to undergo an accelerated growth and expansion. Figure 12-1 illustrates the hypothetical growth and develpment of a psychiatric organization.

One of the most important issues with which the organization is faced in this phase is the competence of the staff and the availability of resources to provide the services and programs to which the organization has made commitments. The successful organization will be making adjustments and corrections of its original goals and plans and, as needed, will innovate concepts and obtain the necessary resources to provide for these innovations.

The increasing complexity of the organization and its accelerated growth during phase II requires a flexible organizational structure. A staff characterized by the quality of its enthusiasm and commitment may be more adaptive during this accelerated growth phase than a staff characterized for its attention to detail or its "productivity."

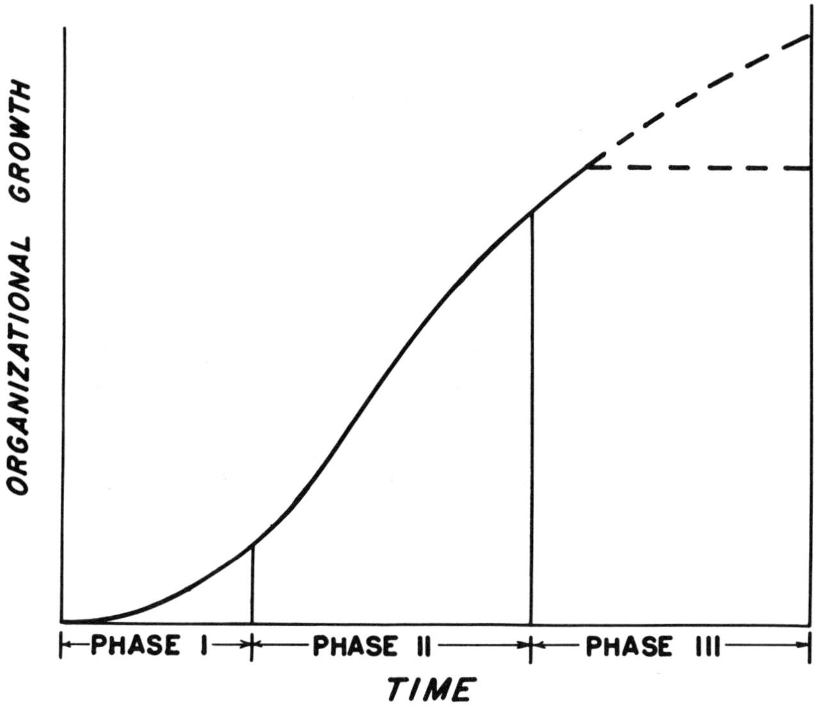

Figure 12-1. A Hypothetical model of phases of organizational growth and development.

The organization during phase II also must compete for scarce resources with other similar organizations to demonstrate that it can achieve the goals and purposes better and more effectively. To a greater or lesser extent, the competition will entail political considerations. The organization must therefore occupy itself with rapidly changing developments within it, concomitantly with developments in its environment, e.g., with economic and political forces.

Phase III: Consolidation and Efficiency

The bifurcation of the growth curve in phase III, shown in Figure 12-1, is meant to illustrate two characteristics of this phase that tend to conflict with one another. These refer to the simultaneous need to consolidate the developments of the organization in order to improve efficiency, shore up the quality of the work, and maintain a continued capacity for growth and change, although at a less accelerated pace. This is one of the critical transition points in the organization's growth and development, on which its continued success depends.

The need for consolidation at this point is due to increased costs as the result of a variety of organizational developments. If one views the time dimension of phase II over a number of years, in the latter part of the phase, the organization would include among its members a higher percentage of senior staff than at the beginning, including many on pensions or who have available other financial privileges that accrue with seniority. In addition, with the development of more consolidated administrative structures, the qualities of enthusiasm and flexibility among the staff that were assets during the accelerated growth of phase II become translated into fiscal liabilities. The staff members who functioned best during the transitional phases of program development and innovation tend to be less productive and efficient when program consolidation is accomplished.

During phase III, the role of middle management becomes crucial if there is to be an improvement in competence and maintenance of quality. This changing role entails a significant recasting of the organizational structures and operations. The delegation of increased decision-making authority to middle-level staff and the development of improved methods for program feedback at all levels, while always important, are critical at this point. The personality characteristics that were effective in the formative phases will be most sorely tested around issues of authority and power. The need for individual changes coupled with the need for organizational changes at this phase contribute to the critical role of middle management in the development and growth of the organization.

Table 12-1 provides a summary overview of the hypothetical phases of organizational growth and development.

THE SYMBOLIC ROLE OF THE LEADER

The formulations to be presented about the members' perception of the symbolic role of the leader during phases of organizational development are extrapolated from the author's work with small groups and from constructs of social scientists, notably Weber,[24] Lewin,[25] and Parsons.[26] The following comments by Myeroff and Larson[27] about Weber's constructs of the role of the charismatic leader at times of social change are relevant.

> The charismatic hero arises during social crises when consensus has broken down and dissent prevails. . . . The vaunted status of the charismatic hero is short lived, however, for pure charisma exists only in the process of originating. . . . In coping with practical problems of administration, his charisma becomes routinized—transferred from his person to his position. When charisma becomes a transferable, objective entity which accrues to a position rather than an individual, Weber designates it as the charisma of office.*

The importance of the role of symbolism during times of change has been noted by Parsons as cited by Edelson:[28]

> Parsons has emphasized that men respond not to things as they are but to the (symbolic) meanings things have for them. . . . The emergent property of a social system is the existence of a common, more or less integrated, system of symbolized meanings shared by its members. Such symbolized meanings include values and the integrative standards or norms, sought ends, and relevant representation of the object-situations derived from values.**

---

*From Meyerhoff BG, Larson WR: The doctor as culture hero: the routinization of charisma. Hum Organization 25:188–191, 1965. With permission.

**From Edelson M: The integration of the behavioral and clinical experience in teaching medical students, in Lidz T, Edelson M (eds): Training Tomorrow's Psychiatrists. New Haven, Yale University Press, 1970 p 17–44. With permission.

Table 12-1

Hypothetical Phases of Organization Growth and Development—Interorganizational and Intraorganizational Characteristics

	Organizational Structure	Organizational Relationship to Supraordinate Bodies	Membership Relationship to the Organization	Interorganizational Conflicts Over Power	Intraorganizational Conflicts Over Power
PHASE I The Beginning	The organization is loosely structured. The members identify with the organization as a whole on the bases of a shared mythology about its goals and purposes.	Official sanction of the sponsoring bodies.	Commitment of the membership to organizational goals and enthusiastic belief in its success. — *Hope* —	The power of the mandating authorities vs. the autonomy of the organization.	Prestige of membership based upon extraorganizational status vs. emergent status in the organization.
PHASE II Accelerated Expansion	The subdivisions are more or les well structured but loosely integrated. The member identifies with his subdivision on the basis of pride in its perceived superiority over the other subdivisions.	Competition with other organizations for recognition of its superiority by the supraordinate bodies, including support by "the body politic."	Conviction of members of a subdivision in its superior achievements and its preeminent contribution to the success of the organization. — *Pride* —	The power of the organization to obtain scarce resources in competition with similar organizations vs. the need for interorganizational collaboration.	Competition among subdivisions vs. the intraorganizational need for cooperation.
PHASE III Consolidation and Efficiency	The organization is integrated through a balance between centralized administrative and decentralized operational functions. The members identify with one another on the basis of pride in their collective, realistic achievements.	The organization becomes established on the basis of the use of its services by consumers and/or effective accountability to supraordinate bodies.	Confidence of a member in his competence and his value to the overall organizational goals and services. — *Respect* —	— — — *Organizational needs and goals versus* — *societal needs and goals*	

Phase I: The Mystique of the Omnipotent Leader

Weber considered the charismatic leader to possess "the gift of grace, vouchsafed by God to an extraordinary individual," a reflection of the Great Man theory of social change that prevailed during Weber's time. Boring[29] contrasts the Great Man theory of history with the deterministic view:

> Great Men are agents of the forces of history that act upon them, that their decisions and the choices of lesser men are determined in part by personal idiosyncrasy, in part by chance, but enough by the cultural stream of opinion and belief for the great trends of history to be distinguishable.*

In a similar vein, I would hold that the charismatic leader, in most instances, primarily is a group-evolved symbolic phenomena characteristic of the early phases of organizational development.

This is not to deny that certain individual characteristics seem to be required of a leader in order to fulfill the group-allocated charismatic role. Considering, however, the extraordinary diversity of individuals who have come to be seen in this light by their organizational membership, to which one can bear witness by a random review of a variety of different organizations, the nature of the predisposing individual characteristics is difficult to identity.

What appears to me to be much more significant than the individual differences among leaders is the differences among organizations for the need of a leadership mystique. The extent of the need and the duration of time that the members of organizations are involved in maintaining the mystique appear to be the result of many intra- and extraorganizational factors. For one thing, the need for the mystique would appear to be proportionate to the lack of definition of the organizational goals and the lack of clarity about the competence of the members or the availability of resources to achieve realistically those goals that are defined or are capable of definition. Any new program that has innovative objectives, which by intent are not readily definable, or any established program undergoing a major change in personnel or goals can be expected to manifest among its members the emotional characteristics of individuals being led by a leader to whom unusual and larger-than-life qualities are ascribed.

The ubiquitous development in early phases of groups, regardless of their size and goals, of a symbolic construct ascribing mythological or idealized qualities to a leader attests to the importance of the emotional relationships between the members of an organization. In an earlier publication, the author commented:

> the members' emotional contributions to the shared group mythology and the related ritualistic behavior appear to serve the common task of the group both in the evolving of a social structure and in providing the data from which the members may achieve their work goal. These goals or task-oriented identifications are of a "functional" nature as the result of the interdependency of group members upon one another, and they refer to mechanisms within the ego that have not been extensively considered in this context in analytic theory.**

*From Boring EG: History, Psychology and Science. New York, Wiley, 1963 p 20. With permission.

**From Kaplan SR: Therapy groups and training groups: similarities and differences. Int J Group Psychother 17:4, 1967, p 473–504. With permission.

Table 12-2 summarizes the hypothetical symbolic constructs of the role of the leader and the members' expressive/instrumental roles and conflicts during phases of organizational development.

Phase II: The Mystique of the Plenipotentiary Administrator

The change of the symbolic role in phase II from "omnipotent leader" to "plenipotentiary administrator" corresponds to Weber's construct of the change from "charisma of person" to "charisma of office." The leadership role of the organization is still perceived as having a larger-than-life quality, but it is focused on an exaggerated perception of the authority of the leadership position. The term *administrator* is used both to indicate the traditional *bete noire* of the professional and to capture the exaggerated plenipotentiary power ascribed to the office of the executive administrator during this phase.

There is a symbolic "progression" in the change from the charisma of person to the charisma of office. As suggested in Table 12-2, this progression is associated in successful organizations with improved clarity of structure and differentiation of functions and more effective competition with other organizations for scarce resources.

The differentiation of functions and role specificity require the formation of subdivisions, which develop unequally. This unequal development of subdivisions results in differences in rewards and frequently an emergence of rivalries within the organization. It is during the accelerated expansion of phase II that the organization is most vulnerable to the disruptive effect of internal rivalries. At this point, it is without the cohesiveness that the charismatic leader provided during phase I, and it has yet to consolidate and balance the integration and differentiation of functions. The vulnerability of the organization will be magnified if there is a simultaneous convergence of external bureaucractic or political conflicts.

Phase III: The Illusion of the Selfless Healer

The use of the symbolic construct of the "selfless healer" as the conjoint model for the roles of the leader *and* membership is to suggest that there are unattainable values that continue in human organizations no matter how invested in their task and how efficient and "productive" the organizational membership. The selfless healer as a role model is meant as a specific reference for the membership of health or mental health care organziations. It is used as an overdetermined symbolic construct that simultaneously represents the realistic pride of the membership in their individual contributions to the work of the organization, the ideology of the organization toward which it must continuously strive in an ever-changing environment as well as the achievement of realistic goals based on the competence of the membership and the soundness of the organizational structure, which the members have evolved through a difficult process over time.

Table 12-2
Hypothetical Phases of Organization Growth and Development—Interorganizational and Intraorganizational Characteristics

	Expressive (Emotional) Roles of Organizational Members	Instrumental (Task) Roles of Organizational Members	Symbolic Role of Formal (or Informal) Organizational Leader(s)	Individual Expression of Organizational Conflict	
				Interpersonal	Role Identity/ Diffusion
PHASE I The Beginning	Dedication to the organization goals *— Faith —*	Initiation of programs and hard work *— Imagination —*	Omnipotent leader *— Mythological —*	Loyalty to profession vs. loyalty to organization *— Dependence —*	Preorganizational role vs. emergent organization role
PHASE II Accelerated Expansion	Dedication to the subdivisions and to the collective goals of the organization as a whole *— Idealism —*	Expansion of programs and extraorganizational promotion of the organization *— Industry —*	Plenipotentiary leaders *— Heroic —*	Personal gain vs. shared achievements *— Power —*	Specialized role vs. "team" role
PHASE III Consolidation and Efficiency	*— Intraorganizational and interorganizational — cooperation and collaboration*		Selfless healers *— Ideological —*	Career ambition vs. organizational growth *— Autonomy —*	Established organizational role vs. reorganizational role

REFERENCES

1. Bion WR: Experiences in Groups. New York, Basic Books, 1961
2. Foulkes SH, Anthony EJ: Group Psychotherapy. London: Penguin Books, 1957
3. Kaplan SR: Therapy groups and training groups: similarities and differences. Int J Group Psychother 17:4,1967, p 473–504
4. Kaplan SR: Psychotherapeutic approaches in working with the disadvantaged, in Goldman G, Millman, D. (eds): Innovations in Psychotherapy. Springfield, Ill, Thomas, 1972
5. Kaplan SR: Dreams and the group setting. Int J Group Psychother 23:188–195, 1973a
6. Kaplan SR: The group dream. Int J Group Psychother 23:4, 1973b, p 421–431
7. Kaplan SR, Roman M: Characteristic responses of therapy groups to the introduction of new members. Int J Group Psychother 11:4, 1961, p 372–381
8. Kaplan SR, Roman M: Phases of development in an adult therapy group. Int J Group Psychother 13: 1, 1963, p 10–26
9. Kaplan SR, Ahmed B: Group strategies with disadvantaged populations: the public mental health setting, In Seligman, M (ed): Group Strategies with Different Populations. Springfield Ill, Thomas, 1977
10. Kaplan SR, Razin A: The psychological substrate of self-help groups. J Operational Psychiatry 9: 2, 1978, p 57–65
11. Kaplan SR, Razin A: The dynamics of group cohesion, in Kellerman H (ed): Group Cohesion: Biological, Psychological and Sociological Perspectives. New York, Grune & Stratton, 1981
12. Kornblith AB, Kaplan SR: Group approaches in drug treatment programs in Lowinson J, Ruiz P (eds): Substance Abuse in the United States: Problems and Prospectives. Baltimore, Williams and Wilkins, 1981
13. Steiner J, Kaplan SR: Out-patient group work-for-pay activity for chronic schizophrenia patients. Am J Psychother 13:3, 1969, p 452–462
14. Peck HB, Kaplan SR, Roman M: Prevention, treatment and social action: a strategy of intervention in a disadvantaged urban area. Am J Orthopsychiatry 36:1, 1966, p 57–69
15. Peck HB, Kaplan SR, and Roman M: Community action programs and the comprehensive mental health center, in Greenblatt M, Emery PE and Glueck BC Jr (eds): Poverty and Mental Health. Psychiatric Research Report, 21 American Psychiatric Association, April, 1967
16. Peck HB, Kaplan SR: Mental health programs for the urban multi-service center, in Shore MF, Mannino FV (eds): Mental Health and the Community: Problems, Programs, and Strategies. New York, Behavioral Publications, 1969
17. Kaplan SR, Boyajian L, Meltzer B: The role of the non-professional worker in disadvantaged areas, in Gruenbaum H (ed): Community Mental Health Practice. Boston, Little, Brown, 1970
18. Kaplan SR, Roman M: The Organization and Delivery of Mental Health Services in the Ghetto: The Lincoln Hospital Experience. New York, Praeger 1973
19. Kaplan SR: The reciprocal roles of the university and the community in the development of community mental health centers, in Atkins RW (ed): How the University Can Aid Community Mental Health. Proceedings of the Scientific Conferences, Department of Psychiatry, School of Medicine and Dentistry, University of Rochester, 1969
20. Kaplan SR: Teaching of community psychiatry in psychiatric residency training programs, in Lidz T, Edelson M (eds): Training Tomorrow's Psychiatrists. New Haven, Yale University Press, 1970
21. Kaplan SR: Characteristic phases of development in organizations, in Millman D, Goldman G (eds): Group Process Today: Evaluation and Perspective. Springfield, Ill, Thomas, 1974
22. Kaplan SR: Psychiatric rehabilitation in the ghetto. Soc Sci Med 10, 1976, p 203–204
23. Kaplan SR: Community participation, in Feldman S (ed): The Administration of Mental Health Services (rev 2nd printing). Springfield, Ill, Thomas 1980
24. Weber M: The Theory of Social and Economic Organizations, trans Henderson LJ and Parsons T, Glencoe, Free Press, 1947
25. Lewin K: Field Theory in Social Science. New York, Harper & Row, 1951
26. Parsons T: The Social System. Glencoe: Free Press, 1951
27. Myerhoff BG, Larson WR: The doctor as culture hero: the routinization of charisma. Hum Organization 25:188–191, 1965
28. Edelson M: The integration of the behavioral and clinical experience in teaching medical students, in Lidz T, Edelson M (eds): Training Tomorrow's Psychiatrists. New Haven, Yale University Press, 1970
29. Boring EG: History, Psychology and Science. New York, Wiley, 1963

PART IV

Leadership and Training

Walter E. Barton, M.D.
Gail M. Barton, M.D., M.P.H.

13

The Psychiatrist–Administrator

Case Problem

M.R., age 28, had been a resident of a state school for the mentally retarded for 8 years. He was profoundly retarded (IQ 20) due to post measles encephalitis. He also had periodic episodes of excitement, diagnosed as Bipolar Disorder, Manic Episode, controlled by lithium carbonate 600 mg tid (blood level 0.5–0.8). M.R.s medication was stopped in order to institute behavior therapy. There was no physician involved in this order to stop the medication. A month later, M.R. became very excited and violent. After injuring four residents and six staff members, he was sent on an emergency order to the state mental hospital. On admission, the lithium was started again, and Haldol® 40 mg/day was given for 4 days, reduced to 30 mg on the fifth day and 10 mg on the sixth. The patient at that time was somnolent and unresponsive on the ward and had not been assaultive during his stay. The court refused to commit the patient for a longer period on a technicality—the court was told that the physician who signed the commitment application had never seen the patient. As a consequence, the patient was returned to the state school for the mentally retarded, where he was somnolent and unresponsive. The staff members at the school were outraged at the "overmedication" and filed a written complaint with the commissioner of mental health.

You have been asked to investigate the incident and to make recommendations to prevent recurrences.

The case problem cited above reports an incident that actually occurred in a state school run by a lay administrator who was well trained in administration in general. Even so, he was unaware of the consequence of stopping lithium, of the need to consult a physician, of requiring examination by a physician to commit, or of the time span necessary to stabilize the dosage of Haldol®. Nor had he perceived the necessity of establishing procedures to control violence in the institution.

There are those who believe that the reasons for insisting that the administrator of a mental health facility to be a clinician are no longer valid. This case would provide a cogent argument to the contrary. It is true that efficient management of an organization today is so complex that formal training in administrative knowledge and skills is essential. We believe, however, that only generic training in administration or health administration is inadequate to handle the unique and complex situations that arise in a mental health facility. We favor the clinician–

executive, one with clinical competence, and we also favor one who has had *formal* training in administration. (See Chapter 14.) Learning administration by one's mistakes or by watching others' mistakes is inefficient, to say the least. There is a discrete body of knowledge that the clinician can garner by taking the time and energy to get it.

WHAT DOES AN ADMINISTRATOR NEED TO KNOW HOW TO DO?

Since the administrator is a leader who is responsible for management functions, the administrator must be able to do the following:

1. Planning: identification of service needs and ways to meet them
2. Organizing: structuring tasks to be done and allocating resources
3. Staffing: determining who will do what in the organization
4. Directing: guiding toward objectives and facilitating performance
5. Controlling: ensuring quality performance and accountability
6. Communicating: sharing experience, receiving, utilizing, and returning information
7. Innovating: taking risks to solve problems in new ways as an agent of change preparing for the future
8. Representing: relating to constituencies essential to the attainment of objectives.[1]

The administrator must also possess the capacity for leadership. Leadership is defined as the development of task orientation to the workers and the capacity to assign roles essential to the total group's performance toward an agreed upon objective.[1] Administrators are expected to make decisions, set priorities, resolve conflicts, coordinate the work of others, expedite task completion, motivate staff to achieve their potential, use power wisely, and delegate authority and responsibility to qualified others.

Suppose you have been assigned the task of developing a program for patients over 65 for the mental health center in which you are the staff psychiatrist. The knowledge you will need is both clinical and administrative. You would need to review clinical data on the problems and issues of aging, the types of mental disorders to be expected in that age group and the therapies generally utilized, and the models of delivering services in the home, clinic, and residential centers.[2–5] The administrative information needed in this case might well be beyond the scope of the clinician's usual reading.[6,7] The planning that would need to be done would require administrative knowledge on how to identify the problems that will be encountered rather than simply imitate "a program" for the elderly. What specifically would one be seeing? Depression, physical incapacity, alcoholism, or poor nutrition? Then one must analyze what solutions would be utilized. In making a needs assessment, one answers such questions as Why is it important?[1] With what frequency does the problem occur in the local area? Are there unrecognized and unmet needs? Do they interfere with function? What resources are available? Which are lacking? How would you remedy deficiencies? Are space and equipment available to house the new program? How is the program to be financed? Is it feasible to proceed at the determined cost?

There are many skills required by an administrator beyond those of planning. One is time management. Nothing is more important for the busy administrator than the skillful use of the scarce commodity—time. It is consumed in putting out the fires of crises. It is wasted in meetings or in reading piles of mail. One must learn to focus on what is most appropriate and give priority to the projects that will attain the most valued objectives. Other projects await their turn. There is an old saying "If you want something done, ask a busy person to do it." It affirms the administrative skill of using time wisely. Some things need doing at once; once done, they are out of the way. Others are delayed to a more appropriate time, and a few are indefinitely postponed.

Timing in a group is also a special skill and is essential in "processing" a group problem. Because groups are often assigned tasks, the leader of the group must be alert to the group process as problems are debated. A solution offered too early is ignored; if offered too late, it is tabled. At the right time, a proposal, including a summarizing statement and recommendations, is well received. Leadership may involve guiding the group toward the proposal or actually proposing it oneself. Conizance of values and time management also influence the administrator's actions. Appreciation of values and their importance is seldom taught. For example, if you believe that the way to motivate workers is to use a carrot and a stick, you may choose a bait that will gain cooperation and punish those who do not or will not try. An alternate approach is to assume workers *wish* to achieve and do their very best and have pride in a favorable outcome. The clinician–administrator will most often find that professional mental health workers usually meet expectations.[8] Therefore, clarity of expectations and a spirit of optimism can go farther than muddled fatalism.

One way to clarify expectations is with a job description. The job description of the administrator should detail the minimal acceptable requirements in education, experience, or in technical skills. It should outline the functions to be performed and the responsibilities and relationships to any superior authority.[9] For example, the chairperson of a department of psychiatry in a university-medical school works under a dean, who in turn relates to the faculty, the president, and the board of trustees. The executive director of a mental health center may be the employee of a citizen governing board. A state mental hospital superintendent, meanwhile, may be under the commissioner of mental health, who in turn is under the secretary of human services, who works under the governor. (See Chapters 4 and 15.)

An understanding and conception of organizational structure is another important element of which the clinician–administrator should be aware. The organizational structure may be a simple operation: a support model or a more complex quintet model with five major subdivisions. In the former, the chief executive has but two major subdivisions that incorporate all organizational activities: clinical service under a psychiatrist and business administration, which includes administrative specialists in personnel, finance, and all other activities that are not defined as "clinical" services. In the quintet model, the five major divisions generally are medical, professional services (laboratory, x-ray, pharmacy, etc.) nursing, business administration, and personnel administration. Of course, there are many variants of these organizational structures.[1]

WHY DO PSYCHIATRISTS AVOID ADMINISTRATIVE POSTS?

Let us now explore why psychiatrists generally avoid administrative posts. Psychiatrists are trained to evaluate, diagnose, and treat the individual patient. They may also work intensively with small groups of patients and be attuned to the process within their unit. They seldom are concerned with the ward as a system with input from the outside or its output into other care systems after the patients leave or with the support systems that allow the ward to function. Funding mechanisms are of concern to them only when the therapists do not get paid for services rendered. The may have little concern for the costs of the service even though the public puts a high priority on soaring health care costs.

Administrative concerns may be seen as paper shuffling. It is true that regulation, evaluation, and accountability generate an enormous number of reports. Psychiatrists may abhor having their work scrutinized for quality by other than their peers and resent any intrusion into the doctor–patient relationship. Psychiatrists, although experts in human behavior, soon discover there are problems in dealing with personnel, labor unions, citizen boards, human service agencies, and the legislative executive and judicial systems for which they ordinarily lack knowledge and skills. The complexities, uncertainties, and frustrations may be sufficient obstacles to encourage a return to clinical practice, where one can be in control.

The better the clinician, however, the more likely the psychiatrist is to be offered a leadership role in running a ward, a unit, or a division. To fill these posts well, training in administration is helpful.

PREPARING FOR ADMINISTRATIVE POSTS

Top executive posts in the mental health field are open to those without formal training in administration. Even though the American Psychiatric Association has given certificates in administrative psychiatry for 30 years after qualifying examinations, as yet few facilities require any certification relating to administrative expertise. The American College of Mental Health Administration was incorporated in 1979 to extend opportunities for training of clinician–executives and to work toward the requirement in job descriptions of mental health administrators for formal training in administration. While there is little incentive to get training now, we believe it can and should be required in the future. (See Chapter 14.)

Psychiatrists and mental health professionals should have at least one course in administration during their residency or professional training years. This would provide an awareness of the special knowledge and skills essential to become a competent administrator. When such an introductory course is combined with assigned management tasks and supervision in administrative duties, the lessons learned and experienced become good practice. For those who will be challenged to seek executive posts, a full year of training in administration is recommended. We believe the curriculum developed by the Task Force on Mental Health/Mental Retardation of the Associated University Programs in Health Administration (AUPHA) contains the essentials for building competence.[10]

The number of short courses available in administration is increasing. Their principle value is to serve as a stimulus for more intensive study and as a guide to practice. There is little evidence that executive training courses make one a good leader. Nor is there evidence that any particular leadership training method consistently improves organizational performance.[12] Perhaps it is not surprising to discover that measurable changes in leadership behavior fail to be significant following short courses, for leadership development is a long-term endeavor requiring long-term training tied to supervised learning experiences.

We believe that leaders can be taught to think, feel, and act in a more rational way. Self-acceptance, assuming responsibility for failure without blaming others, acknowledging the rigors of reality, and utilizing teaching as an integral part of the job training system will make a difference.[11] Essential skills to be acquired include, but are not limited to, decision making, communication, use of time, conflict resolution, and the management of change. Skills are best learned by demonstration, supervised practice, rewarding correct behaviors with repetition, and discussion of the learned behavior. Measurable changes in administrative behavior will occur with these skillbuilding technques.[13]

The possession of knowledge of administrative theory and practice is also vital for the clinician–administrator to acquire. It will greatly assist in the diagnosis of organizational problems. It will also reduce fear of the unknown and the uncertainty that contributes to the administrator's anxiety about capability. Skill development makes the administrator more competent in problem solving. We do know that most successful organizations have able, well-trained leaders.

BARRIERS TO ACHIEVEMENT

Even with good training there are barriers to achieving success in administration. The principal obstacles to administrative success fall under three categories: personal inadequacy, situational factors, and circumstances arising outside the organizational boundaries that influence performance.

Personal Inadequacy

The character of the individual may be the source of failure, just as the values manifested may affect everyday relationships. Greed, dishonesty, intemperance, and immorality are examples of behaviors that can block success. Physical illness may also so deplete an administrator's energy as to sap the zeal for successful day-to-day problem solving. A serious mental disorder may distort reality, estrange staff members, and require the administrator to have temporary relief from duty for treatment time.

The lack of knowledge about administration can be so evident as to make others unwilling to share in what is seen as an impending disaster. Lack of skill may be manifest in indecisiveness and an inability to come to a decision. Communication skills may be so poor as to arouse intense hostility instead of cooperation and "followership."

Cronyism and favoritism may produce an inner circle in tune with one another's needs for consensual reinforcement but out of touch with the real world of the needs of patients and potential input of the other employees. Inflexible traditionalism is another flaw that may thwart necessary change to keep an organization vital and relevent. Power may be abused, and injustice and unfairness may prevail. Unfortunately, high morale and a wholesome working environment cannot be achieved simply by administrative fiat. Sometimes situational factors spoil success as well.

Situational Factors

Factors within the organization that thwart success are unclear goals (nearly always multiple) and lack of role and task definition. Inadequate resources to carry out the mission such as enough qualified staff, money, space, and equipment can prevent any planner from achieving objectives. Faulty structure of the organization, such as span of control, lack of delegation of authority and responsibility, with undercutting and bypassing of decisions made by assigned leaders can create poor morale. The administrator cannot order staff members to be dedicated to organizational goals or command loyalty; it is earned from within and can only work if situational factors are sufficiently synchronized to allow it. Factors outside the organization can also doom an administrator to failure.

Factors Outside Organizational Boundaries

There may be such a lack of understanding of the organization's mission by the public that they refuse to support it. Frequently, a neighborhood totally rejects the plan of a facility for the mentally ill in their neighborhood. A patient's failure to achieve an expected cure may lead to liability actions. A facility that fails to meet perceived standards of quality may be cause for a class-action suit against the administrator's facility. Judicial rulings or legislation may infringe on the administrator's ability to use the best medical judgment and previously accepted therapies. The executive branch may insist on patronage, with jobs for their friends. (See Chapter 15.) They may issue so many regulations that total compliance would divert most of the administrator's and staff's valuable time away from patient service. Resources may be so severely curtailed that they fail to support the organization's legislated mission. Canceling a residency training program's budget quickly puts the administrator in charge of the training out of a job.

ACCEPTING THE CHALLENGE OF BECOMING AN ADMINISTRATOR

The clinician invited to accept the challenge of an administrative post should assess the organization's mission and objectives, his or her personal qualifications, the situation and environment, the structure of authority, the resources available, and the timing of the invitation. (See also Chapter 15.)

If the purpose and objectives of the organization generate an enthusiasm so compelling that you would gladly give the organization priority over what you are doing now, it is worth looking more closely at the offered post. It should be possible to assess the job requirements, your own capabilities for meeting them, and the potential for personal growth.

First, from a personal standpoint, it is important to evaluate the potential site. Does the environment provide what you desire for yourself and family? Are there comfortable living quarters, good schools, your church, cultural opportunities, recreational facilities, people you could enjoy? Are the rewards offered sufficient to maintain or enhance your standard of living?

Next, one looks at the situation within the organization. Are there sufficient resources, quality staff, enough space and equipment? Is the funding sufficient to make it possible to achieve the assigned mission? If the resources currently available, such as staff, are poor, is it possible to replace them? Is it likely that needed funds can be found for building the program?

Then there is the authority structure. It should be scrutinized to learn how disagreements are resolved to ensure that there is authority sufficient to meet the responsibility. Where are there overlapping roles, functions, authority? What happens when the superior authority does not approve a decision?

Lastly, one asks, Is the timing right? Is the organization ready to act on the changes you would make? What are the reasons the job has defeated several others who have held the post? What changes in the situation are feasible to make success possible?

With the above questions answered affirmatively, that is, the offered post offers an exciting challenge, it has an objective you value, it is in a place in which you would like to raise your family, and the situation seems ready for your leadership, with resources available to make success possible, with people around with whom you could enjoy working, then take it!

REFERENCES

1. Barton WE, Barton GM: Mental Health Administration: Principles and Practice. New York, Human Sciences Press, 1982
2. Butler RN: Why Survive? Being Old in America. New York, Harper & Row, 1975
3. Usdin G, Hofling CJ (eds): Aging: The Process and the People. New York, Brunner/Mazel, 1978
4. Busse EW, Pfeiffer, E (eds): Mental Illness in Later Life. Washington, DC, American Psychiatric Association, 1973
5. Glasscote R. Gudeman JE, Miles D: Creative Mental Health Services for the Elderly. Washington, DC, American Psychiatric Association, 1977
6. Littlestone R: Planning, in Feldman S (ed): The Administration of Mental Health Services (ed 2). Springfield, Ill, Thomas, 1980, pp 3–40
7. Massie JL, Douglas J: Managing a Contemporary Introduction (ed 2). Englewood Cliffs, NJ, Prentice-Hall, 1977
8. Austin MJ: Management Simulations: for Mental Health and Human Services Administration. New York, Haworth Press, 1978
9. Metzger N: Personnel Administration in the Health Services Industry: Theory and Practice. New York, Spectrum Publications, 1975
10. Report of the National Task Force on Mental Health/Mental Retardation Administration. Adm Ment Health 6:267–323, Summer 1979
11. Barton WE: Leadership Development. Administration in Mental Health 9:34–40, 1981
12. Fiedler FE: The leadership game: matching the man to the situation, in Fiedler FE, Vroom VH, Argyris C (eds): Organizational Dynamics. New York, Amacon, 1977
13. Cassel RN, Heichberger RL (eds): Leadership Development: Theory and Practice. North Quincy, Mass, Christopher Publishing House, 1975

Seymour R. Kaplan, M.D.

14

Training for Psychiatrist–Administrators

The marked expansion of psychiatric programs since World War II has required many psychiatrists to assume administrative functions. These developments have occurred so rapidly and have involved such a diversity of services and programs that it has been only in recent years that psychiatrist–administrators have come to recognize their shared identity. The development of this book is an example of this recent awareness.

With the recognition of the scope of administrative responsibilities has come the recognition of the need for specialized training programs for psychiatrist–administrators. This chapter will describe an administrative psychiatry fellowship program conducted by the author during the 1970s.* Since the fellowship was a component of the Albert Einstein College of Medicine residency training program, it was developed on an introductory level for young psychiatrists without administrative experience. The curriculum was addressed primarily to full-time trainees, although a number of trainees participated on a part-time basis.

The curriculum consisted of two interrelated components. The major training experience was the "clinical" administrative assignment to a psychiatric service under the administrative authority of the Albert Einstein College of Medicine, Department of Psychiatry. The second component consisted of seminars and workshops that were geared to administrative issues involved in the trainee's clinical assignment. In addition, the individual supervision of trainees by a faculty member had a central teaching role in the curriculum.[1]

THE CLINICAL TRAINING METHOD

The "clinical" teaching method was modeled on the medical training of house staff who are assigned to patient care services necessary for the functioning of the health facility in which they work. The didactic materials were derived from the

*The fellowship program was supported by a grant from the Psychiatric Education Branch, National Institute of Mental Health (NIMH; no. 5TO1 MH14726).

clinical assignments so that theory and practice were closely integrated. Similarly, faculty supervision was based on the trainees' ongoing administrative responsibilities. The appropriate use of the teaching method required training positions with delegated administrative responsibility for the direction, planning, or evaluation functions of the program.

The major clinical training assignment developed for the fellowship program was for the position of a clinical team leader on a psychiatric inpatient service of a general hospital. Two other positions were used for the training of fellows: the assignment to the office of the deputy clinical director of a state hospital and a clinical evaluation assignment in a community mental health center (CMHC). The following section, which includes a discussion of these assignments, contains a detailed description of the specific program and its organizational context in which the clinical team leader assignment was developed as well as the specific functions of the assignment.

The Clinical Team Leader Assignment

The Program

The assignment was for the position of clinical team leader of one of the teams of the hospital division of the Sound View Throgs Neck Community Mental Health Center (SVTN–CMHC). The SVTN–CMHC was established in 1967 upon the award of a federal staffing grant and served a catchment area of approximately 205,000. There were a total of 188 staff members, including 18 psychiatrists, 20 psychologists, 30 social workers, 7 nurses, 11 other professionals (e.g., rehabilitation counselors, special education therapists), and 49 mental health workers, who provided direct services to the patient population and the community at large. Twenty-seven staff members held faculty appointments.

The Organizational Context

The SVTN–CMHC was under the professional sponsorship of the Department of Psychiatry, Albert Einstein College of Medicine. The relationship of the SVTN–CMHC to its superordinate bodies, a complex multiauthority structure typical of psychiatric services affiliated with a medical center in New York City, is illustrated in Figure 14-1.

The administrative organization of the SVTN–CMHC programs was decentralized. There were three outpatient clinics located in each of the three subcatchment areas that comprised the population served by the SVTN center. Each clinic had a community advisory board whose members were represented on the central community advisory board for the overall center. The history and development of the relationship between the SVTN–CMHC and the community advisory boards are described by the author in a prior publication.[2]

The hospital division of the SVTN–CMHC was at the time, one of the major inpatient teaching services for the Einstein basic psychiatric residency program. Eight of the 14 first-year residents were assigned to the hospital division, 4 during each 6 months of their first year of training. The daily inpatient census averaged 25 patients, with a median length of stay of 12 days. The hospital division's

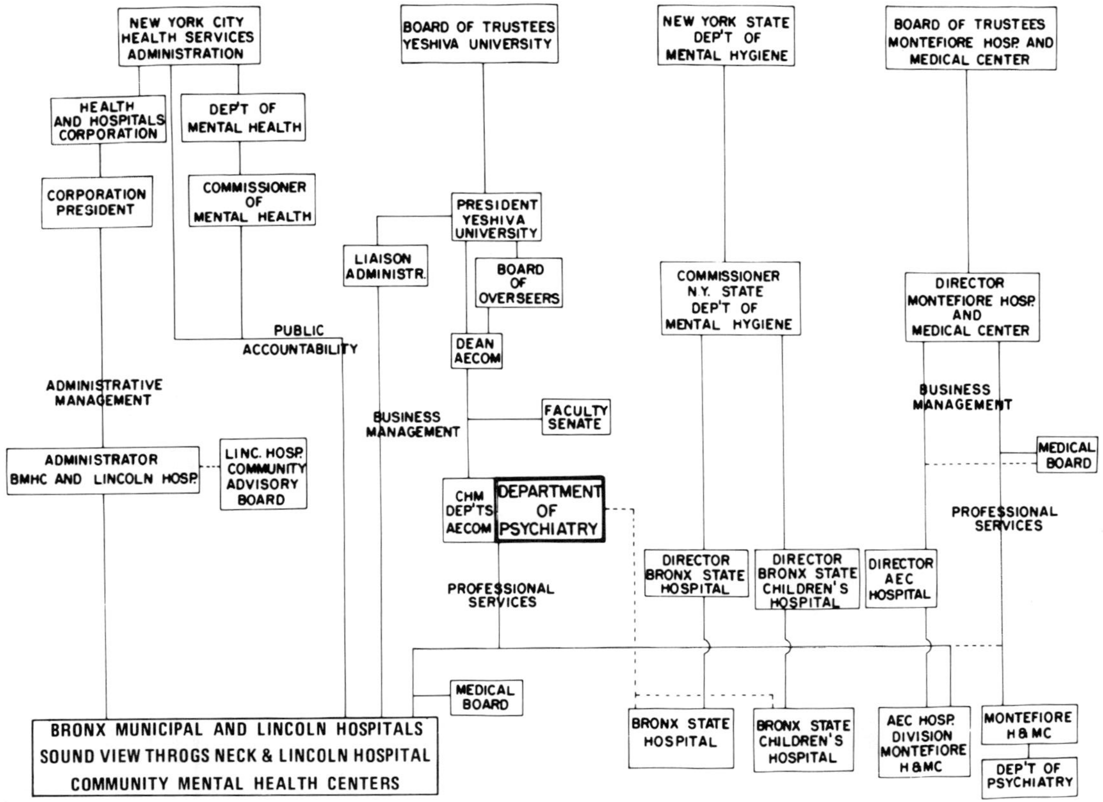

Figure 14-1. Structural relationship of public and private institutions and boards to the Department of Psychiatry of the Albert Einstein College of Medicine (1970).

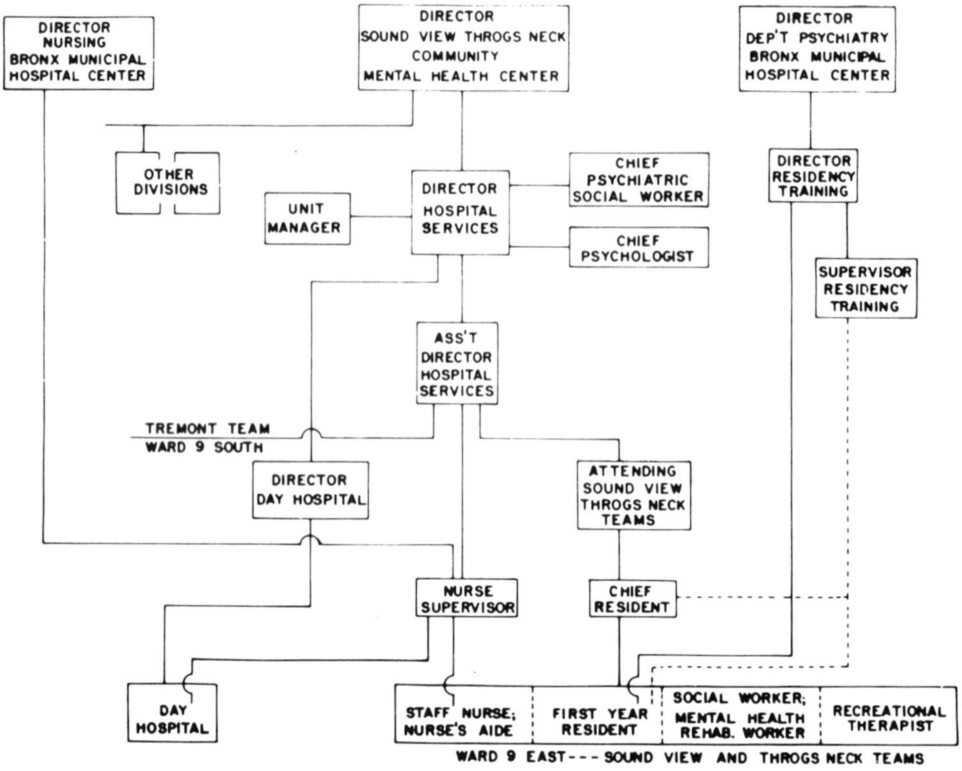

Figure 14-2. The professional organization of a psychiatric inpatient team in a general municipal teaching hospital (the Sound View Throgs Neck Community Mental Health Center Model).

staffing pattern was organized into two multidisciplinary teams, each consisting of an attending psychiatrist, two nurses, a rehabilitation technician, a team liaison from the clinics, two first-year residents, and an activity therapist. The organization of the hospital division was structured to avoid the duplication of administrative functions. For example, the team members did not have the conventional dual authority to the heads of their respective disciplines (i.e., to a chief psychologist or chief social worker). The administrative fellow directed one of the teams and subsumed the functions of the chief resident, whose line authority is illustrated in the organizational structure of the hospital division, shown in Figure 14-2.

The Functions: A "Job Description"

The functions of the clinical team leader assignment are contained in Table 14-1 under a "job description," following the approach used in "management by objectives." (The seminar outline for the study of management by objectives is included below.) The terms used under the job description are *job segments,* which describe each specific task of the job; *performance standards,* which describe the objective of each job segment; and *criteria of performance,* which describe results by which each performance standard is to be evaluated.

The Team Leader as a Social System Clinician

The relevance of the team leader assignment for administrative practices in clinical psychiatry is indicated by its similarity to the concept of "social system clinican."[3] Levinson and Klerman[4] describe this concept in the following quotation:

> It is our thesis that neither a traditional administrative approach nor a purely clinical approach is sufficient for the effective fulfillment of the tasks of organizational leadership. They require a synthesis of executive and clinical modes of functioning. Fuller understanding of the nature and the resolution of these tasks is, we believe, of prime importance in the development of new mental health programs.*

The functions of the team leader, outlined in the job description, included the mixture of clinical and administrative modes of functions, to which Levinson and Klerman refer. It also illustrates the complex authority relationships involved. The team leader was in a subordinate relationship to the director of hospital services; he had line authority over his team members, with whom he also collaborated in decisions concerning the management of patient care; he shared "executive" decisions with other committee members; he had a group leadership role in the patient–staff therapeutic community meetings and in the staff group discussions following the meetings; and he had a preceptorship relationship with psychiatric residents.

The Assignment to the Office of Deputy Clinical Director

This administrative training assignment evolved from the teaching affiliation between the department of psychiatry and the Bronx Psychiatric Center, the state hospital that serves the population treated at the Bronx Municipal Hospital Center. In some respects, this assignment is similar to the traditional field placement in the administrative curriculum of graduate schools. While there are no standard procedures for this type of assignment, it is common practice for the trainee to "shadow" a director, that is, to sit in on meetings attended by the director. It usually is difficult, however, to assign delegated authority for essential tasks in these field placements, particularly for nonmedical trainees.

In this training assignment, developed for the fellowship program, however, we were successful in arranging for meaningful administrative responsibilities. A preliminary draft of the job description, performance standards, and criteria of performance for this assignment is contained in Appendix 14-1. Because of the need to enhance the training opportunities in state hospitals, it is anticipated that the development of this type of fellowship teaching position could be enlarged and expanded upon.

The Clinical Evaluation Assignment

This assignment initially was developed under the sponsorship of the SVTN–CMHC in response to the requirements by municipal agencies for program accountability. The fellow assigned to this position participated in the center's util-

---

*From Levinson DJ, Klerman GL: The clinician-executive. Psychiatry Feb 30:3–15, 1967. Copyright © 1967 by the William Alanson White Psychiatric Foundation, Inc. Reprinted by special permission of the William Alanson White Foundation.

Table 14-1
The Clinical Team Leader Training Assignment in the Fellowship Program in Administrative Psychiatry and Mental Health Planning

	Job Description	Performance Standards (Job Segment #6)
Job Title	Clinical Team Leader	Performance Is up to Standard When:
1. Job Segment:	*Reports to director of the hosital services*	The patient receives a statement of legal right form within 24 hr of admission (form is signed and forwarded to mental health lawyers). This is the responsibility of the nursing staff.
Definition:	Weekly meeting with the director of hospital services to present areas of progress or problems concerning patient care services, personnel, and residency training programs	
2. Job Segment:	*Becomes acting director*	A written initial diagnosis and tentative treatment plan is on the patient's chart within 24 hr of admission and countersigned by chief resident or clinical team leader.
Definition:	When the director of hospital services is absent, the clinical team leader becomes the acting director and assumes temporary responsibility for short-term functions (i.e., budget planning and major personnel changes would be deffered).	The treatment plan is "coordinated" by the patient's therapist, but the entire team assumes responsibility for the various facets of milieu treatment. Progress notes are written daily by the nursing staff (initialled by the therapist) and two to three times weekly by the therapist.
3. Job Segment:	*Represents clinical team at weekly executive committee meetings*	
Definition:	Represents the team in the executive committee regarding clinical matters (ie, issues concerning treatment and patient care assignments); personnel issues (ie, scheduling) and resource allocation (ie, needs for staffing; office space).	The patient improves and plans for outpatient follow-up care formulated and discussed with OPD liaison team members. The patient fails to improve and plans for transfer to the long-term treatment facility for more prolonged inpatient care are formulated.

Job Description		Performance Standards (Job Segment #6)
Job Title	Clinical Team Leader	Performance Is up to Standard When:
4. Job Segment:	*Leads therapeutic community meetings*	
Definition:	On Monday, Wednesday and Friday of each week there is a therapeutic community meeting of 45 minutes' duration attended by all staff and patients, followed by one-half hour "post" attended by the staff. Both meetings are chaired by the clinical team leader.	
5. Job Segment:	*Participates in the residency training program*	CRITERIA OF PERFORMANCE (Job Segment #6)
Definition:	The clinical team leader has teaching and supervisory responsibilities for the first-year residents assigned to his or her team.	Readmissions within 6 months or less to the acute inpatient service are minimized so that no more than one-third of the inpatient census at any one time should be patients who have been hospitalized within the previous six months.
6. Job Segment:	*Supervises and coordinates the team's management of patient care*	
Definition:	Supervises the inpatient team's formulation of the diagnosis, treatment plan, and tentative disposition plan for each patient, within 3–5days of admission. Coordinates the arrangements by the liaison members of the team for services for patients to be discharged and for the transfer of patients requiring long-term treatment.	A yearly follow-up check of discharged patients should find at least 75 percent still engaged in a therapeutic or rehabilitation program.

ization review committee and clinical care committee. The assignment involved an active working membership on the committees as well as liaison functions concerned with the difficult administrative problems of the implementation of review procedures in health institutions. The objective was to enhance the ability of the trainee to implement evaluation procedures rather than to develop skills in evaluation methodologies.

Since its initial development, however, this assignment was subsumed under the training functions of the assignment to the deputy clinical director. With the increasing rigor of the reviews by the Joint Commission on Accreditation of Hospitals, there has been a marked interest in improving capabilities in this area. The inclusion of Chapter 19 and Chapter 21 in this text indicates the recognition of the administrative importance of quality of assurance, accreditation, and regulatory procedures.

SEMINARS

The following discussion of a model curriculum is presented primarily for the purpose of illustrating the teaching format rather than the specific content of the seminars. The format combines experiential and didactic approaches, the former geared as much as possible to the ongoing administrative issues with which the trainee is involved.

Problems of Innovation and Change in Psychiatric Institutions

This seminar utilized comparative case studies to identify the similarities and differences of problems of innovation and change in psychiatric organizations. In keeping with the curricular objectives, the programs used for the comparative case studies were those to which the trainees were assigned or with which they were familiar. Perhaps because this approach is similar to the use of the case study method in clinical training in psychiatry, one encounters few problems in obtaining open and frank discussions.

An effective arrangement was to have the trainees and the directors of the psychiatric services to which they were assigned collaborate in the presentation of the case studies. The review of the psychiatric services being presented, in relation to previous case studies, provided the basis for comparative analyses. Similar parameters were used as the basis for each case study. These included the governance of the psychiatric institution; the organizational structures for the administration of the business activities and for the psychiatric services; and the financial resources available to the institution.

Organizational Dynamics

The teaching materials for this seminar were based on the extrapolation of small group theories to behavior in organization.[5–12] The practical value for the clinical training assignments was in their application to the leadership role of mental health teams and in the relationship between the mental health team, as a group, and its environment. Reading materials about the role of the leader during phases of organizational development were available in the author's publications.[13,14]

Management Theory and Practice

This seminar was adapted from the result-oriented approach to management decisionmaking, often referred to as "management by objectives" (MBO). This management technique involves a systematic appraisal of organizational goals and objectives, specific methods employed to achieve the objectives and general standards and means for evaluating the results at the end of a specific time period.

The job description, performance standards, and criteria of performance described above for the clinical team leader assignment are based on modifications of the technique of MBO. The applicability of MBO to psychiatric services are described in Chapters 1 and 4. Examples of the course content are in Appendix 14-2.

SUPERVISION

Individual supervision of trainees by faculty and by senior administrators in the programs in which the trainees work comprised a major teaching aspect of the clinical training method. Supervisory time often has to be determined by practical work requirements but should be scheduled on a weekly basis.

A "typical" weekly training schedule is illustrated in the outline in Figure 14-3.

DISCUSSION

During the period for which NIMH stipend support was granted (1971–1974), nine fellows were appointed to full-time fellowship positions. Over the 8-year period in which the author conducted the program, there were 30 additional trainees who participated on a part-time basis. The success of the program is indicated in part by the careers of former trainees and faculty. Five have held positions as state or municipal mental health commissioners; several have been directors of state and proprietary hospitals; and most have been, or are, directors of psychiatric departments or heads of service divisions in general hospitals. Over the course of years since initiating the fellowship program, discussions with former trainees and observations of their subsequent career development have indicated areas of limitations of the Einstein program. Notably among these have been inadequate training in the areas of finance and budget and problems with training around the exercise of power and the use of authority.

Limitations of the Einstein Program

Training in Financial and Budgetary Procedures

At a conference held in 1974, to evaluate the Einstein administrative psychiatry fellowship program, former trainees who held high-level administrative positions in governmental agencies noted that a major area in which their training was

	MONDAY	TUESDAY	WEDNESDAY	THURSDAY	FRIDAY
9:00 AM	Supervision (Clinical) Program	Organizational Dynamics Seminar (September-January)	CLINICAL ASSIGNMENT	Case Study Seminar (September-January)	CLINICAL ASSIGNMENT
10:00 AM	CLINICAL ASSIGNMENT	Management Theories and Practices Seminar (February-June)		Administrative Theories and Practices Seminar (February-June)	
10:30 AM		CLINICAL ASSIGNMENT		CLINICAL ASSIGNMENT	
12:00 Noon					
1:00 PM			Supervision (Director of Clinical Program)	Supervision (Director of Fellowship Program)	
2:00 PM			CLINICAL ASSIGNMENT	CLINICAL ASSIGNMENT	
5:00 PM					

Seminar Time: 3 hours/weekly
Supervision Time: 3 hours/weekly

Special Workshops: or Projects — Intergroup Relations; Evaluation Methodology; Others

Figure 14-3. Fellowship in administrative psychiatry and mental health planning—a model weekly schedule.

deficient was in financial and budgetary procedures. In part, this deficiency was due to the fact that the Einstein training assignments were in government-sponsored facilities; the Bronx Municipal Hospital Center, SVTN–CMHC and the Bronx Psychiatric Center. The services in these facilities are financed entirely by contracts with city and state agencies that do not involve the administration in direct billing and collection of fees for services. There was therefore no opportunity for assignment of the trainees to the business office to participate in the financial operations of the programs.

It is questionable, however, whether practical experiences in financial and budgetary procedures could have been developed for young, inexperienced trainees. Moreover, the former trainees did indicate that it is doubtful whether, at the time of their participation, they would have appreciated, or been interested in, an assignment that included working with the business office. Rather, they recommended that arrangements be provided for postfellowship training experiences in financial and budgetary procedures. Whether a fellowship program should provide this continuing experience or other arrangements should be made, it was clear that the training of prospective psychiatric administrators could best be served by a flexible curriculum that extends beyond a formal fellowship curriculum.

Power and the Exercise of Authority

The statement that "power is the ultimate aphrodisiac" has been attributed to Henry Kissinger. A variation on this point of view has been offered by another Harvard faculty member.[15]

> Often the clinician-turned executive is hindered in the exercise of authority by his feeling that an interest in power is intrinsically immoral. . . . Indeed, the predominant view of power in the professions (and especially the mental health professions) is much like the Victorian view of sex. It is seen as vulgar, as a sign of character defect, as something an upstanding professioal would not be interested in or stoop to engage in. A friend of ours who has a serious ego-syntonic interest in being a department chairman and in discussing openly the power issues that usually remain implicit in departmental meetings, reports that he often feels "like a whore in a monastery." His efforts to explore power issues occasion the same response as would the telling of a sexual joke at a ladies' tea party: polite silence followed by a discreet change of subject. The *devaluation* of the interest in and use of power contributes heavily to the misuses and perversions of power that plague our organizational life.*

In a paper describing a curriculum the author developed for teaching community psychiatry in the basic residency program at Einstein, he expressed a similar opinion.[16]

> I agree with the GAP report (about psychiatric leadership) although I would stress the issue of authority and power in teaching programs since I believe it to be the fundamental issue. The understanding of the role of power in the human situation has been generally neglected in residency training and in the theory and practice of psychiatry. It was Freud's difficulty in "negotiating" with his gifted friend and follower, Alfred Adler, that in part resulted in the omission from the main body of

*From Levinson DJ, Klerman, GL: The Clinician-Executive revisited. in Administration in Mental Health. Rockville, Md, NIMH, 1972, p 64–67. With permission.

> psychoanalytic theory of Adler's views about the basic role of power in the dynamics of human behavior. . . . However, it may be that in the final analysis the art of negotiation and (coping with the exercise) of power are matters of life-long experience that cannot be taught.*

The chapters by Barton and Barton (Chapter 13), and, particularly, the observations by Greenblatt (Chapter 15) also include comments regarding the issue of power and the exercise of authority. This issue, however, still is not adequately addressed in our training programs or in the professional community at large.

Recent Developments

Although formal training in basic psychiatric residency programs has not flourished, there have been encouraging developments in the increased interest in the certification examination in administrative psychiatry given by the American Psychiatric Association (APA). As a concomitant to the fellowship program, in 1974, the author initiated a review course for candidates for the examination. Over the course of the next 6 years, over 50 candidates participated in these courses. The increased interest in undertaking them was assisted by the encouragment of Dr. Thomas Tourlentes during his tenure as chairman of the APA committee and as president of the American Association of Psychiatric Administrators. During the 1981–1982 academic year, the review course, based on the syllabus developed by the author, is being conducted by three other departments of psychiatry: the Cornell University Medical Center, under John A. Talbott, M.D.; the University of North Carolina at Chapel Hill, under William Hunter, M.D.; and at Wright State University Medical Center, under Paul Rodenhauser, M.D.

Although it is still uncertain whether there is any substantial change in the traditional ambivalence among medical professionals about the role of the administrator, these developments seem to suggest a lessening of a censorious attitude toward the issue of power and the exercise of authority. It is difficult to see how there can be significant improvements among the medical leadership unless this issue is openly acknowledged and addressed in the professional community at large.

REFERENCES

1. Kaplan SR, Miller S, Altman N, et al: Teaching administrative psychiatry and mental health planning, in Mental Health Administration. Washington, DC, National Institute of Mental Health, 1972, p 30–39
2. Kaplan Sr, Ahmed B. Community participation, in Feldman S (ed): The Administration of Mental Health Services. Springfield, Ill, Thomas, 1980
3. Greenblatt M: The psychiatrist as social system clinician, in Greenblatt M, Levinson DJ, Williams RH (eds.): The Patient and the Mental Hospital. Glencoe, Ill, Free Press, 1957
4. Levinson J, Klerman L: The clinician-executive. Psychiatry Feb 30:3–15, 1967
5. Kaplan SR, Roman M: Characteristic responses of therapy groups to the introduction of new members. Int J Group Psychother, 11: 372–381, 1961
6. Kaplan SR, Roman M: Phases of development in adult therapy groups. Int J Group Psychother 13:10–26, 1963
7. Kaplan SR: Therapy groups and training groups: similarities and differences. Int J Group Psychother 17:473–504, 1967
8. Kaplan SR: Psychotherapeutic approaches in working with the disadvantaged, in Goldman

*From Kaplan SR: Teaching of community psychiatry in psychiatric residency training programs, in Lidz T, Edelson M (eds): Training Tomorrow's Psychiatrists. New Haven, Yale University Press, 1970, p 61–94. With permission.

G, Millman D, eds: Innovations in Psychotherapy. Springfield, Ill, Thomas, 1972
9. Kornblith AB Kaplan SR: Groups and drug programs, in Lowinson J, Ruiz P (eds): Substance Abuse in the US. Baltimore, Williams & Wilkins, 1981
10. Kaplan SR, Razin A: The psychological substrate of self-help groups. *J Operational Psychiatry,* 9:57–69 1978
11. Kaplan SR, Razin A: The dynamics of group cohesion, in Kellerman H (ed): Group Cohesion: Biological, Psychological and Sociological Perspectives. New York, Grune & Stratton, 1981
12. Kaplan SR, Roman M: The Organization and Delivery of Mental Health Services in the Ghetto: The Lincoln Hospital Experience. New York, Praeger, 1973
13. Kaplan SR, Ahmed B. Group strategies with disadvanted populations: the public mental health setting, in Seligman M (ed), Group Strategies with Different Populations. Springfield, Ill, Thomas 1977
14. Kaplan SR: Characteristic phases of development in organizations, in Millman D, Goldman G (eds): Group Process Today: Evaluation and Perspective. Springfield, Ill, Thomas, 1974
15. Levinson DJ, Klerman GL: The clinician-executive revisited, Administration in Mental Health. Rockville, Md, NIMH, 1972, p 64–67
16. Kaplan SR: Teaching of community psychiatry in psychiatric residency training programs, in Lidz T, Edelson M (eds): Training Tomorrow's Psychiatrists. New Haven, Yale University Press, 1970

APPENDIX 14-1.

Selected Examples From Administrative Assignment To The Office Of The Deputy Clinical Director (DDC)

Job Description

Job Title: Clinical Assistant to the DDC

1. JOB SEGMENT: *Reports to the DDC.*
   Definition: Weekly meetings with the DDC to present reports about assigned activities.
2. JOB SEGMENT: *Assists the DDC in his functions as Director of Clinical Program Areas.*
   Definition: Assists the DDC in the preparation of materials for meetings with:
   a. In-patient Unit Chiefs
   b. Directors of Special Clinical Programs
3. JOB SEGMENT: *Assists the DDC in his functions in special program areas.*
   Definition: Assists the DDC in the preparation of materials for the following special program areas:
   a. Incident Reports
   b. Court/legal activities
      • Order of transfer (out-of-borough)
      • Discharge to other boroughs
      • District Attorney's Office
   c. Archives and Inquiries
4. JOB SEGMENT: *Represents the DDC when legally sanctioned in special program areas.*
   Definition: Represents the DDC in Special Areas when it is legally appropriate, and when competence has been demonstrated to the DDC.
5. JOB SEGMENT: *Assists the DDC with other committee functions.*
   Definition: Assists the DDC in the preparation of the materials for the following committees:
   Committee Activities
   a. Accreditation Committee
   b. Personnel Utilization Committee
   c. Institutional Review Committee
   d. Infection Control Committee
   e. Pharmacy and Therapeutic Committee
   f. Mortality Review Committee
6. JOB SEGMENT: *Represents the DDC when legally sanctioned at selected committees.*
   Definition: Represents the DDC when it is legally appropriate and when competence has been demonstrated to the DDC at selected committee meetings.
7. JOB SEGMENT: *Acts as liaison between the DDC and the Coordinator of Training for psychiatric staff*
   Definition: Provides liaison between the DDC and the Coordinator of Training for psychiatrists in the following functions:

a. Arranges for teaching materials for training programs for psychiatrists
b. Organizes special teaching materials recommended by the DDC

Performance Standards

JOB SEGMENT 4

Performance is up to standard when the trainee has demonstrated competence to represent the DDC in special program areas.

JOB SEGMENT 6

Performance is up to standard when the trainee has demonstrated competence to represent the DDC at selected committee meetings.

Criteria of Performance

GENERAL (For all job segments)

Materials prepared by the trainee for the DDC have specific application and are used by the DDC at least 75% of the time.

JOB SEGMENT 4

The trainee demonstrates competence to represent the DDC in special program areas, as indicated by DDC's delegation of major responsibility in at least one special program area and the delegation of some responsibility in at least one other special program area.

JOB SEGMENT 6

The trainee demonstrates competence to represent the DDC at committee metings, as indicated by the DDC's delegation of major responsibility for at least one committee and the delegation of moderate responsibility (conducts 30% of meetings without DDC) for at least two committees.

APPENDIX 14-2.

Seminar Schedule 1971–1972

Sept.	9	Introduction
Sept.	16	Management
Sept.	23	The Table of Organization
Sept.	30	The Table of Organization
Oct.	7	The Individual Setting
Oct.	14	The Individual Setting
Oct.	21	The Job Description
Oct.	28	Job Segments
Nov.	4	Standards of Performance
Nov.	11	Achieving Agreement on Standards
Nov.	18	Agreement Setting Interview
Dec.	2	Evaluating Performance
Dec.	9	Work, Planning and Review Interview
Dec.	10	Planning and Control
Dec.	23	Introduction to Goal Setting
Jan.	6	Management by Objectives
Jan.	13	Organizational Objectives
Jan.	20	Organizational Objectives—cont.
Jan.	27	Key Result Areas
Feb.	3	Key Result Areas—cont.
Feb.	10	Operating Objectives
Feb.	17	Writing Operating Objectives
Feb.	24	Screening Operating Objectives
March	2	The Importance of Outcome Objectives
March	9	Action Goals
March	16	Individual Goals
March	23	Incorporation and By-Laws
March	30	Systems Analysis
April	6	The Role of Government
April	13	Boards: Their Purpose and How to Work With Them
April	20	Policy: What is it? How to Develop It?
April	27	Financial Management: Costs, Budgets, Policy
May	4	Plant, Insurance, Equipment, Audits
May	11	Personnel: Policy, Functions, Evaluation
May	18	Decisionmaking
May	25	Summary and Evaluation of Course

Examples of Curriculum for Specific Topics

Nov. 4 *Topic: Standards of Performance*

Process: Develop standards in the group around selected job segments and descriptions.

Preparation: Bring job descriptions and job segments and have reviewed them.

Handouts:
1. "Writing your performance standards."
2. "Guidelines for supervisor."
3. "Guidelines for observer in standards of performance agreement setting interview."

Dec. 9	*Topic: Work, Planning, and Review Interview* Process: Role Playing and Discussion Preparation: Fill out and bring Work, Planning, and Review Form. Handouts: 1. "Management by Objectives or Appraisal by Results." 2. "Management by Objectives as Applied to a Division on Alcoholism in a State Department of Mental Health." 3. "Management by Objectives: a tool for the Federation Executive."
Jan. 13	*Topic: Organizational Objectives* Process: Discussion and Group Work on Organization Objectives Preparation: Fill out A. "What Is Our Business and What Should It Be." B. "Monitoring the Environment" C. "Changes" D. "Effect of Changes" E. "Organization Objectives" Handouts: "Key Result Areas"
Jan. 27	*Topic: Key Result Areas* Process: Discussion. Preparation: Read "Key Result Areas," determine areas special to your own program, determine if you would not use any of those presented; cite examples. Handout: "Operating Objectives of an Organization."

Milton Greenblatt, M.D.

15

The Politics of Administration

This chapter is written from the perspective of a senior administrator offering advice to a young psychiatrist or mental health worker wishing to become a mental health administrator. The older colleague enlightens the younger person about political aspects of hospital governance, dealing with mental health boards, outside agencies, or constituencies; about the nature of the political system, the kinds of politicians an administrator is likely to meet, the part legislation may play in an administrator's life; and particularly about how to handle pressures of patronage. The senior administrator addresses these issues from experiences gained during his own career in which he administered a state mental hospital, a state mental health system, a Veterans Administration (VA) medical center, and a university teaching hospital.

CLARIFICATION OF TERMS

Before getting into substantive issues, it is useful to clarify the use of a few terms. In this chapter, the term *administration* is an umbrella designation embracing two concepts: (1) *management,* the day-to-day handling of operations to ensure the organization's smooth and efficient running according to guidelines laid down in the recent past; and (2) *leadership,* the necessary planning and implementation to change the organization, to move it from point A to point B, to enhance its growing edges, to modify its overall services in relation to defined goals, perhaps even to change or augment a constituency. Management, therefore, requires the ability to tend to a multitude of details to keep the ship on present course, while leadership necessitates the ability to exert imagination, vision, and entrepreneurial skills, to set progressive expectations, and to move all or parts of a system. The terms *director, executive,* and *superintendent,* as often used in mental health settings, may refer to one or both of these functions.

PREPARATION FOR APPLYING FOR AN ADMINISTRATIVE POST

Before a mental health professional applies for a chief administrative position she or he should ask, Do I really want the job? Am I ready for it? To answer these questions, one must know a great deal about the job; then one must assess and analyze one's own motivation and capacities, including the ability to think in terms of a total system, to work in sometimes ambiguous situations, to relate to multiple persons and organizational functions, to tolerate criticism and frustration, and to sustain large outputs of energy over time. Most importantly, one must ask oneself, What are the organization's goals and expectations, and are they achievable within the framework of my God-given talents?

GOVERNANCE

To answer the above question, one must first learn: What is the pattern of governance of the organization in question, and how well will I fit into it? Who appoints the administrator and to what extent is the appointee beholden to the appointing agency? For example, if appointed by the governor of the state, the length of the administrator's stay in office is likely to be determined by the governor, who probably can remove his appointee at will. In addition, the administrator's term is likely to expire at the end of the governor's term in office. This makes the appointee the governor's subordinate, a part of the executive branch of government, a political-professional person, fair game for criticism and attacks from the opposite party (whatever one's personal affiliations)—and always fair game for the press and any public or private agency that cares to investigate the appointee or his or her operation. Obviously, this is not the type of position for someone interested in job security. If one wants freedom from public attention, scrutiny, and public criticism, such a position should be avoided at all costs. On the other hand, if one is something of a gambler, not easily wounded, and able to enjoy the rough-and-tumble of the political arena, such a job may be quite appealing.

The *pattern of governance* (see also Chapter 4) within the institution usually revolves around the relationship between the administrator and his board. Boards are of two types: (1) advisory and (2) policy making. The category into which a particular board fits depends largely on the size and personality makeup of the board, its history, and its direction as determined by its leadership; but, generally, advisory boards do not appoint personnel, and they meet less frequently and exert less power than policy boards. Since, however, advisory board members usually represent diverse interests and a variety of constituencies and often have powerful connections, they can exert a great deal of informal influence over organizational policy and personnel appointments. The author remembers one board that included a close friend of the governor, a friend of the cardinal, a physician with strong ties to the state medical organization, several prominent businessmen, and representatives of powerful minority groups. They were very conscious of their informal power, and they used it.

The policy board, by contrast, may appoint personnel, including the administrator. It also may have the power to terminate such appointments. It formulates policy that the administrator, functioning mainly as an executive secretary, carries out. It has the ultimate responsibility for the work and welfare of the institution, and if it is to feel secure in its own task, it must at all times have confidence in the ability and effectiveness of the chief administrative officer. Policy boards often work their will by appointing subcommittees to investigate and oversee various functions of the institution.

Because there are many patterns of governance at the board level, aspiring administrators must ascertain the precise characteristics of governance in the institution they are contemplating joining to decide if they want the job, can live with it, or must reject it.

There also are other more subtle considerations to assess concerning the overall effect boards have on the life of the institution. These usually fall into one or more of three categories:

1. Boards may *legitimate* the work of the institution by soliciting and contributing funds or material; offering volunteer services; interpreting the functions of the institution to the community; and supporting the institution in times of stress.
2. Boards may carry out an *auditing or investigatory function* by reviewing programs, progress, budgets, appointments, promotions, relationships inside and outside the institution and by reviewing complaints, grievances, and class or job actions.
3. Boards may exert a *directing or controlling function* by making general policy and planning and supervising its implementation.

The important thing to remember is that whatever the interests of the board may be at any particular time, the board presents a set of expectations for the administrator, which, if fulfilled, leaves him in good standing and, if unfulfilled, can lead to serious stress and strain. It also is well to realize that many boards, whether advisory or policy setting, tend, over time, to adopt more than one of these functions. Indeed, the author believes there is a general tendency for boards to shift emphasis from legitimation to auditing and control. Certainly, individual members of the board, as they become more secure and knowledgeable, want to understand more fully the reasons for decisions and actions, hoping and expecting to become more involved in future decisions and actions. Wise administrators will recognize and acknowledge that board members may know more and have more experience in some aspects of administration than they have and therefore will seek out these persons for advice and counsel. To promote mutual respect, confidence, and trust, a wise administrator will take the initiative to explore talents and role expectations of board members.

CONSTITUENCIES

The constituencies to be served are special and unique to every organization. The commissioner of the department of mental health in a large industrial state, for example, at a minimum, must seek and maintain the good will of the governor, the legislature, the attorney general, the state auditor, the citizens' lobby, the university and professional communities, labor organizations, and the mental health department itself. Beyond that, such a commissioner also must be interested in the good will of federal agencies such as Medicare and Medicaid, various foundations, private contributors, the National Institute of Mental Health (NIMH), and, of course, the Joint Commission on Accreditation of Hospitals (JCAH). It is perhaps appropriate to make a few brief remarks about some of these constituencies.

The Governor

We have already indicated how important it is for the head of a state mental health system to enjoy the good will and respect of the governor. Citizens' and professional groups served by the system want their mental health commissioner to be close to the state's highest elected official and to influence positively the final budget the governor submits to the legislature. In recent years, however, the tendency of states to form cabinet-type governments has downgraded the ability of mental health officials to influence governors directly. Usually, a cabinet member is interposed between the mental health authority and the governor. This official often analyzes and hones the budget before it is sent to the governor.

The cabinet system also may distance the mental health official from the governor in situations in which the mental health department is amalgamated with other departments, such as public health and welfare, in hopes of reducing duplication and effecting economies. Often, under this arrangement, the cabinet officer to whom the mental health authority reports is not an M.D. or even a health professional, which tends further to deprofessionalize and politicize the relationship. The net result is that the mental health department tends to lose its identity, and its purpose become blurred.

In all instances in which an administrator's direct access to a governor is limited, the official must establish and maintain a good working relationship with the cabinet secretary and operating heads of all agencies with which the mental health department does business; otherwise, bureaucratic delays and hindrances, always a source of frustration, may be compounded. The administrator must realize, too, that the competition for scarce resources is ever present and that friendship with other agency heads must be maintained despite the fact that annually or more frequently he or she "goes to the mat" with other directors to fight for manpower and other resources.

The Legislature

The legislature votes on the dispersal of state funds based in large measure on the budget submitted by the governor. The sophisticated administrator, however, knows that many things may happen to the original budget as it gets massaged by the legislature. Items may be added or subtracted. Powerful lawmakers may reshape the budget to reflect special interests of constituents and lobbyists. The job of the mental health authority is made even more difficult because while he or she would like to have his or her budget enhanced without incurring the wrath of the executive branch—which has already made its decision as to how much to allot to that department—legislators from the opposite party may be happy to capitalize on differences that appear between the governor and his agency head.

The job of the agency head is compounded further by the fact that he or she is repeatedly bombarded by individual legislators for jobs, services, or favors for various of the legislators' constituents or friends. The time when aggressive legislators usually push for special consideration is when the budget comes up for final vote. If the agency head plays along with these politicians, he risks getting caught in situations in which he may trade material gain for integrity. The caveat "The best politician is the least politician" is thus often the best rule to follow.

In negotiations with the legislature, the most important figures are likely to be members of the ways and means committee, members of various monitoring or watchdog committees investigating activities of the state, and individual champions of special mental health and/or retardation causes. The agency head is advised to cultivate these individuals, to keep them abreast of departmental plans and activities, and to work out plans to meet mental health needs of their constituents.

Once elected, legislators usually want to stay in office; thus, they set out to augment their power and prestige by supporting popular causes. This requires much public notice and exposure as a reformer or champion. The health professional must realize it is within these constraints that the legislator tries to serve his people; the lofty image of a great statesman may not be a compelling motive.

The mental health authority often appears before legislative committees and hearing bodies to rationalize his or her budget and support, modify, or oppose legislation relating to departmental functioning. New bills for study may be advanced by legislators, private citizens, special interest groups, or by the department itself. Indeed, it is highly desirable (and an indication of departmental alertness and aggressiveness) for the department to take an active legislative role in shaping its destiny rather than to react perpetually to legislative initiatives taken by others.

When legislative negotiations have reached an impasse or bills inimical to departmental functioning threaten to be passed, the agency head may appeal for help to the president of the Senate, or the Speaker of the House. These legislators may understand and accept the department's point of view and often possess extraordinary powers and great technical skill to influence procedures. Should all else fail, a department head should appeal to the governor directly to assert his influence with legislators and/or to exert his veto power.

The Attorney General's Office

The attorney general's office defends state agencies in suits brought against them by individuals or groups. This office also investigates charges of misfeasance or malfeasance against any state employees. Often lawyers have to be consulted by mental health officials on interpretation of law or to provide advice and counsel as to conduct in office of employees who may be vulnerable on a conflict of interest basis. Finally, the attorney general renders invaluable service to the department by developing and elaborating new laws regarding mental health concerns.

The Auditor

The auditor is the citizens' watchdog, whose job it is to make certain that funds of the commonwealth are properly expended and that no one defrauds the public. His regular audits of hospitals and clinics usually are thorough and intensive. But difficulties can arise because the office of auditor is susceptible to political influence; indeed, the auditor may exploit his role as public defender by making extensive use of the media whenever he finds something "wrong." During an election year, this practice has great allure, especially if the auditor wants to be re-elected.

Citizens' Lobby

The citizens' lobby has grown greatly in vigor and power in the last few decades. Several years ago in Massachusetts, citizen advisory councils, area boards, mental health associations, mental retardation associations, associations lobbying for children's services, citizen trustees of various hospital and schools, and "friends" of this or that project numbered in the hundreds. Some of these groups, such as citizen advisory councils to the central mental health administration, were formally part of the state administration in that they were appointed by the governor. Area mental health boards were appointed by the commissioner. Many other groups were entirely independent of the department—for example, the associations of mental health or retardation. These independent groups were viewed by the legislature and the press as more faithfully representing sentiments of the people than groups appointed by government officials.

With recent sharp increases of citizen involvement in policies concerning delivery of health services, new challenges have come to confront the administrator. More voices are heard on behalf of patients than ever before. Many are sharp and strident and often critical of management and professionals. Without these new voices, however, help for the mentally ill still would remain in the background, as it has in centuries past. The challenge to the administrator is to unify the impact of these voices, to keep them from fighting among themselves, thus stalling many worthwhile programs. The challenge is also to bring citizens' views in consonance with professionals' views and to avoid costly and damaging citizen–professional splits. For today citizens want to know more and to have a say in planning programs and allocating funds. They wish to influence priorities, including those concerning research and training.

Citizen influence on executive functions is complemented by another equally important movement: individual citizen involvement as volunteers in direct treatment of mentally ill and retarded persons. I know of no state that as yet has exploited the full potential of citizen volunteers, although their contribution, even at the present time, in terms of hours served and effect on the clinical course of thousands of patients has been massive. One of the most interesting developments has been the student volunteer program, which received sharp impetus in Boston in the 1950s and 1960s and then spread to other cities.

Hiring of volunteer organizers at state and federal levels as a formal part of the mental health structure has given the volunteer movement great encouragement. A task for the administrator, always looking for new resources, is to stimulate and support this volunteer movement, to enhance recruitment and training of volunteers, and to explore new ways to utilize their abundant talents in service to patients.

University and Professional Communities

While universities and professionals should make common cause with departments of mental health, often it is up to the administrator to take the initiative in developing a working alliance with these groups. Over the years many medical schools have come to depend on state and VA mental health facilities to provide adequate clinical material for their students, and to obtain space and funds for research programs. The VA has had a formal policy to develop alliances with medical schools through the special deans' committees; this has worked very well through the years, with consequent upgrading of VA patient care, training, and research. In Michigan and Boston in the early part of the century, the "psychopathic model" of collaboration between state and university was inaugurated, and this, too, has spread.

The task of the administrator is to cultivate and enhance these university relationships, which are not always smooth. For example, *Stars and Stripes,* a publication of veterans' service organizations, frequently sounds the alarm that medical schools are "ripping off" the VA system for research and training purposes while neglecting clinical care for sick veterans. Some administrators of VA hospitals resist sharing power and authority, an implicit part of any collaborative arrangement with a university. The administrator's task is to cultivate a spirit of mutual trust, generosity, and good will between both sides in the greater interest of enhancing education, research, and clinical care in service to patients.

Professionals working in mental health systems also have ties to professional organizations outside those systems. Service providers thus often have two loyalties. The professional organizations to which they belong set standards and structure the nature of interprofessional relationships. In recent years, these organizations have become increasingly involved in political action related to licensure and to reimbursement of professional services by third-party payers. Clinical psychologists, as is well known, are militantly dedicated to achieving parity with psychiatrists in licensure and reimbursement and also are pushing toward a greater say in institutional governance, as well as standards set by JCAH. Here again, the task of the administrator is to see that political activities of professionals outside the organization are not played out within the institution and that tensions and animosities developed on the political front do not imperil the therapeutic climate inside the organization. At the same time, he must be able to make sensitive judgments concerning roles of various professional groups in both governance and hierarchical relations within the hospital.

Labor Organizations

Labor relations are sure to consume a good deal of the executive's time. Complaints and grievances of individual workers will require careful investigation by management to inform the director, who may have to rule on such matters as part of his judicial role. Any of his decisions may be sent to a higher authority or to a labor relations board for review; therefore, the director, in order to consolidate his position and avoid embarrassing reversals, must know his cases very well and should be well supported by legal counsel. If morale in the institution is high and the chief officer has a reputation for fairmindedness, the number of such grievances may be kept to a minimum. If, however, morale is low and workers are angry with management, the number of suits and grievances may climb to the point that management accomplishes almost nothing else than dealing with these problems.

Every complaint should thus receive full and generous attention by supervisory personnel at the lower levels, with every effort made to resolve issues through informal channels. The manner in which the chief executive officer and his lieutenants relate to subordinates tends to carry over in the way subordinate department heads handle their workers. In poorly run organizations, this middle-management echelon may see to it that almost all the time of a major executive is taken up with the unhappy frustrations of line workers. In well-managed organizations, middle management can take full responsibility for morale and worker happiness in their own divisions, freeing up the chief executive to do his important business on behalf of the whole institution. That business is planning, effecting institutional change consistent with desirable goals, and, of course, sustaining and improving staff and patient morale.

Labor groups now play a major role in almost all hospitals. Sometimes there are several such groups, each relating to management through regularly negotiated contracts. Often, management must yield to requests or demands for changed or improved conditions for workers, but it never should yield any of its vital management rights, such as privilege of appointments, setting of goals and standards for patient care, authority over priorities of programs, and ultimate command in times of crisis. Once a contract is reached, however, management must carry out its part of the bargain in good faith; otherwise, it risks strikes, work slowdowns, and job actions. A sophisticated administrator should be aware that workers in pursuit of change can have a significant impact on the organization's operation even in state and federal health institutions in which strikes are outlawed. There are many effective techniques disgruntled employees can use short of an overt strike.

When bargaining with employee groups, it is wise for management to come to the table with some previous negotiating experience or to avail itself of help from experienced negotiators, for labor will mobilize all the talent it needs to get its way. Furthermore, even when threats and accusations are made by labor, management must be strong enough to resist encroachment on its management rights. Remember, however, that a good contract, thoroughly hashed out to the satisfaction of both parties, can be a great asset in dealing with workers and in establishing a favorable climate for treating patients.

The State Department of Mental Health

To a large extent, the above discussion deals with administrative relations with outside groups. Establishing and maintaining good relations within the *institution itself* are just as important. No matter what is going on, the administrator wants to have the support and good will of all his own people at all levels. If he is intent on changing the system, he must have sufficient support so changes will be accepted and remain stable over time. Otherwise, through foot dragging, backlash, and inciting by labor or outside groups, the efforts of the administrator will be vitiated. Much of the ability to win over these constituencies depends on the basic personality and endowment of the leader, but some of it depends on technical knowledge, training, and experience, as well as management style—elements that can be taught and learned.

Finally, in reviewing the several agencies the executive must keep in a happy frame of mind to maintain his position and prosper, it is necessary to mention relations on the *home front.* If the executive's family life is in turmoil or family members are nonsupportive, his office behavior may be impaired, for the enormous demands his job places on his time and energy can easily threaten domestic tranquility. Wife and children may be neglected or drawn into tensions and strivings of the administrator's official life, which they either may be unwilling or unsuited to bear. These are highly personal matters that the administrator must recognize and work out with members of his family. Of all the fronts with which the administrator must be concerned, relations on the home front often are most decisive in determining success or failure on the job and frequently determine the point at which the administrator decides to terminate his or her tenure.

The Media

The media deserves special comment because administrators often do business with it. They would do well to meet representatives of all levels of the media, both editors and reporters. From this contact, they will learn what kinds of information the media expect from them on a regular basis and what plans for public exposure of the institution are afoot—good or bad. The media may want to know about fires, deaths, suicides, new programs or projects, honors conferred on staff—all perhaps to be reported benignly. On the other hand, the media may have complaints against the hospital from patients, families, friends, employees, or legislators that are likely to be reported in such a manner as to promote sales of newspapers. Moreover, not all information will be reported accurately. If and when critics level unfair charges at the institution, tinged with emotionalism and distortion, it behooves the administrator to respond with objective facts and figures. Although the aggrieved may let fly with anger and inaccurate or unjust accusations, it is the job of the administrator to respond with balanced judgment and without malice.

The Administrator as Moderator

From what has been said so far, the reader will infer that the task of the administrator, manager, or leader today emphasizes more than ever before skills of mediation, collaboration, coordination, and the ability to win by charm, expertise, knowledge, or personal charisma the willingness of diverse groups to work together. Gone are the days when administrators sat behind their desks, developing plans and giving orders that usually were followed with little question. Today, administrators must bring people together, present them with issues and problems

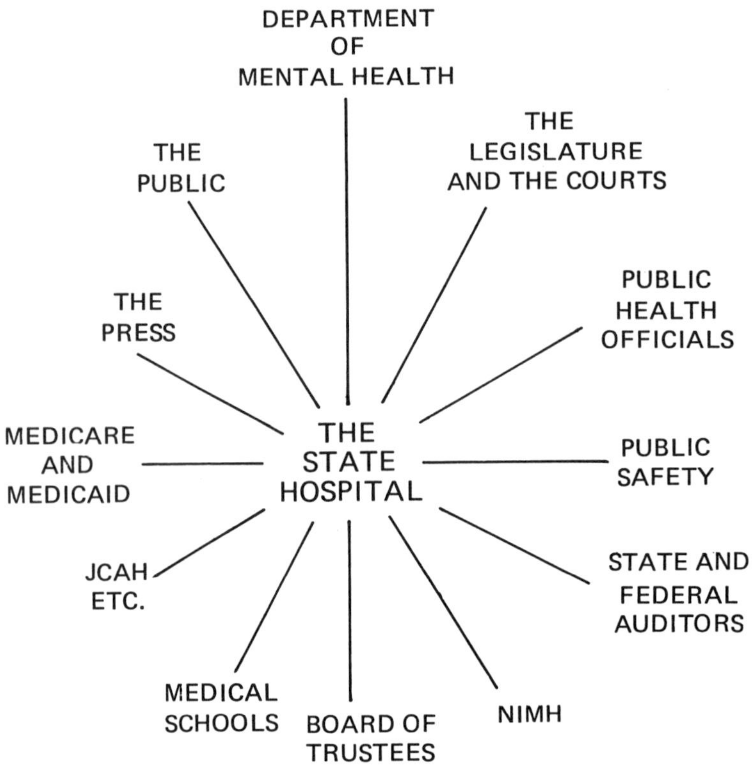

Figure 15-1. The web of accountability.

to be worked out, and invite input from all sources. They then must help fashion a master plan and implement it while keeping their various groups apprised of progress as well as difficulties encountered along the way. It is this moderator-type role that an aspiring administrator must adopt and feel comfortable with in many, if not most, activities, whether his or her title is mental health "director," "superintendent," or "chief executive officer."

Each administrative post is surrounded by a circle of agencies with which the administrator must contend. As from the center of a wheel, spokes emanate from the mental health agency to a variety of other offices or agencies, and the two-way communication between any and all elements constitutes the essence of administrative life. As administrator of a state hospital (Boston State Hospital, 1963–1967), the important offices in the author's life were as represented in Figure 15-1.

The department of mental health and the board of trustees were the author's official appointing officers, although after participating in the appointment, the trustees were mainly advisory. Public health officials inspected the hospital regularly for sanitation and food handling, and public safety officials inspected for adherence to fire prevention standards. State auditors regularly scrutinized books for proper handling of funds and other assets, and federal auditors scrutinized all federal grants. We were heavily involved with local citizens both in relation to their generous volunteer contributions to the hospital and as representatives of the community. Two medical schools utilized the hospital for training and research, bestowing academic titles on some of the staff.

THE POLITICAL SYSTEM AND THE POLITICIANS

An administrator who moves into a political system may be surprised to learn how different that system is from the academic and clinical systems in which he has previously worked. The pursuit of politics is an intensely adversarial game. Opposite parties are in perpetual war for power and control. Each politician belongs to a party that is seeking to diminish, embarrass, or unseat members of the opposite party. In this game, truth and justice sometimes may be sacrificed to personal aggrandizement. Often *ad hominem* charges and accusations take the place of the search for truth, and service to one's constituents takes a back seat to gratifying narcissistic needs. The administrator who aspires to high levels of government is thrust into this world. He must understand how this political system works and realize he cannot change it to a more professionally oriented system such as the one he has been used to. Nor can he discard the values of his own profession and descend to political gutter tactics. Either road may render him ineffective in his primary task of attracting resources and promoting interest on behalf of mentally ill and retarded persons.

The administrator will note that the political system is more or less characterized by three elements: (1) a search for power, (2) an ambience of suspiciousness, and (3) an ambience of materialism.

Power is often the dominant motif of the political system. Power resides in voter strength and in the politician's reputation as able fighter, aggressive champion of the people, and bold reformer. Power is accrued also by membership on important committees, particularly those that allocate resources (ways and means), decide crucial questions (judicial committee), or investigate wrongdoing. Power also is enhanced by increasing one's name recognition; appearances before the public are, thus, all important, and newspaper space and radio and TV time are much coveted. The need for power competes actively with the desire to serve one's constituents and to follow higher ideals of true statesmanship.

In the political system, there is much suspiciousness concerning the motives of the various actors. Each person is assumed to be interested primarily in serving himself or his immediate band of supporters. Higher motives are regarded with skepticism. The climate of suspiciousness is linked with an ambience of materialism. In governmental systems, people seem to work for material gain—money, security, higher position, vacations, and the accoutrements of status—whereas altruism, love of scholarship and learning, search for truth, or dedication to the health and welfare of one's fellow man seem to be more highly valued in hospital and academic settings.

Again, administrators are challenged to accept this state of affairs and to show by their actions that their own value systems remain intact, although they are able to do business with political types who march to another drummer. They cannot, however, be disdainful or supercilious with respect to their political associates, for politicians also believe they are professionals who serve their public well. But in order to do so, they feel they must be able to sustain themselves in a rough-and-tumble world.

Political Types

Working in the psychopolitical sphere, the author learned that although politicians vary greatly in intelligence, education, personality, and motivation, they can be classified into five general categories.

1. The most common brand of politician includes those who have risen through the ranks by subordinating themselves to the machine, becoming useful and experienced in the technology of vote getting, knocking on doors if necessary, and generally serving their party faithfully. They have been brought up in the world of hard knocks and have no illusions about the pathways to power and influence.
2. A second type of politician comes to notice by serving one of the agencies of government that supports the executive branch. He has thereby become an expert in roads, fisheries, welfare, veterans' affairs, and so on, and may have learned about administration by serving as a member of the governor's cabinet. By virtue of effective service and an attractive personality, such an individual may move from the professional ladder to the political ladder—in other words, move from appointive to elective office. Such a person is more likely than other politicians to be sensitive to the problems of a professional department in a political world and therefore may be of special value to a health administrator at the state or federal level. It is important to point out here that rarely do mental health professionals seek elective office in this sense and thus are not usually seen as potential competitors by these professional politicians.
3. A third political type is perhaps rarer than the first two. Reference is made to the man or woman from a distinguished or affluent family with a history of public service who sees a political career as an opportunity for leadership to advance the nation's social welfare. Rather than occupy their time managing the estate accumulated by forebears, becoming an important functionary in a family business, or simply clipping coupons, they aspire in an idealistic way to benefit mankind. Some of these individuals do well in the political arena and eventually rise to positions of political power and prestige. They may be excellent allies to mental health professionals caring for the sick and powerless.
4. Still another category includes those individuals without prior governmental experience or service who become well known by occupying highly visible situations or occupations and who, by personality or charisma, earn the respect and affection of the people. Without formal political credentials, in a hop, skip, and jump, they are elected to political office. This category would include such persons as Ronald Reagan, Ted Kennedy, and John Glenn. Since they do not owe their good fortune to political allies and supporters, they may feel relatively free to pursue a statesman's course. They, too, may therefore be of special assistance to the health administrator.
5. Finally, throughout history, there has existed a special category of politicians to whom might be assigned the designation "defenders of the republic." These are the soldiers who have earned the respect and affection of their

countrymen through their courage, leadership, and success in fighting our nation's battles. Out of affection, a feeling of debt, or belief that administrative skills demonstrated in battle may be transferable to the political scene, the country turns to these leaders in times of peace. George Washington is, of course, the prototype of this group, which includes, as well, Andrew Jackson, William Harrison, Zachary Taylor, Ulysses Grant, Benjamin Harrison, and Dwight Eisenhower. Local heroes of combat also may be honored similarly.

The Politician as an Individual

What is the politician like as an individual? In 1978 we tried to formulate an answer:[1]

> The fact is that politicians *as individuals* are about as easy to get along with as one's professional colleagues. They are generally more open about their feelings, more extroverted, more anxious to do a favor and earn gratitude, more interested in grabbing power, and more open about enjoying the limelight than are our professional colleagues. Their likes and dislikes are more obvious and explicit. If they are out to stab you in the back, they may tell you so to your face. Medical colleagues are more subtle, working their will through the fine politics of the hospital and academic community, where promotions, rank, and honors are the ultimate prizes instead of votes.
>
> The politician is a gambler; the professional wants security. The politician likes camaraderie, drinking in a group, living like a soldier of fortune. The professional is more serious-minded and his conduct and actions are guarded, especially in the social sphere.*

Although it appears that in many ways the politician and the professional are opposites, it is still necessry for them to work together for the public good. It is the politician in the long run who often supplies the professional with sanction to do his job and in many instances with the necessary resources. We should remind ourselves that this liaison is very old and in some situations has reached very high levels of effectiveness.

LEGISLATED THERAPY

In recent years, the treatment of patients as well as the work of doctors and other professionals have come under increasing scrutiny of parents, groups of interested citizens, the press, the legislature, and the courts. Efforts of the legislature to monitor and oversee the work of medical institutions under governmental aegis have led to a spate of laws, rules, and regulations, to which the name "legislated therapy" has been applied. Sometimes these laws appear to be very well thought out and to include an enlightened view of medicine as well as a deep commitment to upgrade the quality of care given the poor and indigent. At other times, the legislature appears to overreact to public uproar, newspaper sensationalism, or unverified charges and accusations made by angry, unconscionable people.

---

*From Greenblatt M: Psychopolitics. New York, Grune & Stratton, 1977, p 19. With permission.

The national legislation developed after 1963, inspired by the Joint Commission on Mental Health and Illness, supported by the American Psychiatric Association, the NIMH, and especially by President John F. Kennedy, set the nation on a "bold new approach" to the treatment of the mentally ill and retarded. The federal legislation was followed by well-laid plans at the state level to depopulate overcrowded state and federal hospitals, to develop transitional facilities and community-based operations, and to mobilize paraprofessionals and indigenous helpers. In many states, great advances were made in upgrading the level of care within hospitals by allocating more funds to mental health facilities, by expanding rights of patients, and by intensifying staff training.

On the other hand, each year at the state level many bills bearing on the function of the mental health department had to be carefully analyzed and followed through by administrators because their passage would have eroded programs or made little or no contribution to improving the mental health system. For example, because a bill prohibiting female employees of the Commonwealth of Massachusetts from lifting weights of more than 50 lbs seriously affected their work with bedridden patients who had to be moved or lifted, opposition by mental health professionals was mounted, and the bill was never passed.

Another bill stipulated that unmarried pregnant females should be committed to a mental hospital for 90 days. Still another bill would have prohibited the housing of patients of both sexes in the same building of a state hospital. One proposal was aimed at prohibiting "outside professional affiliations" of commissioner, assistant commissioners, and superintendents of facilities administered by the department of mental health. Bills have been introduced seriously curtailing the ability of research personnel to do their work. Should such bills pass, they would tend to deprofessionalize a department of mental health and make care and treatment of patients subordinate to vagaries of political intervention. During the author's tenure as commissioner, literally dozens of proposed bills each year could have impaired functioning of the department of mental health. Occasional bills, indeed, were aimed at phasing out the department altogether.

Space does not permit discussion of all the technical maneuvers to get unwanted bills tabled, postponed, relegated to study, held up in the third reading, held over to the next session, or vetoed by the governor. But careful analysis of each bill, consultation with legal talent, advice from experts on political infighting, and constant watchdogging were necessary; and at hearings the department was expected to present a rational and objective point of view on each proposal.

Today the health establishment must share its goals and problems with many other groups, for the public feels its health is too important to be left to doctors or to health professionals generally. Like it or not, the administrator must accept the citizen as a partner in planning for carrying out the advance of medicine.

PATRONAGE

Since administrators control jobs and services provided by their facilities, they inevitably find themselves pressured by persons seeking one or both of these emoluments. Executive watchers are quick to classify administrators as "susceptible to pressure or persuasion," "fair-minded and just," "playing favorites," and so on, and there are those who are ready to capitalize on any manifest weakness or vulnerability. Such persons may be seeking work opportunities, promotions, or special consideration in jobs or preferential treatment for clients who are friends or relatives. When one presides over valued resources, such pressures are inescapable.

Pressure for favors for friends and constituents escalates when unemployment is high and when politicians are gearing up for an election year. A job found may mean a whole family of votes plus a loyal follower who can be solicited to recruit voters on election night. In some states, a formal office exists to do favors for prospective voters. Sometimes designated as the office of State Service, it may function as a place in which a political party dispenses favors to its constituents.

Everything may run reasonably smoothly as long as the office serves mainly as an employment center. Things may be less satisfactory, however, if the State Service office tries to dictate who will be employed, especially against the wishes of a respected superintendent or clinic director. If second-rate people are forced into vacant slots, a hospital's effectiveness can be severely damaged. Even a slight reduction in level of care may lead to more accidents, injuries, suicides, or deaths—with many attendant woes. It is therefore incumbent on the health administrator to stand his ground in support of the "best man or woman" principle even if it means loss of his own job. Indeed, it should be an axiom of state and federal administration that no one should become a candidate to fill a high-level "psychopolitical" job if he or she is likely to become dependent on it. One of the virtues of doctors as top-level administrators is that in such a political crisis they have "doctoring" to fall back on. If one has recourse to other satisfactory employment, one may hold tenaciously to important principles.

If the administrator is running a hospital with a fine reputation or one that is introducing new programs highly desired by the public —programs in alcoholism, drug dependency, or adolescent or children's disorders, for example—the pressure for admission to hospital beds may be extraordinary. Here unwary administrators may fall into several traps: (1) They may yield to political pressures to admit favored citizens out of order, to a preferred ward, or to a preferred doctor or medical team. As a result, they achieve in record time reputations for weakness and unfairness. (2) They may relax their criteria for admissions so as to overload and crowd their wards. This is, indeed, a grievous error, for once staff becomes overburdened, quality of care suffers, staff absenteeism grows, and recruitment of new staff becomes more difficult. This was the plague of the old state hospital. Administrators allowed legislative and public pressures to get the better of them; thus, over the years, hospitals deteriorated, while legislators failed to provide adequate space, staff, or establish new institutions. The simple rule worth following is "Never admit a patient you cannot treat well."

The level of pressure exerted by individuals asking for favoritism concerning patient services varies greatly, but there is always tendency to suggest that a case constitutes an emergency for which there is no alternative but immediate admission to the hospital or clinic. Sometimes the prospective recipient is someone who significantly aided a legislator in the last election. Sometimes it is the legislator's own sick family member for whom the favor is requested.

An administrator can make several serious errors under these conditions:

1. Assign the problem to a person low in the administrative hierarchy and stay out of the action. This is a poor strategy since the petitioner is insulted, gets angry, and becomes vindictive.
2. Refuse to see the patient or to have him seen by a highly qualified person.
3. Appear to be hurried or have other important business to attend to when explaining the best way to treat the patient. (Admission may not always be the best alternative.)
4. Yield to threats.

When requests for favors are handled properly and the situation explained clearly, often the legislator (petitioner), if given sufficient time, will cooperate in finding other alternatives for treating the patient. It is even possible he will come to understand the administrator's problems so well that he thereafter becomes a comrade in arms rather than an angry enemy.

Yet sometimes it is necessary to accommodate to the stern realities of psychopolitical life:

> A total and successful exclusion of all political accommodation can lead to a loss of support, power and [maybe] friendships of prestigious political figures on whom one depends for the successful operation of a [state] service. . . . Never yielding earns one a reputation for rigidity and may isolate the system from access to resources; yet, yielding too often results in a decline of respect from one's professional colleagues and, yes, from politicians, too.*

REFERENCES

1. Greenblatt M: Psychopolitics. New York, Grune & Stratton, 1977, p 19, 57

SUGGESTED READINGS

Argyris C: Interpersonal competence and organizational effectiveness. Irwin-Dorsey Series in Behavioral Science in Business. Homewood, Ill, Irwin-Dorsey Press, 1962

Arnhoff F: Social consequences of policy towards mental illness. Science 188:1277–1281

Arthur RJ: Social psychiatry: an overview. Am J Psychiatry 130:841–849, 1973

Bachrach LL: Deinstitutionalization: An analytical review and social perspective. National Institute of Mental Health, Series D, No. 4, US Department of Health, Education, and Welfare, Publication No. (ADM) 76-351, 1976

Barnard CI: The Function of the Executive. Cambridge, Mass, Harvard University Press, 1948

Barton WE: Administration in Psychiatry. Springfield, Ill, Thomas, 1962

Barton WE: Vanishing American—mental hospital administrators and commissioners. Ment Hosp 13:55–61, 1962

Bennis WG: Changing Organizations. New York, McGraw-Hill, 1966

Black BJ: The workaday world: some problems in return of mental patients to the community, in Greenblatt M, Levinson DJ, Williams RH (eds): The Patient and the Mental Hospital. Glencoe, Ill, Free Press, 1957

Blum RH, Funkhouser ML: Legislators' view of alcoholism. Q J Studies Alcohol 26:666–669, 1965

Bockover JS: Moral Treatment in Community Mental Health. New York, Springer, 1972

Brooks GW: Opening a rehabilitation house, in Greenblatt M, Simon B (eds): Rehabilitation of the Mentally Ill: Social and Economic Aspects. Publication No. 58. Washington D.C., American Association for the Advancement of Science, 1959

*From Greenblatt M: Psychopolitics. New York, Grune & Stratton, 1977, p 57. With permission.

Bryan WA: Administrative Psychiatry. New York, Norton, 1936
Budson RD: Legal dimensions of the psychiatric halfway house. Community Ment Health J 11:316–324, 1975
Budson RD: The Psychiatric Halfway House: Multiple Systems and Individual Program. Pittsburgh, University of Pittsburgh Press, 1978
Cannon MS: The Halfway House as an Alternative to Hospitalization. Division of Biometry, Survey and Reports Branch. Washington D.C., National Institute of Mental Health, 1974
Caplan G: Principles of Preventive Psychiatry. New York, Basic Books, 1964
Caudill W: Social processes in a collective disturbance, in Greenblatt M, Levinson DJ, Williams RH (eds): The Patient and the Mental Hospital. Glencoe, Ill, Free Press, 1957
Chafetz ME: People and process—a psychopolitical case study. Psychiat Ann 6:108–119, 1976
Christie R, Geis FL: Studies in Machiavelliansim. New York, Academic Press, 1970
Ennis B: The impact of litigation on the future of the state hospital, in Zusman J, Bertsch EF (eds): The Future Role of the State Hospital. Lexington, Mass, Lexington Books, 1975
Feldman S, Goldstein C, Offit J: Mental Health Administration: An Annotated Bibliography. Washington D.C., Department of Health, Education, and Welfare, 1980
Gilbert DC, Levinson DJ: "Custodialism" and "humanism" in mental hospital structure and in staff ideology, in Greenblatt M, Levinson DJ, Williams RD (eds): The Patient and the Mental Hospital. Glencoe, Ill, Free Press, 1957
Goffman E: On the characteristics of total institutions, in Asylums: Essays on the Social Situation of Mental Patients and Other Inmates. New York, Anchor Books, 1961
Greenblatt M: The psychiatrist as social system clinician, in Greenblatt M, Levinson DJ, William RH (eds): The Patient and the Mental Hospital. Glencoe, Ill, Free Press, 1957, pp 317–326
Greenblatt M. Introduction, in Greenblatt M, Emery PE, Glueck BC, Jr (eds): Poverty and Mental Health. Washington D.C., American Psychiatric Association, 1967
Greenblatt M: Historical forces affecting the closing of state mental hospitals, in Proceedings of a Conference on the Closing of State Mental Hospital, "Where is my home?" Prepared by Plog Research, Inc., and Stanford Research Institute, April 1974, pp 3–17
Greenblatt M: Administrative psychiatry, in Freedman AM, Kaplan HI, Sadock, BJ (eds): Comprehensive Textbook of Psychiatry—II. Baltimore, Williams & Wilkins, 1975, pp 2443–2454
Greenblatt M, Glazier E: Some major issues in the closing of the hospitals, in Ahmed PI, Plog SC (eds): State Mental Hospitals: What Happens When They Close? New York, Plenum, 1976, pp 127–139
Greenblatt M, Levinson DJ, William RH (eds): The Patient and the Mental Hospital. Glencoe, Ill, Free Press, 1957
Greenblatt M, Sharaf MR, Stone EM: Dynamics of Institutional Change. Pittsburgh, University of Pittsburgh Press, 1971
Greenblatt M, Orleans SO: Illustrious psychiatric administrators. Am J Psychiatry 134:626–630, 1977
Greenblatt M, York RH, Brown EL: From Custodial to Therapeutic Patient Care in Mental Hospitals. New York, Russell Sage Foundation, 1955
Halleck SL: The Politics of Therapy. New York, Science House, 1971
Hodgson RC, Levinson DJ, Zalesnik A: The Executive Role Constellation. Cambridge, Mass, Harvard Business School, Division of Research, 1965
Hollingshead AB, Redlich FC: Social Class and Mental Illness. New York, Wiley, 1958
Joint Commission on Mental Illness and Health: Action for Mental Health. New York, Basic Books, 1961
Jones M: The Therapeutic Community. New York, Basic Books, 1953
Kernberg OF: Leadership and organizational functioning: organizational regression. I J Group Psychother 28:3–25, 1978
Kotin J, Sharaf M: Management succession and administrative style. Psychiatry 30:237–248, 1967
Lasswell HD: Psychopathology and Politics. New York, Viking Press, 1960, pp 74–77
Levinson DJ, Klerman, GL: The clinician-executive. Some problematic issues for the psychiatrist in mental health organizations. Psychiatry 30:3–15, 1967
McGregor D: The Human Side of Enterprise. New York, McGraw-Hill, 1960
Pattison EM: Young psychiatrist administrators. Presented at the 125th Annual Meeting, American Psychiatric Association, May 1972
Reese WG: An essay on administration. Am J Psychiatry 128:10, 1972

Cesar L. Benarroche, M.D.
Boris M. Astrachan, M.D.

16

Interprofessional Role Relationships

Facility administrators are concerned with structuring the division of labor in order to accomplish tasks and with arranging for the division of authority in order to monitor and enhance the quality of work. These efforts are complicated in professional organizations in which members of various disciplinary groups retain significant individual autonomy and may even compete with members of other groups for control over the nature of work.

In mental health organizations, the development of multidisciplinary teams for the evaluation and treatment of the mentally ill has had a salutary impact on the accessibility, quality, and range of services delivered. This continuing evolution has been plagued, however, by role blurring, high status rivalry, impaired decision making, low satisfaction, and perturbed patient care.[1,2] More recently, it has been suggested that "the roles of psychiatry are sometimes seen as diffuse by colleagues in the medical and academic community. It is not always clear where psychiatry leaves off and other non-medical mental health professions begin."[3]

Freidson[4] has described medicine's preeminent role among the health professions and the manner in which it defines its own work as well as the domain of other health professions by virtue of medicine's emphasis on its scientific base, ethical codes, intensive training, and internal monitoring.

Work in mental health settings is influenced by the complex relationships that exist and evolve among the various professional groups. To some extent, these relationships are affected by group membership characteristics (e.g., physicians tend to be male, white, of upper-middle-class background; nurses tend to be female, to have a higher percentage of minority group members than physicians, and to be of lower-middle-class backgrounds), diverse clinical and theoretical perspectives, and interpersonal and group dynamics.

The most critical issues for the administrator in defining interprofessional relationships in mental health organizations, however, are role related and include (1) the legal and ethical responsibilities of the interacting professionals; (2) the definition of psychiatric tasks and perspectives and clarity about the capacity of the various professions to function autonomously in each area; and (3) an awareness of the impact of organizational systems on the shaping of role transactions.

The authors will explore interprofessional role relationships first by defining some models for such relationships. We then present an overview of the task framework that we have evolved[5] that may facilitate the analysis of the role relationships in organized settings. Finally, we address some particularly confounded role relationships like the so-called medical backup, the psychotherapy supervisor, and the clinician–administrator. We write from the perspective of psychiatrists, but we believe that our analytic framework is generally useful to understanding such relationships.

MODELS OF INTERPROFESSIONAL RELATIONSHIPS

Interprofessional role relationships can be classified as bureaucratic, technical (collaborative, consultative, and supervisory), and prescriptive.

Bureaucratic Relationship

This is a hierarchical, administrative interaction aimed at the superintending or management of affairs within an organizational setting. In the mental health field, decisions about hiring or firing, scheduling, assignment of tasks, elaboration and implementation of policies, including patient-care-related ones (i.e., type and number of patients to be treated, nature and frequency of charting activities), all fall into this category.

Technical Relationships

These relationships are defined by the reciprocal responsibilities of the relating professionals, the nature of their tasks, and the extent to which they can, within the context of law and by virtue of training and experience, function independently (see Figure 16-1).

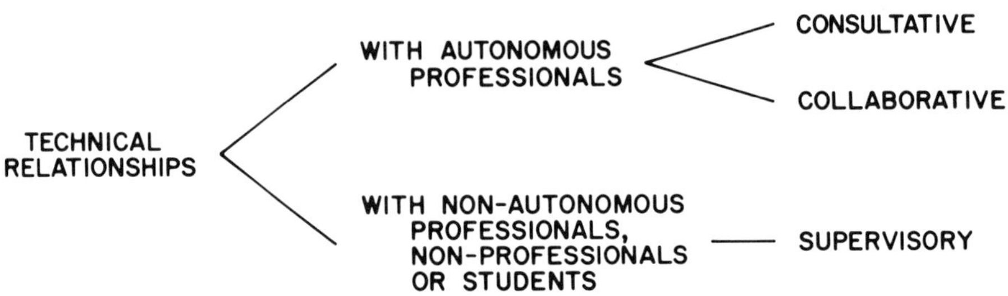

Figure 16-1 Nature of technical relationships.

Consultative Relationship

In this model (see Figure 16-2), an independent professional is responsible for patient care and requests assistance from another independent professional (e.g., two physicians, two psychologists, or a physician requesting psychological consul-

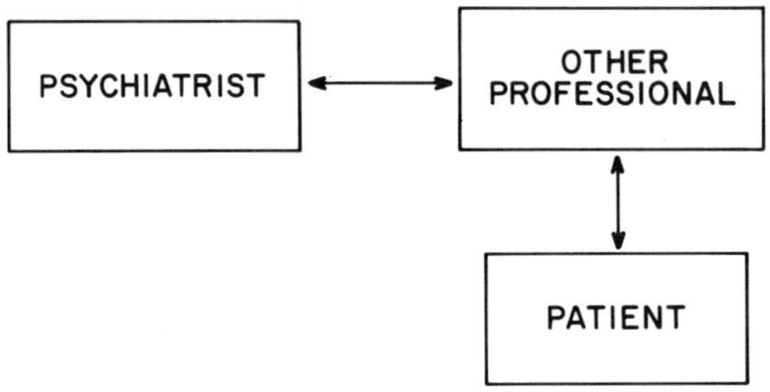

Figure 16-2. Consultative relationship.

tation, etc.). The consultant may or may not see the patient, but the client is the other professional, and the consultant usually does not leave orders (unless this has been previously agreed upon), but rather makes an assessment of the patient focusing on a particular area of expertise (e.g., psychopharmacological evaluation or casework). The patient usually pays directly or indirectly for the consultation, but the recommendations are made not to the patient but to the professional requesting the consultation, who is not required to follow the advice. (See also Chapter 1.)

Obviously, this model works if the professionals respect one another and are reasonably comfortable about one another's competency and ethical standards. When a consultant believes that inadequate care is being given, he has a responsibility both to the professional who asked for help and to the patient, but the responsibility to the patient must transcend that to the consultee.

Collaborative Relationship

In this form of interaction, two professionals, each capable of independent function within defined technical areas, have individual relationships to a patient (see Figure 16-3).

Each professional is independently responsible for the exercise of his or her skills insofar as they apply to the care of the patient (e.g., a therapist–administrator split in a hospital setting; a psychologist providing psychotherapy; a psychiatrist, medical backup). Each professional has responsibilities to the patient, and the patient must be fully informed of the nature of those responsibilities. If either professional has questions about the nature of care delivered, there is a joint

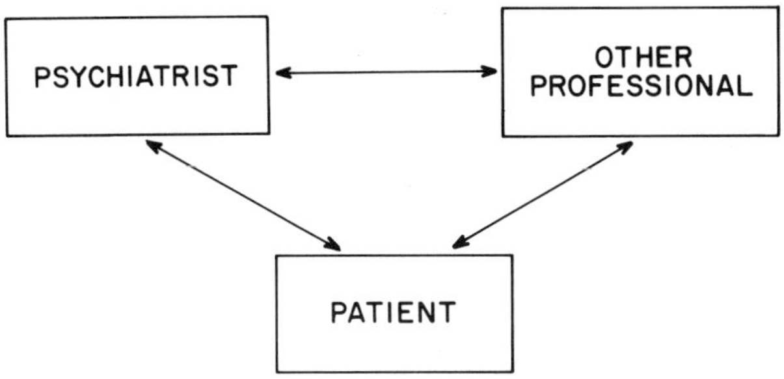

Figure 16-3. Collaborative relationship.

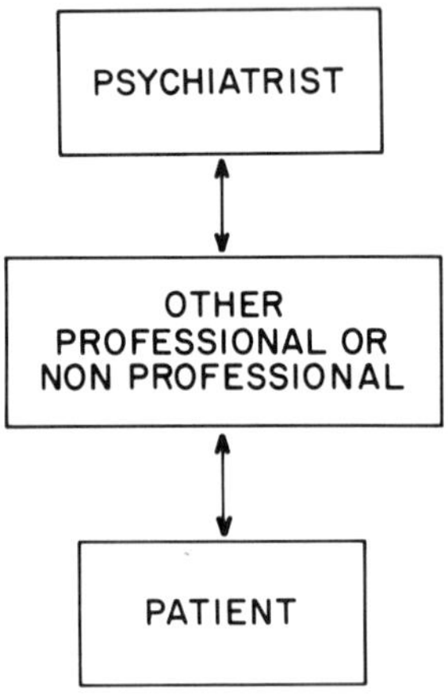

Figure 16-4. Supervisory relationship.

responsibility to try and resolve issues in the collaboration. Once again, the primary responsibility must be to the patient.

Supervisory Relationship

In this type of interaction, one professional has responsibility for the work of another professional, nonprofessional, or student (see Figure 16-4). This responsibility may exist within disciplinary channels or may cross disciplinary boundaries. The supervisee may be an employee of the supervisor or of an institution, but the reciprocal roles are defined within an organizational context. The employing organization (or professional) has responsibility for determining the skill levels of supervisee and supervisor as well as for ensuring adequate lines of communication between the administration and the supervisors. By definition, the supervisor provides professional direction and ongoing active guidance. Most professionals, however, view supervision as an important educational intervention but express discomfort about its administrative component.[6] The physician who supervises is responsible (both ethically and legally) for the quality of the services delivered due to the *actual or apparent control* that he or she exercises over the supervisee.[7] Consequently, the supervisor must ensure that the patient is informed about the existence and nature of the supervisory relationship as well as of any subsequent changes in the supervisory contract.

When training is an *additional* objective of supervision, the supervisor, without abrogating his or her full responsibility for the treatment provided, must modulate the degree of directiveness in the relationship in order to foster the clinical competency of the trainee. Although this modulation of guidance may seem to suggest collaborative or consultative models, didactic supervisors always retain responsibility for adequate treatment implementation and may incur a "vicarious liability."[7] When the professional is sufficiently trained and qualified so as to be responsible individually for the care of the patient both clinically and from a medicolegal perspective, the appropriate model for interprofessional relationship is ongoing consultation and not supervision.

Relationship by Prescription

The prototypical model of interprofessional role relationships is that of the doctor and the nurse within the general hospital. This unique type of interaction has both bureaucratic and technical qualities and is rooted historically in the relationship of nursing to medicine and in the hierarchical structure of nursing. Within the hospital or organized health care institution, the physician usually acts as an independent practitioner who has responsibility for the diagnosis and treatment of patients. The nurse functions within a hierarchical professional structure that is responsible for patient management and care. Individual nurses are charged with carrying out medical orders in ways that are defined by nursing practice acts and institutional nursing procedures. The physician who writes an order usually does not seek to define the actions of a particular nurse. Rather, his or her orders will be processed by nurses functioning in a defined hierarchical structure. In these activities, nurses engage in complex and highly technical diagnostic and therapeutic tasks. In the reciprocal relationship of physician and nurse, each retains responsibility for carrying out his or her specific patient care obligations. Furthermore, the nurse has a duty to question physician orders when he or she believes carrying out those orders may be injurious to the patient.

Psychiatrists and nurses become very familiar with this type of relationship during their medical and nursing training. The incorporation of other mental health professionals into the medical-nursing teams has at times led to inappropriate attempts to replicate the physician–nurse relationship among members of other disciplines. Moreover, the evolution of the role of a nurse clinician as an autonomous professional has required some readjustment of role expectations from both physician and nurses.

ROLE RELATIONSHIPS IN ORGANIZATIONAL SETTINGS

The association between intrastaff conflict and perturbed patient care has long been acknowledged.[8,9] The failure to acknowledge, understand, and accommodate explicitly to the multiple and sometimes overlapping bureaucratic, technical, and prescriptive relationships plays a significant role in intrastaff tensions. The use of inappropriate models for role relationships may lead to confusion about the delegation of authority and responsibility, to the delegation of responsibility without authority, to the abrogation of responsibility and/or authority, and even to staff "burnout."

Many psychiatric facilities routinely confound bureaucratic, technical, and prescriptive relationships. With some legitimacy, psychiatric administrators insist that the structure of the treatment environment significantly impacts on patient care and thus requires direct management. Psychiatrist–administrators therefore attempt to require direct accountability of disciplinary chiefs to unit or service directors for their discipline-based unit treatment activities. In this manner, bureaucratic authority is superimosed on technical and prescriptive relationships.

Outpatient settings regularly confound various forms of authority. Typically, there is almost an blind assumption of responsibility for monitoring patient care by the bureaucratic leadership. In such cases, the outpatient unit director is responsible for the care provided by other professionals, trainees, and nonprofessionals who receive only limited supervision (usually directed toward a very small percentage of their total case load) and administrative guidance by senior staff. In many settings, particularly those affiliated with training programs, some of the work is supervised (primarily for educational purposes) by professionals who are not integrally connected with the unit, who perceive their work as performed within a consultative framework, and who do not routinely interact with the unit administration. Administrative monitoring, training, and direction of treatment may thus be quite separated and responsibility for patient care may become dangerously diffuse. Professionals have at times assumed that their supervision of allied health workers is primarily an educational function and thus have ignored major administrative issues with serious consequences.[10]

Ignoring either the monitoring or didactic aspects of supervision or excessively emphasizing one at the expense of the other may lead to limited or even impeded patient care and serious administrative problems. Clinicians who assume that the patient is a collaborator in the treatment process view therapy as a private, circumscribed activity. Supervision that seeks monitoring is then predictably perceived as an interference in the therapy (or as a diabolical method of evaluating staff performance) that inevitably strains the supervisory relationship. Clinical supervisors do have real responsibility for assessing the competency and the capacity for adequate clinical work of supervisees. Ignoring this responsibility may allow for the perpetuation of poor clinical practice.

PSYCHIATRIC TASKS AND PERSPECTIVES

It may be that greater clarity about professional tasks will facilitate attempts to order interprofessional role relationships more adequately. In prior work, we have defined four major tasks of psychiatry and identified the perspectives required of each task.[5,11] These tasks are interconnected but separable. They are all within the legitimate domain of practice. The tasks and their related perspectives are as follows:

1. Diagnosing, curing, and limiting *illness*—the *medical* perspective
2. Reducing *defect* and enabling those with defect to live more normal lives—the *rehabilitative perspective*
3. Controlling *socially deviant behavior*—the *societal-legal perspective*
4. Fostering *growth and competence*—the *educative-developmental perspective*

The Medical Perspective

Central to work from the medical perspective is the concept of *disease*. Those who are served are identified as patients. The work of this area is to evaluate and diagnose the patient's illness and to provide appropriate treatment. Major concepts include differential diagnosis, symptomatology, pathology, and natural course. In addition to schizophrenia, the major affective disorders and other psychoses, conditions that have been conceptualized and treated as illness by psychiatry, include organic brain syndromes, psychosomatic disorders, and the acute stage of the neuroses and addictions.

In the medical context, overall care of patients is the physician's responsibility. When many individuals are involved in the care of the patient, as in the hospital setting, the physician heads the treatment team and coordinates and supervises the work of other health professionals and allied health workers. Medicine is the prepotent profession in the treatment of disease, although its influence on other groups is limited by established rules and protocols. Integration of curing efforts is by the physician's prescription.

The physician may request consultation from other physicians or other professionals (e.g., psychologist, social worker), and he or she may collaborate in patient care, but the physician retains responsibility for diagnosis and treatment. Other professionals may practice independently in the hospital setting within the framework of their disciplinary expertise and established hospital policy. The admitting physician, however, retains overall responsibility for patient care. Nursing in the general hospital traditionally is responsible for maintaining the environment and providing patient care. In the psychiatric facility, this responsibility is shared to some extent.

The Rehabilitative Perspective

Within a rehabilitative perspective, the primary condition to be dealt with is an *adaptive defect.* A defect is an impairment in functioning. It may have various sources such as genetic, biochemical, traumatic or prenatal disorders, developmental failures, etc. Disease and defect are often interrelated, but they are conceptually distinct. Disease refers to a *disordered organic state,* while defect refers to *inadequate functioning.* Many patients, following acute medical treatment, have some residual defect and require treatment in order to prevent further deterioration, restore functioning, and improve the level of adaptation, In psychiatry, this is often the case with patients suffering from chronic psychotic conditions, chronic organic brain syndromes, symptom neuroses, severe character neuroses, psychosomatic disorders, sexual disorders, and mental retardation.

Medicine plays a major and quite legitimate role in the field of rehabilitation, but it has no monopoly. Several other professions have established roles in this area. In most medical practice, much of the work of rehabilitation is delegated by physicians to others. Following medical diagnosis and acute treatment, specific defects are thus identified and various rehabilitative therapies prescribed. For example, during the treatment of a patient with a stroke, the attending neurologist might request that a psychologist collaborate in treatment designed to rehabilitate the patient.

In psychiatry, the situation is more complicated. A good deal of conflict within psychiatry and between psychiatry and other mental health professions is sustained by widespread confusion about the nature of rehabilitation. Psychiatric patients may require a great many rehabilitative services orchestrated to meet specific needs. Diverse medical, psychological, social, and vocational rehabilitative activities, however, are often combined within a single organizational structure in ways that are confusing to both staff and patients.

In psychiatry, two major rehabilitative approaches have evolved based on theoretical and clinical views about the nature of the defect and the preferred treatment strategies. In the first approach, rehabilitative work follows medical treatment. Its goal is to reduce or correct for defect. The physician prescribes and then may act as a somewhat removed consultant or may directly assume major clinical-administrative responsibilities: diagnosing, prescribing, and coordinating the many diverse elements of a medical treatment program.

A second rehabilitative approach regards psychiatric disorder–defect as developmental in origin. The major goal of the rehabilitative approach that has evolved to deal with such defect is to uncover the developmental bases, to reduce the extent, and to enable the patient to live more effectively with the residual defect. In this approach, psychiatrists engage primarily in psychological and sociopsychological rehabilitation.

In this context, psychotherapy is the major rehabilitative therapy, and it is extensively delivered by nonpsychiatrist professionals: psychologists, psychiatric social workers, nurse clinicians; by professional trainees; and by nonprofessionals. The professional groups identified above spend more time engaged in psychotherapy than in other clinical activities.[12,13] Their work in this area seems to account for much of the interprofessional role blurring and turf battles, particularly since rehabilitative activities, even those strongly identified with medical care, permit—or even encourage—a number of diverse approaches (e.g., optometry vs. ophthalmology, podiatry and orthopedics). Once the focus of treatment has shifted to limitation of defect and/or restoration of function, diverse professionals may act as primary agents in the therapeutic process, with the physician as consultant or even absent from the ongoing treatment program.

Rehabilitative specialists may supervise nonprofessionals who will have major responsibility for the care of the patient (e.g., the psychotherapy of a mental health worker may be supervised by a qualified psychologist, social worker, psychiatrist, etc.), but if ongoing medical treatment or consultation is required, arrangements must be made for the physician to meet regularly with the treatment team so that lines of responsibility and accountability may be kept clean.

The Societal-Legal Perspective

Every society defines the kinds of behavior that it values or tolerates as normative as well as the kinds of behavior that it regards as socially deviant. In our society, psychiatry is often called on by the legal-correctional system in its efforts to control those forms of social deviance that are considered to be the result of mental illness or impairment. The social control task of psychiatry involves treatment of any individual who is committed or diverted to psychiatric care by the legal system. This includes persons with psychotic or severe neurotic disorders who are committed to treatment; those charged with or tried for criminal behavior but diverted to the psychiatric system following a judgment of not guilty for reasons of insanity; those with drug addiction; many forms of sexual deviation; alcoholism; and antisocial character disorders. The state, instead of punishing, intervenes in order to alter behavior. The client's status is, however, extraordinarily limited, and frequently treatment is coercive rather than voluntary.

The relationship of law to psychiatry is complex and unclear. Most work in this task area is rehabilitative in aim. There are, however, inherent tensions between coercion and rehabilitation. Coercion has been most consistently applied in the rehabilitation of drug and alcohol problems. It is less frequent in the rehabilitation of other types of patients. Although we cajole our "treatment resistant" patients in many ways, the ethical standards of practitioners are violated by resort to coercion.

In this area, distinctions between acute medical treatment and rehabilitation have serious implications for practice. The physician has a responsibility to treat patients, to preserve life even if the patient is charged with heinous crimes and is not rehabilitatable. Although we might wish for an equivalent societal commitment to rehabilitation, society has identified no general rights in this area. Within a societal-legal perspective, practitioners may need to act as advocates (on behalf of prospective patients) for the potential efficacy of their endeavors. Clearly, the most problematic interprofessional relationships in this area are between rehabilitation specialists and those other professionals representing the legal-correctional system.

The Educative-Developmental Perspective

From an "educative-developmental" perspective, potential users of service are identified as clients and are regarded as individuals engaged in a search to express their individual capacities more completely. There is emphasis on psychological concepts and individual growth. Although the language of psychopathology may be used here (e.g., clients are sometimes identified as having neurotic symptoms or personality disorders), diagnosis in the formal medical-psychiatric sense is not relevant and may be inhibiting to the work. The primary task is not to treat an illness but to enhance the individual's potential for development. Treatment devolves from an educative philosophy with exploration of *impeded growth*. In this task area, the client is regarded as a person whose psychological growth has been arrested in certain respects but who is capable of attaining full adult growth and maturity. The psychiatrist brings to this work the authority and prestige of medicine, a primary commitment to the patient's interest, and an insistence on ethical practice. The role of educator–healer requires that the therapist be identified as responsible, reliable, and accountable. Professions tend to be granted such trust. Since this perspective is not inherently medical, care also may be provided by clinical and educational psychologists, social workers, nurse clinicians, and other mental health workers.

The clinician does not initiate relationships to other professionals. That is the responsibility of the client. Interprofessional role relationships, if any, are defined by the client.

CONFOUNDED ROLE RELATIONSHIPS

The roles of the medical backup, psychotherapy supervisor, and clinician administrator are typical examples of ambiguously defined, conflict-laden role relationships. The mutual role responsibilities are rarely delineated, and it is often unclear whether it is up to the organization, the professionals involved, or even those who receive services to decide on some informal clarification of the scope of activities of the professionals.

Medical Backup

There is extraordinary variation in this role in psychiatric and mental health organizations. Clinical staff generally expect that the psychiatrist will participate in the assessment and treatment of patients' medical problems (or will arrange for appropriate referral) and will be responsible for the evaluation and monitoring of psychopharmacological therapies. But the "medical backup" role often expands into a variety of other activities, including organizationally required societal-legal tasks that may include assessments for involuntary commitments, evaluations to help determine eligibility for public aid or rehabilitation services, preparation of psychiatric reports for third-party payers, forensic assessments; management tasks, including assessment of and arrangement for the physical containment or isolation of violent or self-injurious patients; and other technical services, like the provision of a second opinion to other mental health workers for diagnostic or treatment purposes.

When a psychiatrist serves as a medical backup, the goal of the interprofessional association is good patient care. In order to assume that responsibility, the physician has to identify (1) the framework in which care will be delivered (from a medical, rehabilitative, or educative-developmental perspective); within each perspective there are varying degrees of autonomy possible for other professionals, and consequently the nature of the appropriate interprofessional relationships may also vary; (2) the training, clinical experience, and credentials of the associated professionals; (3) the patient's characteristics; and (4) the organizational structure of the institution in which care is being delivered (including specifics about lines of accountability for treatment integration and monitoring). Medical backup thus implies a flexible role that has to be adapted to specific circumstances, to the nature and membership of therapeutic teams, and to the demands of organizational settings. Depending on these variables, the psychiatric backup may be involved in prescriptive, collaborative, consultative, or supervisory relationships. Administrators must insist that the role of "medical backup" be defined in ways that protect patient care, identify accountability relationships, allow for the legitimate discharge of medical responsibility, and permit the appropriate level of autonomous or supervised practice of the other professional.

The role of medical backup is further complicated when the primary clinician is not a professional and receives therapy supervision from a different professional than the psychiatrist acting as medical backup. This has potentially major consequences for accountability. In such circumstances, the psychiatrist may have to interact directly (and frequently) with the other professional (as a collaborator) or, if such is not possible, may have to insist on directly assuming responsibility for patient care activities. In this circumstance, the psychiatrist must insist on direct supervisory responsibility over the nonprofessional. This clearly leads to difficulties, as the other supervisory professional will experience serious constriction of his or her authority.

The authority of the nonmedical supervisor is at times undercut when the psychiatrist is the medical backup for a psychiatric nurse. For example, in the case of a nurse (supervised by a psychologist) who is treating a schizophrenic outpatient, a combination of consultative and prescriptive relationships is established when a nurse calls the psychiatrist, indicates that the patient is exhibiting a dystonic reaction, and the physician orders an anticholinergic agent. In this case, the special interrelationship between nurses and physicians allows for this unique transaction that has the potential problem of making the psychologist feel excluded and bypassed.

The medical backup role is often a confounded one because it encompasses a variety of interdisciplinary models of relating around a multiplicity of tasks.

Psychotherapy Supervision

While the medical backup role lacks definition in the areas of agreed upon relationships and tasks, confusion in regard to the role of psychotherapy supervisor reflects the juxtaposition of differing perspectives of care in the treatment of an individual patient and the ambiguous assumption of responsibility for the course of treatment by the therapy supervisor. When the clinician being supervised has the capacity for independet professional functioning and the task of supervision is primarily educational, the appropriate model is consultative (even when the word supervision is used).

Psychotherapy can be conducted within the framework of any of the perspectives previously defined. Supervisors who prefer to work in a specific perspective, however, may tailor their supervision of particular cases more to the dictates of their preferred theory than to the needs of patients.

Clinicians who supervise from an educational-developmental perspective view psychotherapy as the pre-eminent mode of intervention and somatic treatments as rather crude, second-rate, or even "last-resort" types of approaches. Adherents to this perspective predictably conceptualize and conduct supervision utilizing a similar framework whereby supervision is seen as a growth-inducing endeavor for the supervisee and the patient (generally in that order). Learning is then emphasized, and active interventions like the direct observation of psychotherapy sessions are frowned on as intrusive or as potential impediments to the supervisee's maturation. This model of supervision tends to ignore the issue of responsibility of the supervisor for serious errors in patient care management, since in this area supervisors perceive themselves as educators, who owe no legal duty of care to students.[7]

Physicians supervising psychotherapy within a medical perspective are often confused about the extent of their responsibilities. They are aware of the fact that they share responsibility for the diagnosis and treatment of the patient's disease, but their relationship with other professionals (i.e., clinical unit administrators, nonmedical supervisors of clinicians providing other modalities of treatment to the same patient) is often confused. The psychiatrist who supervises primarily within the context of a medical perspective may all too frequently feel compelled to assume a supervisory role toward others involved in the treatment program. For example, the psychiatrist supervisor of a nonmedical clinician treating a manipulative borderline patient who is demanding minor tranquilizers, may become involved directly with the physician providing medical backup and seek to coordinate the multiple aspects of the treatment. This type of supervision may become so active as to limit learning and to interfere with unit managerial responsibilities.

Supervision within a rehabilitative perspective is best suited to integrate the values of responsibility for patient care and the facilitation of supervisee learning. Within a rehabilitative model, the psychiatrist engages in collaborative, consultative, or supervisory relationships with other professionals during the process of evaluation and treatment planning of disease or defect. Following the assessment, rehabilitative efforts ensue that may certainly include psychotherapy. Within this perspective, psychiatrists may choose to refer patients for psychotherapeutic services that may be provided legitimately by independent mental health professionals or nonprofessionals supervised by them. The advantage of this framework for psychotherapy supervision is that it permits a clearer delineation of tasks and the division of labor regarding patient care.

Regardless of the supervisor's theoretical perspective, the process of psychotherapy supervision poses a number of difficult technical and organizational problems that do not have simple solutions. In those situations in which supervisors are legally accountable for the psychotherapy delivered by the supervisee (e.g., the supervisee is not capable of independent professional functioning), the supervisor must have a thorough knowledge of the treatment being delivered. This is not an easy task given the supervisor's almost exclusive reliance on the supervisee's verbal reports of the psychotherapeutic transactions. Muslin and Thurnblad[14] found that the percentage of relevant clinical themes omitted by medical students in clinical supervision was a staggering 54 percent (range 24–90 percent) and, furthermore, that an average of 8 percent of the themes reported were distorted. Although it is probable that these figures would be less dramatic if more experienced student therapists (e.g., advanced psychiatric residents) were studied, they underscore the need for more direct observation of sessions or the more widespread use of audio or visual recordings to ensure reliable monitoring. It may also be necessary to elaborate guidelines regarding the number of hours and frequency of supervision needed for differing patient caseloads and supervisee's experience.

Clinical Administrative Supervision

Predictably, the role of clinical-administrative supervisor shares the complexities and ambiguities of both clinical and administrative responsibilities. Typically, this is the role that evolves in small clinical units in which the bureaucratic leader (the unit director) also has responsibility for the overall clinical coordination of patient care and/or for psychotherapy supervision. The confounded aspects of this role derive from three major sources: (1) the multiplicity of roles inherent to it, (2) the impact of bureaucratic authority on clinical functions and vice versa, and (3) the dynamic group processes that arise within staff organizations. The clinical-administrative supervisor is perceived and functions as a jack-of-all-trades; he or she swiftly alternates between or combines bureaucratic, technical, prescriptive, medical backup (if a physician), and psychotherapy supervisory functions. In one sentence, the professional becomes a reassuring, sometimes paternalistic or authoritarian trouble-shooter. This assimilation of the whole gamut of interprofessional roles and relationships is usually taxing and confusing to all parties involved. Individual leadership styles and interests determine the predominant adoption of a particular set of role relationships in most transactions, usually at the expense of others that might be more appropriate to specific circumstances. For example, staff leaders who feel a need for close monitoring or control of a unit may spend most of their clinically related meetings (i.e., patient "rounds") discussing administrative or policy-related issues.

Those who have been supervised at some point or another by supervisors who also held administrative authority over us must remember the complex set of fantasies that this combined role sparks in the mind of the supervisee. The open discussion of countertransferential issues is generally avoided for fear that the supervisor may use personal disclosures for administrative purposes. Candid acknowledgment of clinicians' perturbed relationships with other supervisors, medical backups, or colleagues treating the same patient are also inhibited or concealed by this threat of breach of confidentiality. On the other hand, the administrative authority of a supervisor may be undermined by the excessive idealization or devaluation of his or her skills demonstrated in clinical supervision. When the clinical-administrative supervisor is not a physician, a number of other issues immediately arise, such as, for example, the nature of the relationship of the administrator to the staff psychiatrists. In crisis situations, nonmedical clinical-administrative supervisors often defer to the physician, a situation that produces further ambiguities regarding lines of accountability and delegation of responsibilities. Finally, group dynamics play a significant role in distorting the perception of clinical bureaucratic leaders. Concepts of underlying, regressive basic assumptions in group life are invariably present in staff organizations.[15] There are many who believe that the confounded aspects of this multidimensional role invariably compromise the performance of clinician–leaders.

The separation of the clinical and administrative functions does not automatically guarantee problem-free leadership since the risks of inadequate communication among the people involved are high. When a delegation of tasks is impracticable, we believe it is helpful to periodically review the overall mutual expectations and objectives of the different supervisory relationships.

CONCLUSION

Mental health providers at times comment that "dealing with patients is far easier than dealing with staff." Interprofessional relationships are extraordinarily difficult to conceptualize and manage. We take the position that if attempts are not made to do so, patient care is perturbed and perhaps even noxious.

In this chapter, an attempt has been made to provide several interrelated ways of looking at structured relationships. Our conceptual framework is based on a set of clearly defined relationship models that implicitly outline degrees of responsibility among staff members and toward patients, an enunciation of the tasks and perspectives of psychiatric practice and examples of key problematic roles that necessitate intensive review and clarification since they remain, as yet, most confounded. The explicit articulation of mutually perceived and agreed upon roles among professionals and nonprofessionals coupled with fully informed patients may aid in clarifying these complicated interactions among members of mental health teams.

REFERENCES

1. Schulberg H, Baker F: Professional Roles and Relations, Schulberg H, Baker F (eds): The Mental Hospital and Human Services. New York, Behavioral Publications, 1978, p 201
2. Whittington H: People make programs: Personnel management, in Feldman S (ed): The Administration of Mental Health Services. Springfield, Ill, Thomas, 1973, p 56
3. Adams J, Marston R: Medicine, Psychiatry and the Future. Panel presentation at the APA Annual Meeting, San Francisco, May 5, 1980
4. Friedson E: Profession of Medicine: A Study of the Sociology of Applied Knowledge, New York, Dodd, Mead, 1970
5. Astrachan B, Levinson D, Adler D: The impact of national health insurance on psychiatric tasks and practice. Arch Gen Psychiat 33:785–794, 1976
6. Scott WR: Reactions to supervision in a heteronomous professional organization. Adm Sci Q 10:65–81, 1965
7. Slovenko R: Legal issues in psychotherapy supervision, in Hess A (ed): Psychotherapy Supervision: Theory, Research and Practice. New York, Wiley, 1980, p 453
8. Stanton A, Schwartz M: The Mental Hospital: A Study of Institutional Participation in Psychiatric Illness and Treatment. New York, Basic Books, 1954
9. Henry J: The Formal Social Structure of a Psychiatric Hospital. Psychiatry, 17:139–151, 1954
10. Kaplan SR, Roman M: The Organization and Delivery of Mental Health Services: The Lincoln Hospital Experience. New York, Praeger, 1973
11. Adler D, Astrachan B, Levinson D: A framework for the analysis of theoretical and therapeutic approaches to schizophrenia. Psychiatry 44:1–12, 1981
12. House W, Miller S, Schalchter R: Role definitions among mental health professionals. Compr Psychiatry 19:469–477, 1978
13. Blum JD, Redlich F: Mental health practitioners: old stereotypes and new realities. Arch Gen Psychiat 37:1247, 1980
14. Muslin H, Thurnblad J: The fate of the clinical interview: an observational study. Am J Psychiat 138:822–825, 1981
15. Bion W: Experiences in Groups. London: Tavistock, 1961

Richard Scott Webster, Ph.D.
Susan W. Talbott, M.B.A., R.N.
Erica Loutsch, M.D.

17

Administrative Development

During the 1980s, psychiatric facilities will have to demonstrate increased accountability. In addition, the delivery of patient care must be improved. To these ends, improvement in individual and organizational management is essential. Management development and training for psychiatric professionals are considered critical for effective facility management.

The authors propose using modular, job-related, ongoing management development programs tailored to the needs of individual administrators and their institutions. The authors believe the ideas presented here will help the psychiatric facility management team develop such programs.

The authors believe the evidence is clear: improved functioning in organizations comes about only when top management initiates and supports a program of administrative development. Programs that encompass principles of effective adult learning help administrators improve their knowledge and skills. (See Chapter 14). When these programs engage the attention of the chief administrator and his or her work group (the "management team"), the chances of success are greatly increased.

Humans have undertaken specialized roles in small groups for at least 2 million years,[1] perhaps for as many as 8–15 million. Human capacity for cooperative work in small groups has developed over more than 40,000 generations. It seems reasonable to take advantage of this conditioning and to recognize our readiness to work together in pursuit, not like animals for the day's meal but for the trust, intimacy, and subtlety that characterize effective work groups in modern human organizations.[2]

Against this backdrop of prehistory, confirmed by research in organizations over the past 50 or 60 years, the authors propose the following ideas:

1. Effective programs of administrative development have basic characteristics that can be adopted by any organization that is committed to improving its functioning.
2. These characteristics are developed most effectively when people work on them with their colleagues and coworkers, in natural working groups, at or near the workplace.

The authors wish to thank Judith Nicholson for her contributions concerning adult learning and for critical reading of the manuscript.

3. Development of administrative skills is enhanced when adult learning principles are recognized and applied.
4. Evaluation of program efforts is necessary and can be accomplished in a cost-effective manner.

LEARNING BY DOING: CHANGING THE ORGANIZATION FROM WITHIN

The opportunities available for administrative improvement are all around us.

The case discussed below describes the process of change through reorganization and staff development in a small children's public mental hospital. While the changes were primarily developed through trial and error, a planned program of administrative improvement resulted. What was done in this case can be done anywhere, given the commitment, interest, knowledge, and skills (*the vision*) of the effective psychiatrist–administrator.

"Psychiatric Hospital A" began as a childrens' unit in an adult state hospital. The organization was that of a classical state hospital, e.g., hierarchieal, pyramidal, authoritarian. Each discipline had its own departmental structure, and there was very little communication across departmental lines. Professionals and paraprofessionals did "their own thing" in almost total isolation from each other. The lack of communication among professionals and between professionals and ward staff interfered with the childrens' treatment, prolonged their stay in the hospital, and alienated their families. The community viewed the unit as a dumping ground for the most severe and hopeless cases.

As a result of pressure from dissatisfied staff and charges by the media that children were being brutalized, the following changes were made from above: a new administrator was appointed, the unit became an independent hospital and moved to a new building, and more resources, both equipment and personnel, were provided.

The new administrator was faced with the task of reorganizing the hospital so that it would fulfill the needs of the patients, provide job satisfaction for the staff, and meet the expectations of the community and the controlling government agency.

The Process

The first few months were used to gather information and interview staff (individually and in small and large groups). During these meetings, several potential leaders emerged, and goals and objectives began to be formulated. Chief among these was the desire for an organizational structure that would be less rigid and authoritarian and would encourage maximum staff participation in decision making and interdisciplinary communication.

A few months later, the hospital was totally reorganized, with the interdisciplinary team as the basic unit of organization. Four teams were established, each responsible for developing and implementing treatment programs for a group of children. The children, in turn, were assigned to a team according to age as well as developmental and educational levels. Each child was assigned a team member who would be responsible for coordinating his treatment. An individual treatment plan was set up for each child at a clinical team meeting. Goals were established in several areas: educational, social, psychiatric, familial, and so on.

Results

Two years later, the median length of hospitalization had been reduced by 50 percent. More children were returning home instead of needing further residential treatment. Staff morale had improved, and the center was perceived in the community as a placement of choice rather than the end of the line.

Issues of Staff Development

The reorganization was not accomplished smoothly and without difficulty. Team leaders were chosen from existing staff because of their commitment to the overall goals, their enthusiasm, and their willingness to assume additional responsibility without extra pay. It was soon evident that in order for team leaders to function in expanded and/or new roles, they would need a great deal of training and support.

Initially, the director, business officer, and personnel manager met almost daily with the team leaders. The purpose of these meetings was to formulate plans and define goals and objectives for the institution as a whole, to secure feedback from each team leader as to how these overall goals should be adapted to the particular characteristics and needs of their teams, and to discuss actual and anticipated difficulties.

Support for team leaders was also provided by outside consultants. They conducted management training seminars and day-long retreats for the entire staff. The retreats were intended to work out some of the interpersonal difficulties that arose from new role expectations. Some of the professional staff found it difficult to function with the interdisciplinary model and felt a loss of professional identity. This was felt most acutely by those who had been heads of their respective disciplines.

After many meetings during which the merits of the interdiscipinary versus the departmental model were discussed at length, a compromise was reached. Members of each discipline met on a regular basis with their department head to discuss concerns unique to their profession. These meetings were also used to identify continuing education needs and to assess quality control efforts. Soon the department heads found a new role within the interdisciplinary structure. They were charged with maintaining professional standards, providing specialized in-service training, and serving as consultants to the administrator and the teams.

CHARACTERISTICS OF EFFECTIVE ORGANIZATIONS

The authors believe that all human organizations and their administrators, staff members, and constituent work groups are likely to work more effectively when the following administrative and management practices are followed:

1. Open communication
2. Good teamwork
3. Widespread participation in decision making
4. Encouragement of individual initiative
5. Mutual support
6. Clear goals and objectives
7. Use of written policies, procedures, and standards
8. Feedback about actual versus planned performance

These eight practices form the basis of the administrative development program described and illustrated in this chapter.

Managers face similar challenges whether they are managing large or small units in health care organizations. As Peter Drucker so simply puts it: "Managers are responsible for directing vision and resources towards achieving greatest results.[3]

Administrative development is most effective when each organization and its constituent work groups are encouraged to undertake an administrative development program in response to its own needs and priorities.

TEAM DEVELOPMENT FOR IMPROVED PATIENT CARE

"Work group" effectiveness is illustrated in another example the way in which each team at "Psychiatric Hospital B" was encouraged to develop programs to meet the particular needs of its patients. Within a few months after a team development program was started, several innovative programs were instituted, based on careful evaluation, by team leaders and the psychiatrist–administrator, of the needs of the patients, staff team members, and community.

For example, the team serving the younger age group found that their inpatient beds were not being filled, while there was a waiting list for day care. After careful study of their census, meetings with several community-based referral agencies, and consultation with the administrator, they developed an expanded day care program.

Another example: the adolescent team found that the length of stay for their patients was slowly increasing. A task force was formed to investigate the situation and explore possible solutions. Linkages were developed with several groups homes, and youngsters were able to be discharged sooner. Under a strictly authoritarian, hierarchical structure, these solutions would not have been possible or would have taken much longer. Staff might not have had access to information such as the low census and increased length of stay. They would not have been encouraged or motivated to seek a solution, and strict adherence to professional roles would not have encouraged the development of new programs.

WORK GROUPS: A PRIMARY FOCUS

The administrative development program described (and advocated) here emphasizes the key role of work groups in accomplishing organizational improvement and change. Figure 17-1 illustrates the point that most administrators are leaders of one work group, while also members of a second.[4]

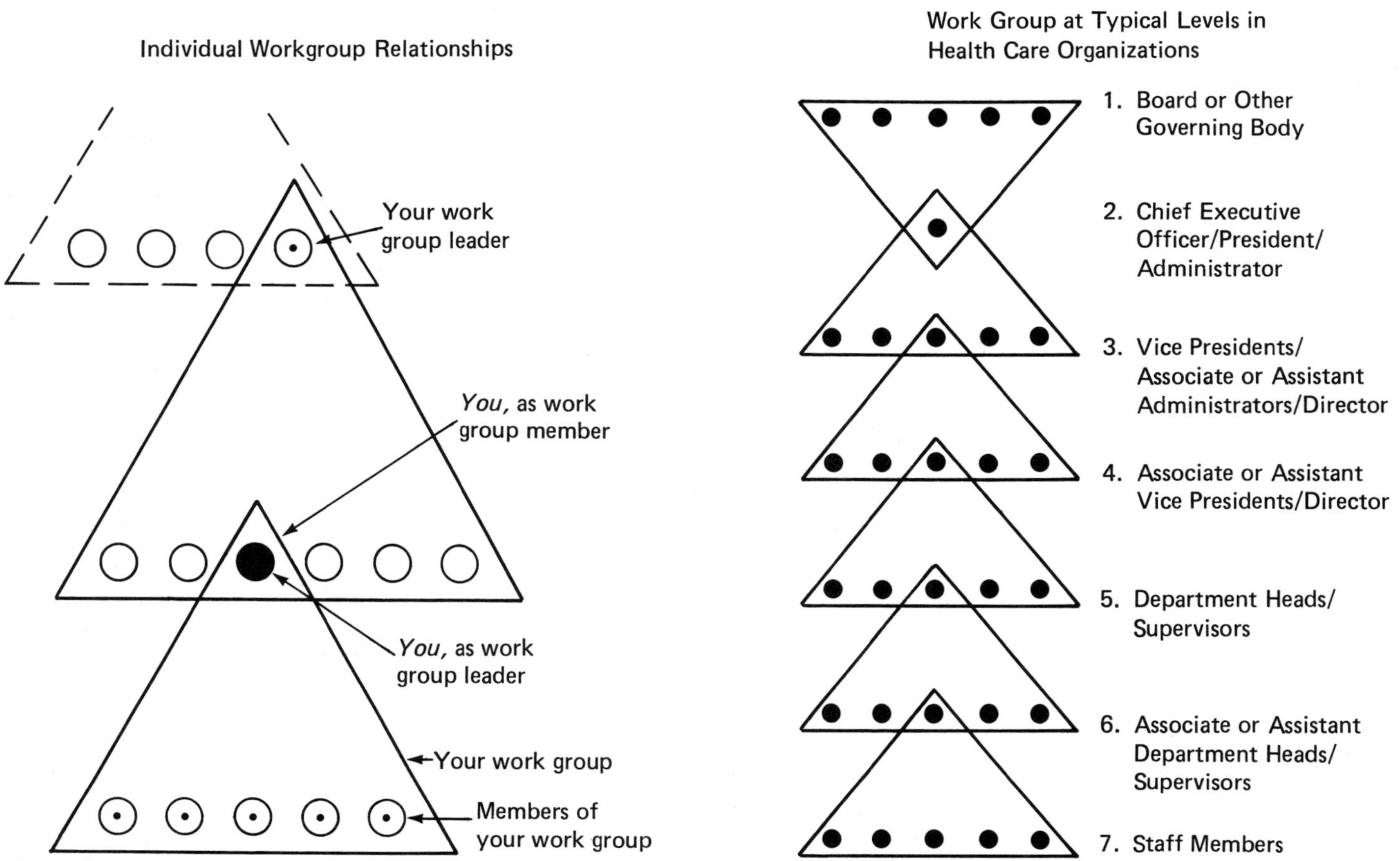

Figure 17-1. Work groups.[4] Adapted from Likert R: New Patterns of Management. New York, McGraw-Hill, 1961.

Work groups are described by the following characteristics and conditions:

1. Members of work groups usually have similar job responsibilities. They may come together in staff or problem-solving meetings.
2. The work group leader is a member of the work group at the next higher level in the organization.
3. Group leaders act as "linking pins" between work groups. They have important responsibilities for transmitting information throughout the organization: upward, downward, and laterally.
4. Information is the "fluid" in the organization's management system. It is the basic resource for accomplishing improvements as well as the basis of new knowledge and for problem-solving activities on which organizational improvement and renewal depend.
5. Many organizations have based improvement and renewal efforts on work group participation. Such groups can include only group leaders or group members or leaders and members working together.
6. Effective work groups must be of a size (four to nine members) that enables frequent and productive communication.
7. Work groups provide every administrator with the opportunity to practice participative management. This requires the involvement of individual human beings in the concerns and decisions that affect them *and* the well-being of their organization.

Using Subgroups to Solve a Problem of Team Size

One of the difficulties faced by a small task-oriented groups or teams is that as the organization grows, communication between teams becomes more difficult. It can even be more difficult *within* teams as they add members.

At "Psychiatric Hospital C", as the patient population and the staff increased, communication among team members and between teams became more difficult and cumbersome. In response to these communication problems, smaller clinical teams were established. Each miniteam included only the clinical staff who worked directly with a group of patients. Discussions at miniteam meetings were centered around treatment planning and *ad hoc* emergency issues related to their patients. The whole team continued to meet as a larger group to deal with programmatic and administrative issues and for clinical conferences.

FEEDBACK: A CRITICAL FACTOR

Administrators must recognize the importance of feedback and provide the means for both administrators and staff members to provide feedback comfortably and effectively.[5] Feedback needs to be provided at several levels, as illustrated in Figure 17-2:

1. Feedback is required to keep individuals (and organizations) informed about their performance and is one means of bringing about desired changes. As illustrated by "Feedback 1" (Figure 17-2), the organization usually provides

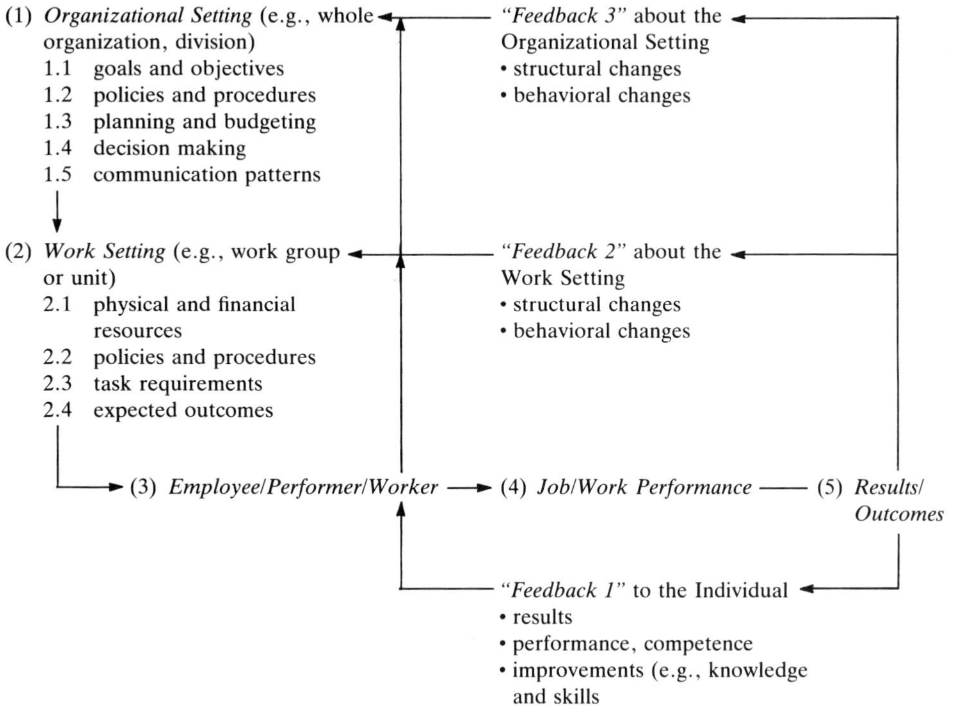

Figure 17-2. Feedback for improving performance: individual, work group, and organizational. Adapted from Kepner Tregoe seminar materials. See also Rummler, GA: Human performance problems and their solutions. Human Resource Management, vol. 11, no. 4, Winter, 1972, 2–10.

some feedback to individuals about their job or work performance through a performance evaluation program.

2. The organizational factors affect the work setting and together have a major impact on an individual's ability to perform. For example, a procedures manual prepared by the business office may facilitate fiscal control while frustrating staff members efforts to get supplies or equipment for patients when and where needed, in a *timely* way!
3. "Feedback 2," about the work setting, and "Feedback 3" about the organizational factors, occur rarely or not at all. Feedback from workers is not used in most organizations to help make needed improvements in the work setting or within the organization.

To continue with the example of the business office, staff are rarely motivated to ask *how* procedures can be changed to facilitate patient care. The authors would suggest that every administrator ask himself the following questions:

1. Should staff in the business office ask questions of the clinical staff?
2. Should frustrated clinical staff members be heard?
3. How can these problems in communication be identified and solved?
4. Are standard procedures being retained simply because they are familiar?

Management by (Group) Objectives: Patient Treatment Planning and Feedback[6]

Feedback to patients about their therapeutic progress is rarely discussed in the literature even though the Joint Commission on Accreditation of Hospitals (JCAH) strongly recommends patient participation in treatment planning.

One way this information can be shared with patients is through the treatment plan. At "Children's Psychiatric Hospital D," an individual treatment plan was developed for each child. This plan specified goals in several areas, e.g., behavior at home, in school, and with peers and relationship with the family. The child and family participated in preparing the plan and the subsequent monthly evaluation. Behavioral objectives were set up for patients who wanted to obtain weekend privileges, trips, and so on. Clearly defined goals and expectations are easier for patients to relate to than the usual and vague announcement that the patient will go home when the doctors think he or she is well enough.

Staff Evaluation and Feedback: Individual Development

Feedback about individual performance was provided at "Psychiatric Hospital E" by periodic evaluations. These were done by the supervisor and discussed with each employee. At the same time that the standard civil service forms were completed, other areas of particular relevance were also dealt with. Topics included the employee's ability to communicate with other team members, his interaction with patients and their families, and his ability to initiate and implement changes.

Supervisors were also responsible for informing staff members of such career development opportunities as civil service examinations, access to training seminars, and educational leaves.

Staff Evaluation and Feedback: Impact on the Organization

At "Psychiatric Hospital E" a monthly census was prepared listing the following data for each team: number of admissions and discharges per month, average length of stay, patient dispositions (back to the family or to another agency), day hospital attendance, and critical incidents. This information sheet provided clinical staff with pertinent patient information *and* served as an incentive by promoting healthy competition among teams.

Performance data, particularly when distributed regularly over months or years, provides information, educates, builds a basis for comparison (trend data), and provokes ideas for improvement. The concept of the self-fulfilling prophecy suggests that we get what we *ex*pect, but we would argue that we get what we *in*spect.

ACTION PLANNING: KEY TO CHANGE

An administrative development program that includes action planning as part of work group meetings gives individuals the opportunity to provide feedback to superiors. Work groups (or other problem-solving groups) can identify, discuss, and recommend improvements. Their recommendations can be acted on by the work group or communicated to appropriate persons in the organization.

Sixty to 90 percent of improvement priorities identified by individuals and work groups relate to the work setting or the organizational factors rather than to individual performance.[7] There is considerable evidence that most people could do their jobs better, with existing knowledge and skills, *if* work settings and organizational factors were improved. Feedback 2 and Feedback 3 can provide information on the basis for making these improvements.

For example, poor communication (and coordination) of patient care plans can add to patients' length of stay and increase costs. No one individual is to blame; "the system" (the work setting or organizational factors) *does* need to be changed.

Key questions for the psychiatric administrator's work group (team) include the following:

1. Can and will our organization seek, accept, and use information from individuals and work groups?
2. Are we ready to examine the organizational and work settings as sources for improvement ideas?
3. Are we willing to examine and improve our feedback system?

Feedback from the Worker to the Organization for Action Planning

Among the most difficult problems faced by psychiatric administrators are poor motivation, low morale, and rapid turnover of a key paraprofessional staff group—psychiatric aides.

Since this group spends the largest amount of time with patients, they are an essential part of the therapeutic environment. At "Psychiatric Hospital F," the psychiatric aides were found to be alienated from the professional staff. They felt "dumped on," morale was poor, and absenteeism rates were high.

To deal with the situation, psychiatric aides were encouraged to voice their concerns at team mettings, in individual interviews, and at hospital-wide staff meetings. From this feedback, it was clear that the psychiatric aides felt that policies and procedures were being imposed without any concern for their impact, that they were being unjustly accused of brutalizing patients, and that incident reviews were often used by the administration to harass them. A consensus was arrived at that psychiatric aides needed to be heard and subsequently to feel that they could effect change in the hospital.

Several aides, elected by their peers, were appointed to the hospital's committees on policy, education, and incident review. After several months, there was evidence that morale had improved, that there was a better understanding of the need for incident review and investigation, and that policies and procedures were better understood and more readily complied with. On the one hand, educational opportunities, such as leave with pay for training, became more widely and more often used. On the otherhand, peer pressure resulted in fewer incidents and a lower absenteeism rate.

ADMINISTRATIVE DEVELOPMENT: THE ADULT LEARNER

Effective administrative development programs must respond to the learning style and needs of the adult learner.[7-9] Important elements are those of:

1. "Ownership" and control of the administrative development program by the organization's administration and staff. This includes the use of outside consultants as catalysts, energy sources, and idea generators. Planning and management of the administrative development program should remain within the organization and an administrative development task force appointed to coordinate the program.
2. Identification of the organization's needs and consideration of appropriate responses.
3. Focus on work groups.
4. Feedback to individuals, work groups, *and* the organization.
5. Experiential learning opportunities for individuals in seminar/workshop sessions.
6. The "four Ts" of administrative development: targets, time, transfer, and tests. "Targets" are the organization's needs, its administrative development objectives. "Time is the scarcest resource. "Transfer" from the development (learning) setting to the job setting is required to bring about change. "Tests" must be undertaken to evaluate changes and assess effectiveness of the administrative development program.

OBJECTIVES OF THE ADMINISTRATIVE DEVELOPMENT PROGRAM

An effective administrative development program deals with administrators' responsibilities for setting goals, obtaining and allocating resources, working effectively with others, and above all, achieving results.

In order to carry out these responsibilities, there are activities (including processes, tasks, and skills) that must be mastered and used to accomplish more effective administration.

Any psychiatric administrator who aims to develop a program to meet organizational and individual needs is urged to consider the following objectives:

1. *Direct* the program to meet the *unique* needs of the organization as determined by the people who work there.
2. *Attend to time and cost.* Take into consideration the efficient use of staff time and the effective use of the scarce resources available for administrative improvement.
3. *Coordinate* the administrative development program with the staff numbers' job activities so that they can use new knowledge and skills on the job.
4. *Emphasize* the benefits that derive from transfer of knowledge and skills to the job setting from each seminar/workshop session and follow-up meeting.

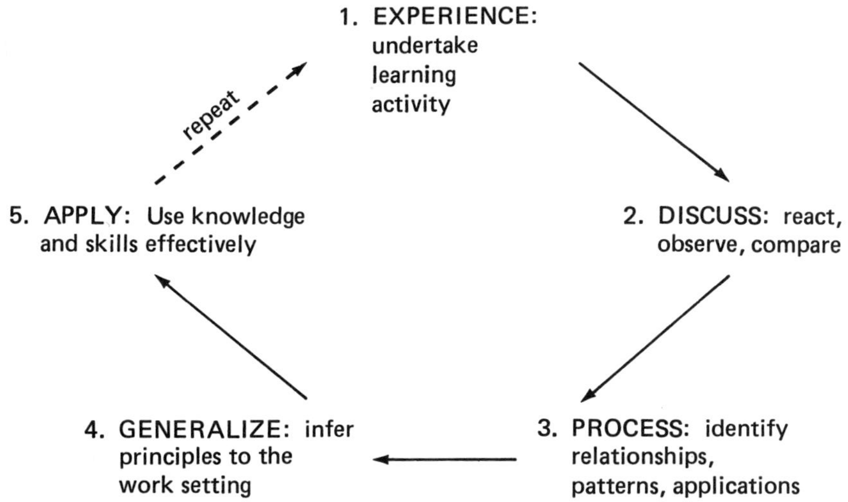

Figure 17-3. The experiential learning cycle. Adapted with permission from Pfeiffer and Jones: Annual Handbook for Group Facilitators. San Diego, CA, University Associates. 1975 and 1980.

5. *Integrate* the organizational improvement goals with the individual's professional development (and personal development whenever possible and appropriate) so that individuals can see the link between organizational and individual development.
6. *Design* the program to incorporate the experiential learning cycle (Fig. 17-3) and other elements that promote adult learning.
7. *Focus* on one primary objective: administrative development, i.e., positive change on the job, through increased individual effectiveness, leading to increased organizational effectiveness.
8. *Establish* the administrative development program as an ongoing program. This approach is most likely to effect real improvements in work group, individual, and organizational functioning.
9. *Evaluate* the program. Provide performance feedback from workshop and other sessions to those involved.

DETERMINING ORGANIZATIONAL NEEDS

The first objective of an effective administrative development program is to identify the unique needs of the organization and the participating teams (units or work groups) within it. Needs assessment can be as simple as interviewing the chief executive and other key managers. Needs assessment must be conducted at the level of detail and intensity appropriate to the circumstances. Administrative reports, for example, can sometimes identify a need for research and development activities. More complex needs assessment alternatives include survey-guided needs assessment[10] or use of focus groups.

Problem Solving Through Participation

At "Psychiatric Hospital G," staff members became concerned about the increase in aggressive patient behavior on one unit. Clearly there was a need to assess the situation and deal with the problem. A small research project to study aggressive patient behavior using five psychiatric aides as research assistants was initiated. The group was headed by the director and a principal investigator.

The research consisted of rating patients' aggressive behaviors as observed on the unit. The participation of all the ward staff was needed to accomplish this.

Rating forms were developed by the research group and were introduced to the ward staff by the psychiatric aide research assistants. They also instructed their colleagues in observing the patients' behaviors and using the rating forms. Although the research project had to be interrupted after 6 months, some interesting side effects resulted:

1. The psychiatric aides who participated became more aware of the patients' aggressive behaviors and interacted with them more appropriately.
2. Several aides became interested in learning more about diagnosis and treatment of mental illness and requested in-service training.
3. Two members of the research group volunteered to attend a course on self-defense at another hospital and then helped organize a similar program at "Psychiatric Hospital G.".
4. The participants reported that as a result of the project, their jobs had become more interesting.

An in-service training program was started with topics suggested by the psychiatric aides. Attendance at this program was much better than at previous ones, probably because the material presented was addressed to the specific needs of the workers, *as perceived by them.*

Why Administrative Development for Psychiatric Facility Leaders?

The role of the psychiatric administrator is to create an environment that will enable the staff to function effectively. The Cummings state that in order to do this "he must serve two masters, he must mediate between the agents of the society and the institution, and balance the needs of both.[11]

Levinson and Klerman point out that most psychiatrists have had little or no preparation for dealing with issues of organizational life.[12] Having been trained to effect change mostly in a dyadic doctor/patient relationship, the psychiatrist is faced with being dependent on staff performance in order to attain program goals.

According to Whittington, mental health organizations are highly complex systems, not comparable to most structures in the business world.[13] Members come from different and highly specialized backgrounds, with high expectations for themselves, their colleagues, and their patients. They do not fit easily into team membership in work groups. Furthermore, the end product is hard to define.

In these circumstances, the need for work focused on recognition and improvement of administrative skills can hardly be overemphasized.

THE ADMINISTRATIVE DEVELOPMENT PROGRAM

Administrative development is, or should be, an ongoing process. Time pressures, work priorities, and marketplace competition require that improvements be made. These same factors can also create resistance to development and positive change.

Administrative development is usually most effective when the program is carried out within the organization by a task group of staff members, with outside support. Figure 7-4 illustrates the central position of the administrative development program task force within the organization.

The program is usually most effective if an outside consultant works with the program task force and its coordinator(s). (Experience has shown that two persons, as coordinators, are usually most effective.) The objective is to empower the task force, with top management support, to take primary responsibility for administrative development.

Program coordinator(s) usually meet with an outside consultant to plan for the following:

1. Program leadership within the organization
2. Program announcement and orientation activities
3. Needs assessment and program priority setting
4. Leadership of seminar/workshops
5. Seminar/workshop follow-up to accomplish positive change on the job

While each of these tasks can be done by outside consultants, results are usually better, and program costs far lower, when primary responsibility is assumed by a task force and its leader or coleaders.

Organizational Change Required

Substantial change is usually required in the organization to establish and carry out an effective administrative development program.[14]

1. Top management must recognize the need and act.
2. A task force must be appointed, given a mandate, and be supported by the chief executive and his work group.
3. Scarce resources (time, energy, and money) must be committed.
4. Continuing attention must be given to the program in the face of relentless forces to maintain the status quo (including limited time, scarce resources, skeptical staff, and vested interests).

It is usually possible to effect constructive change by taking the following steps:

1. The administrator's work group makes a commitment to a more open system and participative organization; at least they examine the hypothesis that such an organization will deliver improved services to patients, help contain costs, and provide higher levels of human satisfaction. Activities include reading, discussion, seeking and accepting results-oriented criticism of the status quo, and forming the operational basis for change.

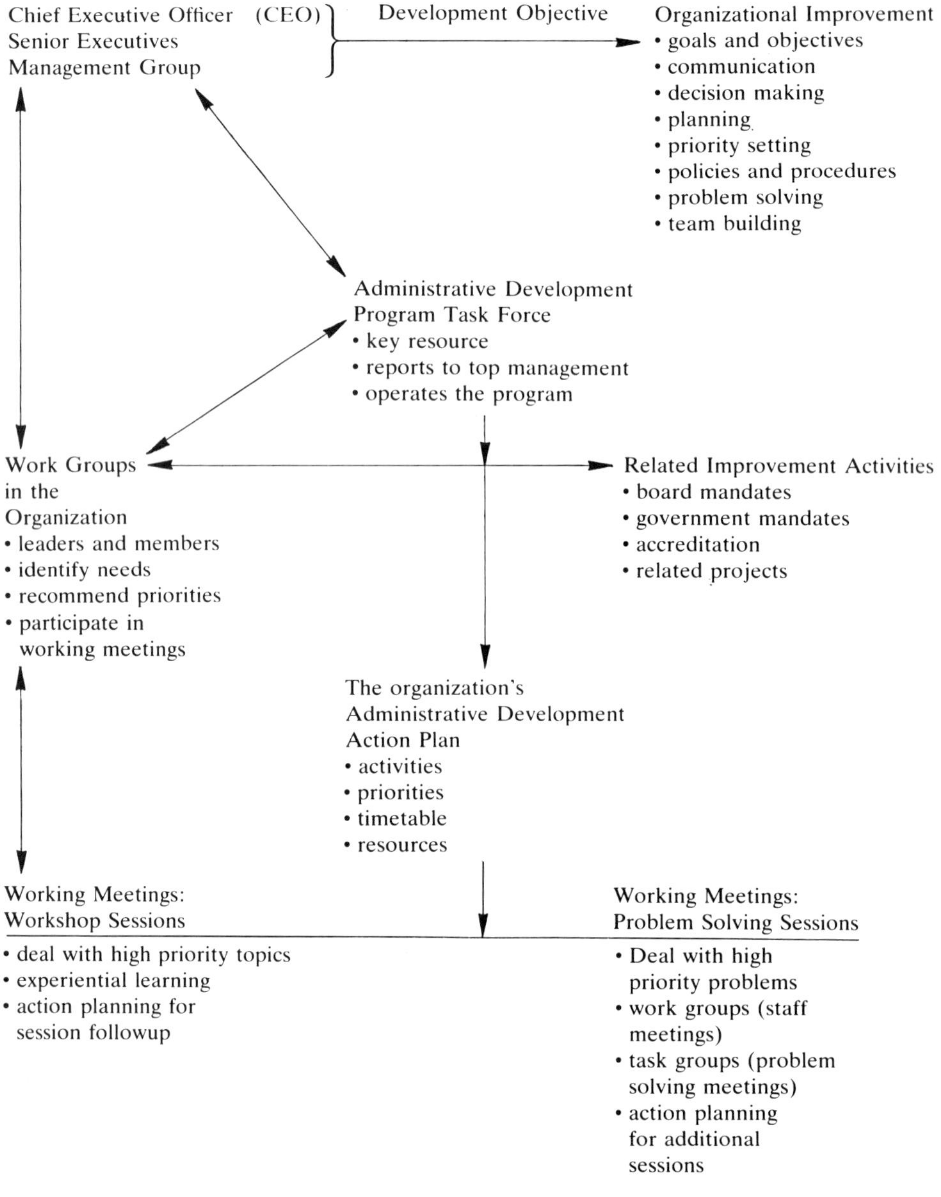

Figure 17-4. Administrative development program: process and relationships.

2. The organization's philosophy, mission statement, goals, and objectives must be reviewed, or if they do not already exist, they must be written.
3. A management philosophy must be defined. This is a task for the administrator and his work group, usually with the help of an outside consultant.
4. Implementation of steps 2 and 3 involves making changes in organizational

structure (peoples' task assignments and reporting relationships) and incentives.

5. Staff must be helped to accept and adjust to change while being encouraged to develop higher skill levels in interpersonal relations and communications. If change is to occur, leadership and commitment must come from the chief administrator and his work group and "cascade" downward throughout the organization. The absence of *real* commitment and support from the top work group will be quickly recognized, noted, and acted on. Result? The program will fail.
6. Close observation of interpersonal relationships, management activities, and staff morale will help the administrator and his work group determine if the objectives stated and assumed in steps 1 through 4 have been reached and that the changes have "taken."
7. Problems of the "old" organization must be dealt with. These may include the following:
   a. Involving the union(s), by determining win-win solutions to problems their members have
   b. Stabilizing employment, helping to assure workers that the organization cares about them, values their knowledge and skills, and seeks to establish a climate and conditions that will help individuals to grow
   c. Improving evaluation and promotion plans and systems
   d. Broadening and lengthening career paths
8. Trust must continue to be built so that the employees throughout the organization will come to believe over time that *real* change is desired and conditions *have* changed, and that the "system" *does* indeed care about them and *wants* to help them succeed and grow on the job.
9. Opportunities must continue to be sought for linking administrative development to organizational improvement and positive change. Consider the following:
   a. Using performance reporting systems that inform, educate, motivate, *and* provide the basis for necessary control
   b. Initiating problem-solving strategies, based in work groups, that involve asking worker groups for ideas and improvement strategies
   c. Forming more autonomous working teams (groups)
   d. Using work-group based problems wherever possible
   e. Discussing *real* operating (and cost-related) problems with employees
   f. Focusing on work-related issues and avoiding paternalism

It must be remembered that change from bureaucratic to participative organizations (from "A" to "Z") starts at the top and works down throughout the organization and takes a considerable amount of time to accomplish.

> The process of participative management, once begun, is largely self-sustaining because it appeals to the basic values of all employees. And in fact the process promotes greater productivity and efficiency through better coordination and will flourish unless intentionally stopped by a disenchanted or threatened union or by top management.*

---

*From Ouchi W: Theory Z: How American Business Can Meet the Japanese Challenge. Reading, Mass, Addison-Wesley, 1981, p 129. With permission.

Program Design

The administrative development program described here is based on widely accepted findings about change and development in human groups. The program includes the use of in-house seminar/workshops and the follow-up sessions they generate.

The program is designed this way because:

1. The administrators and staff members in most health care organizations do not have extensive preparation for administrative work.
2. When seminar/workshops are conducted at or near the work site, more work groups, and work group members, can participate. The organization's needs are better served when people who work together are able to undertake professional development activities together.
3. Organizational objectives (targets) are more likely to be met; real and current job-related problems are more likely to be dealt with; and there is a greater probability that seminar/workshop sessions will result in positive change on the job (transfer).
4. Follow-up meetings are also easier to arrange for additional work on the topic(s) covered and for applying knowledge and skills to solving problems or otherwise improving the organization's functioning and services.

Seminar/workshop sessions and the follow-up sessions they generate are usually more effective when held as "working meetings", conducted within the organization or nearby. Workshop leadership can be provided by outside consultants or the organization's own training or in-service staff.

Proper program design assures that sessions can be lead or co-lead by the organization's own staff members, if that is desired. Most staff members who want to can become effective session leaders or co-leaders. Leadership preparation includes organizational approval, participation in sessions led by others, completion of a session leadership workshop, and coleadership experience within the organization.

Experiential learning materials are available on many administrative topics. These materials can be used for seminar/workshops, each dealing with a major administrative topic. The organization's own staff members can learn to use these materials and function as facilitators rather than as content experts.

Action planning for follow-up should be an integral part of each seminar/workshop, taking 20–33 percent of the session time. When properly designed and presented, the initial session on each topic usually generates follow-up sessions to deal further with action plans that are specific to the needs and problems identified by the participants.

Properly designed session materials include basic concepts, discussion materials, and other content. Sessions provide practical work with the content, problem identification and problem-solving activities, and action planning for session follow-up. Action planning is the basis for transferring results *from* the seminar/workshop *to* the job.

Several desirable outcomes result when administrative development programs are conducted as close as possible to the work setting:

1. Program priorities are set within the organization, leading to increased feelings of staff involvement and participant responsibility.
2. Organizational priorities (targets) are constantly in view; participants focus on *their* organization's objectives.
3. Participating work groups, leaders, and members become involved and familiar with the program.
4. The administrative development program becomes known, recognized, and accepted throughout the organization.
5. The dislocation costs (time, travel, tuition) of off-site programs are sharply reduced.
6. More people can participate, increasing the probability of a "critical mass" of program awareness, knowledge, involvement, and therefore support of program objectives.

Program Priorities

Assessment of organizational needs, by whatever method is most appropriate, usually identifies a rather limited set of high-priority needs.

As noted earlier, the majority of these needs are usually related to organizational improvements that enable people to do their jobs better. Staff commonly express a need for the following:

1. Clear goals and objectives
2. Policies and procedures that are written, current, reasonable, and that enhance individual performance
3. Planning and budgeting systems that invite *real* input from work groups
4. Decision-making and problem-solving systems that do the same
5. Communication and feedback systems that are open enough to allow (encourage) messages about organizational improvement to reach the "right ears" and adequate to create and report positive changes.

Kraft said: "During this century the major development in organizational theory has been the discovery of the human being."[15] Chief administrators and their work groups will do well to recognize and respond to this idea. If they do, they can more effectively build organizations by capitalizing on the trust, intimacy and subtlety necessary to obtain the best the staff has to give.[2]

It is often easiest to approach organizational improvement opportunities (and opportunities are often the "backside" of a problem) through seminar/workshops dealing with specific administrative topics. For example, effective action planning during topic-focused sessions shifts emphasis to job-related problems related to the topic. This process combines the knowledge and skill-building objectives of topical sessions with the job-related problem-solving objectives that attract participants to the sessions. The results are synergistic and mutually beneficial. In fact, an administrator can expect to see positive change in individuals, work groups, and the organization following the successful implementation of an administrative development program. For example:

1. Individuals have (and use) additional knowledge and skills related to their administrative responsibilities.

2. Work group members get together on real problems related to their job responsibilities and the administrative topic under discussion.
3. The organization (e.g., session leader[s], program task force, work group leaders) benefits from the attention and concern for improvement in the quality of work life.

Program Topics

Administrative development program materials are needed to address high-priority topics, identified by needs assessment activities. Work groups at all levels, from top management to unit-based patient care teams, have indicated a need to work on some or all of the following administrative topics:

1. Better meetings
2. Career development
3. Communication
4. Decision making and problem solving
5. Leadership
6. Management concepts
7. Managing conflict
8. Managing time and stress
9. Organizational change
10. Team building

Other topics that are sometimes helpful include the following:

1. Marketing
2. Negotiating
3. Organizational functioning, e.g., planning, budgeting, organizing staffing, and evaluating.

When topical materials are available to the administrative development program task force, it is usually easier to undertake programs for meeting administrative needs. As described above, a program of seminar/workshops, based on an assessment of individual, work group, and organizational needs, adds to knowledge and skills and also generates action plans for dealing with job-related problems.

PROGRAM RESULTS AND EVALUATION

The basic objective of any administrative development program is to help accomplish positive change on the job.

As this chapter tries to make clear, reaching this objective is as much affected by beliefs and attitudes of the chief administrator (and his work group) as by the administrative development program they create.

The objective is more likely to be met if the administrative development program gives appropriate attention to the "four Ts" of organization improvement: targets, time, transfer, and tests.[2,16] Attainment of these four conditions for maximum program effectiveness can be measured by many forms of evaluation. Time and cost constraints often dictate use of simple, low-cost measures of performance and productivity.

Desirable characteristics of program effectiveness tests include the following:

1. Low cost
2. Work group based
3. Low complexity and time consumption
4. Relationship to performance data already collected
5. Continuation over time, to obtain time series (trend) data.

Examples of cost effective tests include:

1. Number of problems brought to and solved by work groups, problem-solving groups, and the administrative development program task force
2. Satisfaction of group members, as measured by surveys of work group performance
3. Satisfaction of group leaders
4. Improvement in work group performance
5. Improvement in work group job satisfaction, as measured by work group member's reports, client or patient reports, or the observation of senior administrators within the organization
6. Improvement in factor scores, when assessment of job influence and support factors are used as part of needs assessment

Formative evaluation, for improving program performance "in course", is usually more useful than summative (retrospective) evaluation. Evaluation, properly designed and undertaken as part of the administrative development program is, in itself, an administrative development technique. Participants learn (by doing) that performance measurement and program justification are required and that these help to obtain needed resources.

REFERENCES

1. Jay A: Corporation Man. 1967. New York, Random House, 1971
2. Ouchi W: Theory Z: How American Business Can Meet the Japanese Challenge. Reading, Mass, Addison-Wesley, 1981, p 5–10, 129
3. Drucker PF: Management: Tasks, Responsibilities, Practices. New York, Harper & Row, 1974, p 17
4. Likert R: New Patterns of Management. New York, McGraw-Hill, 1961
5. Rummler GA: Human performance problems and their solutions. Hum Resource Management 11:2–10, 1972
6. Likert R, Fisher MS: MBGO: putting some team spirit into MBO. Personnel 54:40–47, 1977
7. Kidd JR: How Adults Learn. Chicago, Ill, Follett, 1973
8. Knowles M: The Adult Learner: A Neglected Species. Houston, Texas, Gulf, 1979
9. Knowles M: The Modern Practice of Adult Education: From Pedagogy to Andragogy. Chicago, Ill, Follett, 1980
10. Bowers DG, & Franklin JL: Survey-Guided Development I: Data-Based Organizational Change. La Jolla, Calif, University Associates, 1977
11. Cumming J, Cumming E: Ego and Milieu. New Yor, Atherton Press, 1969, p 113
12. Levinson DT, Klerman GL: The clinician executive: some problematic issues for the psychiatrist in mental health organizations. Psychiatry 30:6, 1967
13. Wittington HG: People make programs: personnel management, in Feldman, S (ed): The Administration of Mental Health Services (ed 2). Springfield, Ill, Thomas, 1980
14. Bennis WG, Benne KD, Chin R, Corey KE: The Planning of Change (ed 3). New York, Holt, Rinehart, and Winston, 1976
15. Kraft A: Behavioral and Organizational Theories, Chapter 10 in this volume.
16. Mahoney FX: Targets, time, and transfer: keys to management training impact. Personnel 57:25–34, 1980

Stuart L. Keill, M.D.

18

Planning Psychiatric Services

PLANNING OF MENTAL HEALTH SERVICES

At a time when the President's Commission on Mental Health[1] reports that each year 3 percent of the population (or 6 million people) of our nation uses specialized mental health programs while we face decreasing financial support and possibly medical health resources as well, skillful planning is needed more than ever before to assure that effective, efficient, and nonduplicative mental health services are available to the population at large. Increasingly, the well-trained clinical psychiatrist is required to plan for a new service or for a change in an existing service. Most have found themselves in this position involuntarily and without prior interest or training in such a process. Often, the resultant planning is reactive rather than proactive, well intentioned, but often either flawed or inefficient.

There are some similarities between the planning of mental health services and generic planning.[2] Human services differ from those providing a "product,"[3] and the administration of mental health services is in many ways unique, involving as it does at every level the important interaction of personalities serving and being served. This interaction affects the "product" or service, the primary client, the secondary client, and the effectiveness and efficiency of the organization as a whole.[4,5]

This chapter provides the clinician with a practical guide that can be utilized planning a range of services such as a major new comprehensive community mental health program in a heretofore unserved area, a small service component of a larger system such as an additional clinic, or an expansion in an inpatient unit. If the resultant plan is to be a useful, relevant, and acceptable one, it will usually involve attention to personnel, organizational structure, policies and procedures, architecture, equipment, and fiscal matters.*

The author wishes to express his gratitude to Sylvia Clarke, MSW, consultant to the Department of Social Work Services at the Mt. Sinai Hospital in New York City. She has been a valued collaborator for a number of years in the planning of a number of mental health services and has particularly helped in the restructuring and clarification of this manuscript.

*As Levinson and Klerman note,[6] increasing the size and complexity of the organization affects the clinical concerns with which the executive is involved. Similarly, in the implementation phase, the

There are a number of excellent, detailed texts and outlines on the planning process that may be consulted for further information.[2,7–9] There are also some superb and complete bibliographies, one of which[10] lists much of the major literature up to about 1976, and another[11] that contains over 5000 references from the two-decade period ending in 1978. These references are comprehensive; there are a number of references relating to specific points in this chapter for the individual who wishes to pursue those aspects of the planning process.

The information in this chapter and the appended references will be meaningless if utilized in a vacuum. As with the mastery of any skill, it is essential first to become comfortable with the body of knowledge and then to proceed to develop the related skills in the actual practice of the activity. It is hoped that the reader will find this outline useful as an additional navigating device as he sets forth on the often turbulent but gratifying sea of planning.

The Planning Process

The stimulus for planning is often external to the individual or the unit. External stimuli may include such forces as a directive from someone in higher authority, changes in the social system; clear community need and/or demands, sudden availability of governmental funds for a particular target group, or changes in the methods we have to deal with mental illness. The introduction of reserpine and Thorazine, the spread of the open hospital and therapeutic milieu concepts, and the increasing costs of inpatient care in the past led dramatically and sometimes painfully to the need to alter programs.

Internal stimuli for planning programs include such factors as particular staff interests or "burnout," the introduction of a new staff member to the unit, or a breakdown in functional capacity of the unit.

Selecting and Orienting a Planning Group

The first stage in any process initiated in response to the stimulus is to *designate a planning group*. Depending on the complexity of the organization to be changed, a small ward or a major regional comprehensive program, the size and level of the group can vary but should include at least several components: (1) representatives from the professional and paraprofessional staff currently providing services, (2) representatives from consumers of the existing and/or potential services, (3) representatives from the group to which the unit is accountable (commissioner, director, superior), and (4) and objective outside consultant with some planning experience. A staff member should be designated as the person to coordinate the meetings, secure appropriate data, and perform other functions to further the work of the committee. In no case should the staff person on the committee be assigned responsibility as a "director of planning." This individual should assist, coordinate, and initiate but never be the single creator of the plan.[8]

---

size and complexity of the organization determine the level at which the psychiatrist relates to nonmedical clinicians. For example, depending on the size of the population served, he may relate to the clinical social worker, to the director of the hospital's department of social work services, or to the deputy commissioner of welfare.

Where the goal is modest, i.e., to expand a clinic or change the nature of an inpatient population, the committee may be made up of four or five individuals who may complete this task in 2–3 weeks. In planning a larger operation, i.e., a new hospital program or a community mental health center, the process will take many months. When planning services for a community population consisting of tens of thousands, there should be several clinical professionals who represent various disciplines involved: paraprofessionals; consumers and representatives of families of consumers; individuals with knowledge of personnel and budget matters; representatives of the executive branch of the governing board of the hospital; representatives and/or of the community to be served; and some representative of the local government planning authority. Especially in the larger groups, the makeup of the committee should include some individuals who carry political weight in the community so that both the community and the planning committee can be reasonably comfortable about the fact that they are headed in the same direction.

Once the group has been convened and agrees on general structure and purpose, an initial *orientation process* is necessary in order to provide a basic frame of reference for all members. This may involve bringing in one or more outside "experts" and/or circulating to the group brief references pertinent to the planning process, mental health delivery systems, and epidemiology that can then be discussed at the early meetings. There are a number of such references that are useful.[12–19]

It is essential to include in the content of the committee members' orientation both the inevitability of change in any system and the need for long-range planning. While unexpected changes in the system cannot be avoided, long-range planning provides direction and a constructive means of dealing with change. Short-term planning is useful only if seen within the context of long-range consequences.

Channels for communication to key persons outside the committee should be structured in order to minimize anxiety and maximize acceptance on the part of the rest of the staff and others who will be affected by the plan. Committee members must be aware of what the administrative group is planning. It would be inconsistent and discouraging for the committee to plan for an improvement in an inpatient unit if the director of the hospital was planning to convert the space to short-term surgical beds. Similarly, involvement with the local governmental mental health authority is meaningless if that group intends to abdicate its responsibility for mental health services to the state and/or the federal government within a year.

Defining the Mission of the Organization

The committee should spend time obtaining relevant input and discussing the primary *mission of the organization* and its parent body. The committee should acquaint itself with history, present philosophy, practice, and direction of the organization. The mission may be to provide a full range of health services to a local or broader population or to provide short-term inpatient care in the context of a nonambulatory health facility; or it may be to provide brief supportive services, including ambulatory and inpatient care to a defined population, i.e., students and faculty of the university, residents of a defined geographical area, or even all individuals with a "service-connected disability."

It is important for the success of the plan that goals not conflict with the mission of the parent body. If the mission is to provide acute health services to anyone seeking it who can afford to pay, it would be inappropriate as a goal for the inpatient unit to attempt to provide alternate housing for chronically disabled patients. While the community may think, as was particularly the case in the 1960s and early 1970s, that one of their main mental health priorities should be to provide expanded job opportunities and improved housing, direct provision of these resources cannot be seen as a major responsibility of a general hospital whose interests are in expanding its clinical psychiatric services. It legitimately might be interested, however, in expanding its activities as mental health consultants to agencies that properly would be charged with the goal of providing such services.

The interests and skills of the existing personnel and the resources may be important considerations when linked with current political, philosophical, and fiscal issues. For example, a large general hospital in an urban area, with a governing body committed to matters of public concern, and a program with a strong reputation for quality and efficient inpatient care of acute psychiatric patients might wish, when faced with under-utilized space, to plan for services for the more chronic mentally ill. These could include both inpatient care and alternatives to inpatient care such as partial hospitalization, crisis intervention, and local agreements with facilities providing sheltered housing arrangements.

All aspects of the mission, including comprehensiveness, preventive care, education, and research must be studied and the philosophy of the organization, the nature of its services, and the groups to be served determined. The mission should be specific enough to be helpful if it is not to run into unanticipated complications. It should be reviewed periodically with the participants, the consumers, and the governing bodies to test its feasibility and acceptability.

Needs Assessment

Having defined the mission, the population to be served and the overall area of services to be provided, the next step is the conduct of a *needs assessment.* At the beginning, it is worthwhile for the planning committee to spend time becoming familiar with the process and means by which such useful material is collected. [20,21] The committee must become knowledgeable and familiar with the ecology and demography of the area to be served and the concerns of those its population. This will include not only the psychiatric needs such as the prevalence of major illness and incidence of successful suicide attempts but also the social problems that have a high correlation with mental illness, such as out-of-wedlock children, inadequate housing, prevalence of delinquency, unemployment rate, and so on. Goldsmith and Unger[22] outlined a number of social factors related to mental health needs and utilized them in a study of catchment areas in Maryland. There are other good introductions to the process,[23–26] and the author especially recommends Rosen's[27] work from the Biometry Branch of the National Institute of Mental Health (NIMH). This kind of study will provide date not only about the characteristics of the individuals residing within the area to be served but also about the ecology of the community that highlights those social and environmental issues closely related to mental health disorders in both cause and effect. At present, approximately 16 percent of health systems agencies (HSA) programs and resources are devoted to primary mental health programs[28] and can provide adequate data relevant to the local condition. A practical aid in such efforts is the NIMH work of Rosen, Lawrence, Goldsmith, et al.,[29] which gives actual examples of how it may be utilized.

It is important to note that the reliability of data will vary depending on the goal of the agency collecting the data, the size of the population studied, and the techniques used in its collection. An awareness of the problem of weighing the comparable validity of several sources of data needs to be encouraged. It is somewhat like weighing apples, nuts, and seeds in one container.

The committee members should study data about specific kinds of mental health needs and about the relationship between resources and demands. While the field of epidemiology is far from perfected, an understanding of its principles will make it possible for the committee both to understand their own activities better and to educate others as the plan develops. Sophisticated knowledge about distribution of disease, defects, and disabilities and the variety of factors that affect the manifestation of such conditions (i.e., epidemiology) is essential. The Weissman[30] study would be a good place to begin. There are a number of reference works[31–34] that combine national data on varieties of pathology and trends in the utilization of resources with which to deal with them. Almost any of the mental health statistical notes from the National Institute of Mental Health, which have been issued frequently since 1967, are also of interest.[35]

Additional information useful to the committee in its work on needs assessment work can be found in studies of the likelihood of undetected mental illness in communities. A particularly complete example of this is Srole's *Mental Health in the Metropolis: The Midtown Manhattan Study*.[36] There are other more recent and briefer references to this subject.[37] Studies of the resources available, of course, need to be adapted to local needs because of the wide disparity between the kinds of resources available in urban and rural areas.[38,39]

It is particularly important to look at specific needs for programs. Are there special groups within the community that are not being served? Is there an unusually high incidence or prevalence of mental illness? Are there clearly observable gaps in the network of services? It is, of course, important to follow up the delineation of a particular need with a study of possible causes. For example, a common complaint is that there are an inadequate number of beds to serve the catchment area. The cause of this must be studied. Are there too many readmissions? Is there an inadequate number of alternative services so that admission becomes the only answer? The old saw that "if your only tool is a hammer, everything begins to look like a nail" is often the case in the demands for increased beds. It may be that inpatient care is, for a number of reasons, too leisurely and patients are kept too long. The goals of the inpatient service may be directed toward long-term reconstruction rather than short-term redirection. In some cases, the reverse is true; the beds are empty. One questions, then, why the underutilization? Are there improved services in other areas? Was the original planning poor?

The means of learning about the problems of existing resources are varied, and some are relatively simple. One can begin by studying which patients come to the facility and their motivation. What are their diagnoses, and what kinds of treatment are made available to them? How effective and efficient is the existing system?

A particularly sensitive part of a needs assessment for a program involving anything other than a relatively small internal organization program revision is the use of some kind of community survey. The techniques for such a survey vary but should include such factors as ongoing communication with creditable representatives of the community at large, political figures, social club officers, religious groups, and so on. It will be particularly important to secure information from them, but also, though this is sometimes referred perjoratively to as co-optation, to involve them in using their considerable power both to overcome obstacles to secure the needed programs and to avoid resistance and major hostility on the part of uninformed community groups. In collaboration with these figures, it is worthwhile to schedule community meetings open to the public in order to address the problems, to give some indication of the committee's commitment to and concern for the community, and to request their assistance. It may be useful, although no always necessary, to have a written[40] or verbal survey by telephone or street interviews with members of the community to determine needs, perceived needs, and perceived image of the existing and changed services.

Lest the reader be intimidated by the scope of data analysis implied in the preceding paragraphs, one can be assured that even in the planning major comprehensive mental health facilities, the wheel need not be reinvented. Many data are already available. A specific example is the question of appropriate number of beds for the defined service area. One HSA determined that .45 beds|1000 would be an adequate number to supply all of the acute and intermediate inpatient mental health needs for a population with primary psychiatric illness[41] in a representative community.

Contact with the state office of mental health early in the assessment process will often bring in a wealth of information about the social indices, the health/mental health needs, and the resources of the particular service area with which the planners are concerned. County and city mental health offices can be of additional help not only in providing data but in providing ongoing consultation and even emotional support, when needed, at no cost other than a willingness to increase somewhat the processes of mental health planning. At a minimum, these governmental agencies will be able to provide data on the incidence and prevalence of the psychiatric disabilities in the area and some indication of which segments of the area population are at highest risk. Often, they may be able to provide a reasonably accurate estimate of the resources. It is important that programs that are planned do not overlap or duplicate existing programs. Since there is some indication[42] that a very significant proportion of the Veterans Administration health services are duplicative of other local services and in some instances seem to be somewhat less efficient, the question points to the ever-important role of politics in determination of professional programming.

The principles of needs assessment, of course, apply throughout the world[43] although clearly there are socioeconomic and resource differences between various sections of the United States and other countries.

Defining the Goals and Priorities

Once the extent and variety of needs are determined, the planning committee is ready to move to the next step in the planning process, which is *definiting the goals and priorities* and scheduling of a preliminary timetable. At this point, it is often useful for the committee to give thought to a structure such as management by objectives as a means of achieving this end. Robins provides a good introduction to the concept.[44]

The goals may be determined by the particular program interests of the community, of the media, or of individuals on the staff.[45–47] The goals or the priority may be to provide one service to a wide geographical area or comprehensive services to a smaller one. It is important that the area or the first area selected be realistic.[48] If the area to be served is too large, the result can be disastrous from the standpoint of the collapse of the services and the anger of the consumer and the public. One could choose to study as the area of service the world,[49] the continental United States,[1,35] an entire state, a large city, or a community within it. There have been a number of studies comparing the different problems and resources of a state[50,51] and a large city.[36,52–54]

Planning for a relatively small, defined service area for which comprehensive services may be provided can be a gratifying experience and one that can set the tone for future planning for expanded services.[55] There are a number of values in selecting a discrete area as a target. If one selects an area that has a limited, easily measured population accessible to the services to be provided, it then is easier to assess the causes of the difficulties, the impact of the solutions, as well as to increase the likelihood of support of the consumers and the local individuals involved. The area served can be as small as a few blocks in an urban area, a census tract, or health area. The catchment area system instituted in conjunction with the Community Mental Health Centers Act is probably too large and complicated for beginning planning activity.

Determining Existent and Expected Financial and Personnel Resources

The committee then begins to examine the balance of available resources through other existing services and the reasonable availability of additional personnel, architectural, and fiscal resources that can be made available through various sources. Studies of timing and availability of these resources must be made. Will there be a sufficient number of young psychiatrists[56] to staff the expanded unit if expansion is planned? If the plan is to provide services to the chronic mentally ill, will there be adequate housing facilities, staff, and resources to care for them in the community, and will the agencies in the community be willing to accept them? If there is to be a new emphasis on the care of the geriatric psychiatric patient, will the necessary resources for comprehensive health needs of this group be available? If the goal is to expand services to children and their families, will the local school system and the mental health association be able and willing to assist in the network of services?

It is obvious that major concerns of governmental figures, the community, and the media are likely to affect the waxing and waning of public monies for particular kinds of programs during the 2- or 3-year period after the inception of the plan.[57,58] Will the public government focus be on services for children or the aged? Will the concern be on accountability and fiscal constraints? Will the spotlight be on inadequate care of the chronically ill and the resulting damage to the communities and patients as well? Will the federal policy on mental health care change? Will the pressure be to provide service at the cost of teaching and research programs or variations of this balance? Is universal health insurance imminent, and is it likely to affect the way services are provided and paid for? Are there likely to be new modalities of treatment that will affect the utilization of programs? Will the role of members of the mental health team of psychiatrists, clinical nurse specialists, social workers, psychologists, and activities therapists change, and will these changes have an impact on costs of services? Will there be a change in the funding bodies' wish to serve certain service areas' interest? Each of these factors may require some directional changes in planning over a course of time.

Redefining the Goals and Priorities

Having completed an evaluation of the present and expected resources, the committee should now *redefine its goals and priorities* in the face of reality. It is quite possible that with the committee's realistic knowledge of the availability of space and personnel resources, only minor changes need be made in previous statements of goals and priorities.

Articulating and Presenting the Plan and Timetable for Approval

At this point, the committee should be prepared to *articulate the plan* and *prepare to make presentations* in its defense. The presentation should include a restatement of the mission, an outline of needs assessment data that supports the conclusions of the planning committee, a statement of the goals, a timetable for implementation of the plan, an anticipated budget on a timed basis, and a section on the presumed availability of resources to make the plan possible.

There are a number of necessary constituencies to whom the plan should be presented. Their number and complexity will vary depending on the size and the location of the program to be implemented. At the very least, the audience should include the staff that will be involved in the implementation of the plan and the supervising or governing body of the larger organization of which the plan would be a part. This may be the director of clinical services in a hospital in which the plan is an expansion of an inpatient unit; the executive director or the governing board of a hospital in which a major expansion of comprehensive services is planned; or the executive branch of county or state government, which will be asked to approve or disapprove the inclusion of this segment in the large governmental plan and possibly provide a major proportion of the funding.

Plans that will affect larger areas of the community also should be presented at open hearings so that members of the community can respond both as individual consumers and as representatives of special groups. In such cases, it is also helpful to have a discussion prior to the open community presentation with other provider agencies within the network of services on whom the plan will be dependent for success.

Some clinicians may object that this process is largely "political." One should note that political strategies are essential to the success of almost every phase of administration. They are irrelevant only if the goals and objectives of the plan are irrelevant since such strategies test the strengths and weaknesses of support and consolidate the former. The committee must be prepared to receive considerable criticism, even attack, from a number of those to whom the plan is being presented. It is important that the committee avoid defensiveness and counterattack, since these may lead to further unnecessary and avoidable resistance. It is also likely that some of these audiences will provide substantial information that may enhance the possibility of success of the plan. As it makes its presentations, the committee should remain flexible so that reasonable and necessary changes stemming from these presentations may be incorporated in the plan. Such a stance will help avoid demoralization of the committee and possible collapse of the major portions of the plan.

Implementing the Plan, Evaluation Structure, and a Staff Development Program

Once approval is secured, the next step is *implementation of the plan.* Completion of the formal written plan and its budget and timetable is, of course, no assurance that the difficulties are ended. It may well be that the planning committee itself may be dissolved and replaced by an administrative staff to implement the carefully designed plan. Given the inevitability of change, long- and short-range planning cannot predict all the forces that might develop to impede progress. By its nature, it can give some direction and some stability to the development of the program. While many obstacles seem to have been resolved at the time of the articulation of the "final" plan, other obstacles will usually develop. A wide variety of factors may have major positive or negative effects on the program.[59] There may be such issues as professional and jurisdictional conflict; changing governmental policies and data; new legislative or judicial restrictions on the delivery of services of other provider agencies; changing philosophical framework in the mental health, public health, and social welfare fields; and major changes in the availability of professional staff. Keeping in mind the long-term goals enunciated in the plan, it will be possible to deal with the impediments more flexibly. The implementation staff should always be prepared for modification based on these factors and be prepared with options when the inevitable obstacles present themselves. It is important to keep the staff and the community aware of these changes to avoid a sense of dissatisfaction or conviction that the plan was "pie in the sky."

In addition to being prepared for short-term planning in response to obstacles, the implementation staff must concern itself as well with (1) the need for ongoing evaluation of the timeliness and effectiveness of the implementation processes and (2) the creation of the necessary staff development for the staff.

While it is by no means simple, the implementation phase often is the most rewarding aspect of the creation of a new or improved psychiatric service. Such rewards can only occur, however, if each of the preceding steps have taken place with adequate attention to reliable data, open communication among all of the participants outside the core planning group, and with a realistic, even if never entirely accurate, concept of the future directions of area and its service needs.

ROLE OF THE CITIZEN IN GOVERNANCE

Adding a somewhat simplified but practical outline of the mental health services planning process, some comments are in order about a specific force that may influence the planning process at any stage of its development. It is important to utilize to the fullest the advantages in these influences and to avoid some of the disadvantages that they may pose. The phenomenon is the role of the citizen board in the planning and management of mental health programs.

Special Aspects

To the planner of a small inpatient unit, the question of governance and accountability may be relatively simple. This individual need explain the plan only to his immediate administrative supervisor, his peers, and in some cases to his other team members, his patients, and their families. As the magnitude of the program to be administered grows, the manager of the program may be accountable to a host of other health professionals and interested members of the public, such as the directors of hospitals or clinics, their citizen boards, executives of the local, state and federal mental health authorities, the media, politicians, and, increasingly, the courts. The members of the planning committee will be well advised to become familiar with the requirements of these groups in the particular area that the program is to be delivered; as mentioned earlier, be prepared to utilize their support and information and to deal flexibly and consistently with their objections. To the great surprise of some professionals, their support can be helpful and their objections are often valid.

The question of *patients' rights* and *patient advocacy* is covered in detail in the now defunct Mental Health Systems Act.[60] The act outlines a "bill of rights" for mental health patients but stops short of requiring its inclusion in individual comprehensive programs and urges the states to make it a state requirement. The planning committee must be attentive to these matters since the list includes a number of areas that open the way to a potential and massive increase in the number of legal suits around patient care. While suits cannot be totally avoided, attention to them in designing the plan for the service may minimize them to some extent.

The rights are wide ranging and include assurances of procedures supportive of the individual's personal liberty, including the patient's right (1) to have an individualized written treatment plan; (2) to participate in the planning of the services to be provided, to know the objectives of treatment, their justification, and possible adverse effects, the reasons for limitations of visitors, the obtaining of his informed voluntary written consent; (3) not to participate in experimentation; (4) to observe restrictions on restraint and seclusion; (5) to a humane treatment environment; (6) to confidentiality; (7) to access to his mental health care records; (8) to privacy; (9) to a grievance procedure; (10) to protection from reprisal following the grievance procedure; and (11) to appropriate referral to other agencies. They also include the suggestion for advocacy programs to protect the rights of the mentally ill individuals and the family and to educate the public.

For years, mental health professionals and service planners have expressed reactions ranging from concern to outrage at what is viewed as the encroachment by the nonprofessional citizen on what had been professional prerogatives. In the United States, however, the tradition of citizen involvement in the governance of human service agencies goes back several centuries. It was traditional for well-intentioned, prominent, usually wealthy members of the community to bank together to provide services for "the deserving poor," the "orphan and widow in failing health," and the "infirm elderly." Generally, such groups provided funds and selected professional administrators and providers to run the program. Sophistication on the part of board members of such agencies increased over the years. Beginning in the 1960s, partly as a result of the Community Mental Health Centers Act of 1963, governmental mandates have become increasingly specific and provided for actual governance by citizens representing the community served by mental health providers. This is currently exemplified by the Mental Health Systems Act.

While some providers within the system express dismay at this, most of the literature related to the subject has been, either guardedly or enthusiastically, positive.[61–63] It is true that some professionals have left the public service system and given as their primary reason the need to deal with sometimes uninformed and "difficult" community representatives. A number of authors, however, have described advantages of this structure and have suggested techniques for improving the symbiotic relationship between the citizen, management, and provider.[64–66]

While the process may slow the pace of the development of plans and increase the expense of their implementation, it is consistent with the American philosophy of citizens' freedom to participate in decisions affecting them and consistent with the current trends toward open communication between government, delivery systems, and the public. It is an essential and challenging experience for any mental health professional and may be approached in various ways. A reasonably comfortable way to begin is with the existing, usually sophisticated, mental health citizen group such as the local or national Mental Health Association. While the individuals and the professional staff at these agencies are no less dedicated to quality and human rights than more militant groups, they have a better understanding of the problems of professionals and the difficulties of the bureaucracy. Many of them, too, may be helpful in reaching larger community groups. They may also help to sponsor hearings to provide information and seek input from the community at large.

When one is starting from scratch, there is a natural history of such interreactions. The early phases of community advisory or governing groups tend to be dominated by articulate individuals who have collected a series of injustices about the public system generally and the mental health system specifically. With some patience, however, the group can be broadened to include other interested citizens whose primary purpose is to improve the mental health system rather than to wreak vengeance for past injustices. This group gradually assumes control of the board, which is then better balanced. Continued careful and open work between the professionals and administrators and these groups will include an ongoing mutual education toward understanding each other's points of view to the point where there can be partnership in the interests of improved mental health services. An early area of clarification to the education of the board members consists of differentiating "what you want" from "what you need" as practical considerations.

The responsibilities and authority of *community boards* vary from one area of the country to another but will often include a number of standard components. They may be mandated to serve as the legal authority for the service. They usually participate in the delineation of goals and objectives of the program. They provide a valuable articulation of expectations on the part of the citizen constituency in the area served. They can provide, particularly in the political sector, a potent force to secure governmental funding: Through their own contacts and power, they may improve coordination with other sometimes reluctant service providers, and in many cases in some of the more advanced programs, they can be active in the education of staff. They may also be effective in acting forcefully to provide supportive outside services, such as housing, in the face of localized community opposition.

As with any other aspect of program planning and implementation, it is important to build in a structure for evaluating the effectiveness of governing boards. Dorwart[66] reported on one technique for comparing the effectiveness of governing boards. Steckler and Herzog[65] have described, with tongue in cheek, a somewhat simplistic but probably effective way of dealing with the board.

In conclusion, citizen participation in the management of community mental health programs appears to be here to stay. Littlestone[9] makes the point that "merging of corporate planning and community organization should be helpful." Harnessing the community representatives' appetite for acquiring knowledge and skills to the professionals dedication, knowledge, and skills can make for a powerful and effective program. It is inevitable that both sides will sometimes agree and sometimes disagree with objectives, methods and priorities, and cast of characters, but the negotiation of these differences can be of benefit to all concerned.

A FINAL NOTE

Possibly the most important point to emphasize is the importance of utilizing existing resources. An attempt to build a monolithic system can in no way fulfill all the needs of the community. Ginzberg[67] notes:

> When a sector of society finds it is handicapped in accomplishing its goals, it tends to reach out and aims to do more. A patient may require social services such as finding a new apartment, getting the patient a suitable job that does; it does not follow that a hospital health system must extend its boundaries until it has its own social welfare housing and employment units. The relative isolation that has characterized medicine in the past suggests that significant gains lie ahead if proper linkages can be established with such important systems such as education and manpower training, employment, social welfare, and transportation.*

*From Ginzberg E: Urban Health Services; The Case of New York. New York, Columbia University Press, 1971. With permission.

For the mental health system, the author would add that the linkages with the correctional system and the quantity of planning data available from the governmental agencies are also important. Like Knowles,[68] the author's particular bias is that the mental health system should be an integral part of a comprehensive health system. This has the added advantage of discouraging a mind/body dualism.

REFERENCES

1. President's Commission on Mental Health, vol. I. Springfield, Va, U.S. Department of Commerce, 1978
2. Steiner GA: Top Management Planning. London, Macmillan, 1969
3. Mayer RR: Social Science and Institutional Change. DHEW Publication, ADM 78–627. Washington, DC, US Government Printing Office, 1979
4. Feldman S: Mental health administration: an appraisal, in Feldman S (ed): The Administration of Mental Health Services. Springfield, Ill, Thomas, 1980, pp XXII–XXI
5. Barton AK: A problem policy program model for planning community mental health services. J Community Psychol 6:37–41, 1978
6. Levinson DJ, Klerman, GL: The clinician executive. Adm Ment Health 1:53–67, 1971
7. Yarvis RM, Edwards DW: Planning: The Design of Mental Health Programs. Sacramento, Calif, Pyramid Systems, 1980
8. Peters JP: A Guide to Strategic Planning for Hospitals. Chicago, Ill, American Hospital Association, 1979
9. Littlestone R: Planning in mental health, in Feldman S (ed): The Administration of Mental Health Services. Springfield, Ill, Thomas, 1980
10. Kramer M: Some perspectives on the role of bio-statistics and epidemiology for the prevention and control of mental disorders. Milbank Mem Fund Q 53:279–335, 1975
11. Yarvis RM: The Resource Guide for Mental Health. Sacramento, Calif, Pyramid Systems, 1979
12. Becker RE: The organization and management of community mental health services. Community Ment Health J 8:292–302, 1972
13. Beigel A: Planning for the development of a community mental health center I, catchment area, administration, continuity of care, staffing and funding. Community Ment Health J 6:267–275, 1970
14. Beigel A: Planning for the development of a community mental health center II, planning of services. Community Ment Health J 6:356–365, 1970
15. Diamond H, Santore A: Basic tasks in developing a community mental health center. Hosp Community Psychiatry 25:232–234, 1974
16. Miller FT: Trends in community mental health programming. Am J Community Psychol 6:191–200, 1978
17. Osterweil J: Mental health planning: prelude to comprehensive health planning. Bull N Y Acad Med 44:194–198, 1966
18. Bachrach LL: Developing objectives in community mental health planning. Am J Public Health 64:1162–1163, 1974
19. Tarail M: Current and future issues in community mental health. Psychiatr Q 52:27–37, 1980
20. Longest J, Konan M, Tweed D: A Study of Deficiencies and Differentials in the Distribution of Mental Health Resources and Facilities. DHEW Publication No. ADM 79-517. Washington, DC, US Government Printing Office, 1976
21. Marrs LW, Helge DI: The role of needs assessment in program planning and evaluation. J Spec Educ 12:143–151, 1978
22. Goldsmith HF, Unger EL: Social Area Analysis: Procedures and Illustrative Applications Based upon the Mental Health Demographic Profile System. US Bureau of Census—Census Tract Papers, Series GE40, 1973
23. Warheit GJ, Holzer CE, Robbins L: Social indicators and mental health planning: an empirical case study. Community Ment Health J 15:94–103, 1979
24. Wedge RF: A Review of the Literature on the Early Identification of Delinquent Prone Children. Sacramento, Calif, California Youth Authority, 1978
25. Evans JL, Leger GJ: Canadian victimization surveys: a discussion paper. Can J Criminol 21:166–'83, 1979
26. Weissman MM, Myers JK, Harding PS: Psychiatric disorders in the United States

urban community: 1975–76. Am J Psychiatry 135:459–462, 1978
27. Rosen BM: A Model for Estimating Mental Health Needs Using 1970 Census Socioeconomic Data. NIMH, DHEW Publication No. ADM 74-63. Washington, DC, US Government Printing Office, 1974
28. Keill SL: The HSA and psychiatrists. Bull Am Ps A 22:1–4, 1980
29. Rosen BM, Lawrence L, Goldsmith HF, et al: Mental Health Demographic Profile System Description: Purpose, Contents and Sampler of Uses. NIMH, DHEW Publication No. ADM 76-263. Washington DC, US Government Printing Office, 1975
30. Weissman MM, Klerman GL: Epidemiology of mental disorders: emerging trends in the United States. Arch Gen Psychiatry 35:705–711, 1978
31. Jones KR, Vischi TR: Impact of alcohol, drug abuse in mental health treatment on medical care utilization. J Am Public Health Association 17, 1979
32. Vischi TR, Jones KR, Shank EL, et al: The Alcohol, Drug Abuse, and Mental Health National Data Book. ADAMHA Publication No. 80-938. Washington, DC, Office of Program Planning Coordination, 1980
33. Bachrach LL: Psychiatric Bed Needs: An Anlytic Review. NIMH Series D, No. 2, DHEW Publication ADM 79-205. Washington, DC, US Government Printing Office, 1979
34. Regier DA, Goldberg ID, Taube CA: The de facto U.S. mental health services system: a public health perspective. Arch Gen Psychiatry 35:685–693, 1978
35. National Institute of Mental Health, Mental Health Statistical Note No. 129. Staff-Patient Ratios in Selected Inpatient Mental Health Facilities—January 1974. Bethesda, Md, National Institute of Mental Health, 1976
36. Srole L: Mental Health in the Metropolis: The Midtown Manhattan Study. New York, McGraw-Hill, 1962
37. Mendelsohn FS, Egri G, Dohrenwend BP; Diagnosis of non-patients in the general community. Arch Gen Psychiatry 135:1163–1167, 1978
38. Knesper DJ: Psychiatric manpower for state mental hospitals. Arch Gen Psychiatry 35:19–26, 1978
39. Straker M, Cummings J: Staffing patterns and team composition. Hosp Community Psychiatry 29:243–244, 1978
40. May AR: Mental Health Services in Europe: Review of Data Collected in Response to a WHO Questionnaire. Geneva, World Health Organization, 1976
41. Keill SL: Psychiatric care: a new role for hospitals? Hospitals 54:67–70, 1980
42. National Academy of Sciences National Research Council: Study of Health Care for American Veterans, a Report for the Committee on Veterans' Affairs of the United States Senate. Washington, DC, US Government Printing Office, 1977
43. Molina-Gusman G: Third world experiences in health planning. Int J Health Services 9:139–150, 1979
44. Robins A: Management-by-objectives for community mental health programs. Hosp Community Psychiatry 25:228–231, 1974
45. Herz MI: Prevention of chronicity in schizophrenia. Psychiatr Ann 8:35–47, 1978
46. Gruenberg EM, Archer J: Abandonment of responsibility for the seriously mentally ill. Milbank Mem Fund Q 57:485–506, 1979
47. Bachrach LL: Deinstitutionalization: An Analytical Review and Sociological Perspective. DHEW Publication No. ADM 76-351. National Institute of Mental Health, Washington, DC, 1976
48. Freedman DX: The president's commission: realistic remedies for neglect. Arch Gen Psychiatry 35:675–676, 1978
49. World Health Statistics Quarterly: Mental Health Planning. Geneva, World Health Organization, 1979, p 32
50. Sauber SR: State planning of mental health services. Am J Community Psychology 4:35–45, 1976
51. American Hospital Association Recommendations for Financing Mental Health Care in the United States. Chicago, Ill, American Hospital Association, 1973
52. Srole L: Measurements and classifications in socio-psychiatric epidemiology: midtown Manhattan study I and midtown Manhattan restudy II, 1974. J Health and Social Behavior, 16:347–364, 1975
53. Srole L, Fisher A: Mental Health in the Metropolis, Book I. New York, Harper & Row, 1975
54. Srole L, Fisher A: Mental Health in the Metropolis, Book II. New York, Harper & Row, 1975
55. Mazer M: A psychiatric and parapsychiatric register for an island community. Arch Gen Psychiatry 14:366–371, 1966
56. Ginzberg E: Economic changes and physician-patient relations. Bull N Y Acad Med 57:29–35, 1981
57. Kramer M: Psychiatric Services and the

Changing Institutional Scene, 1950–1985. DHEW Publication No. ADM 77-43. Washington, DC, US Government Printing Office, 1977
58. Leininger M: Health care delivery systems for tomorrow: possibilities and guidelines. Health Care Dimensions 2:83–94, 1975
59. Furman SF: Obstacles to the development of community mental health programs. Am J Orthopsychiatry 36:230–232, 1966
60. Mental Health Systems Act: Washington, DC, US Government Printing Office, 1980
61. Bolman WM: Community control of the community mental health center: II case examples. Am J Psychiatry 129:181–186, 1972
62. Enelow AJ, Weston WD: Cooperation or chaos: the mental health administrator's dilemma. Am J Orthopsychiatry 42:603–609, 1972
63. Ruiz P: Consumer participation in mental health programs. Hosp Community Psychiatry 24:38–39, 1973
64. Borus JF, Klerman GL: Consumer-professional collaboration for evaluation of neighborhood mental health programs. Hosp Community Psychiatry 27:401–404, 1976
65. Steckler AB, Herzog WT: How to keep your mandated citizen board out of your hair and off your back: a guide for executive directors. Am J Public Health 69:809–812, 1979
66. Dorwart RA, Meyers WR, Norman EC: Effective citizen participation in mental health: comparative case studies. Public Health Reports 94:268–274, 1979
67. Ginzberg E: Urban Health Services: The Case of New York. New York, Columbia University Press, 1971
68. Knowles JH: The role of the hospital: the ambulatory clinic. Bull N Y Acad Med 41:4–17, 1965

SUGGESTED READING

Gibson, RW: The use of financing to control the delivery of services. Psychiatr Ann 4:22–41, 1974

Silber, SC: Strategies for developing multisource funding for community mental health centers. Hosp Community Psychiatry 25:221–224, 1974

Boaz, RF: Equity in paying for health care services under a national insurance system. Milbank Memorial Fund Quarterly 53:337, 1975

Thomas J. Conklin, M.D.

19

Quality Assurance

QUALITY ASSURANCE

Quality assurance is a broad concept that encompasses a variety of patient-related review and monitoring activities. Quality assurance can be defined as a method of maintaining and improving the quality of patient care as well as a method of accountability to the patient, third-party payers, and outside reviewing bodies. The process of quality assurance is not new. It has been evolving in various forms and degrees since the appearance of hospitals. The present quality assurance standard is the result of the evolvement of regulatory processes and increased consumer knowledge of the health care industry.

THE BEGINNING OF ORGANIZED QUALITY ASSURANCE

Federal Regulations

The 1960s ushered in the beginning of organized quality control in health care. The passage of the Social Security Act (Public Law 89-97) in 1965 established the Medicare and Medicaid programs. Each hospital was required to develop a utilization review plan and establish a committee of the medical staff to oversee and control the utilization of services provided in their institutions. This internal review procedure failed to ensure adequately that the medical care rendered to Medicare and Medicaid patients met the standards of necessity and quality and resulted in a great expenditure of physicians' time.[1]

Rising health care cost, the question of fiscal accountability, and inequitable access to health care were concerns in the early 1970s and resulted in greater expectations for accountability and assurance of quality health care.

In 1972, Congress passed Public Law 92-603, which amended the Social Security Act and is known as the professional standards review organization (PSRO) law. The law is based on former Sen. Walter S. Bennet's concept that only physicians are qualified to evaluate the necessity and quality of medical care.

Physicians were required to form and operate local nonprofit organizations to review the quality of medical care delivered to beneficiaries of the Medicare and Medicaid programs in hospitals. The PSRO hospital review is based on three major mechanisms: (1) concurrent review of admissions and continued stay, based on a predetermined length of stay, (2) medical care evaluation studies, and (3) collection of data on medical practices and patient profiles for analysis.[2] Norms, standards, and criteria are used in the PSRO process. Local norms, standards, and criteria may be utilized provided they are approved by the professional standards review council in the PSRO area. The responsibility of performing reviews may be delegated by the PSRO to the medical staff of hospitals. The ultimate responsibility for all review decisions is retained, however, by the PSRO.[3] As the PSRO review program was established, the Medicare conditions of participation were amended, and new utilization review regulations for all hospitals were initiated. These regulations provided that utilization review employ a system of review and medical care evaluation studies compatible with that used in the PSRO program.[4]

Joint Commission on Accreditation of Hospitals

Concomitant with legislation enacted by the federal government, the Joint Commission on Accreditation of Hospitals (JCAH) formed a separate specific accreditation program for psychiatric facilities, and in 1972, standards for psychiatric facilities were included in the *Accreditation manual.* Medical audit became a JCAH requirement in 1974. The audit methodology, called the performance evaluation procedure for auditing and improving patient care (PEP), is a retrospective, primarily outcome-oriented approach designed to identify and correct problems in patient care.

A quality professional services section was added to the *JCAH Accreditation manual* in 1976. Quantitative requirements were associated with this standard, and all psychiatric facilities seeking accreditation were mandated to have two audits completed and two audits in progress in the interim between surveys.[5] The JCAH standards continued to be revised and updated, and the *Consolidated Standards for Child, Adolescent, and Adult Psychiatric, Alcoholism and Drug Abuse Programs* was issued in 1979.

The review and monitoring mechanisms previously described have been under constant scrutiny. The major thrust of PSRO and utilization review has been toward cost containment. The prohibitive expense of maintaining PSRO, however, is defeating the purpose for which this review system was intended. Legislation has been enacted that will phase out the PSROs by 1983 and may eliminate the utilization review requirements of the present law.

CURRENT CONCEPT—MULTIDIMENSIONAL QUALITY ASSURANCE

In contrast to hospitals' quality assurance programs in the 1970s (See Fig. 19-1), an expanded, multidimensional quality assurance program is now required by the JCAH and by the federal government. This quality assurance standard

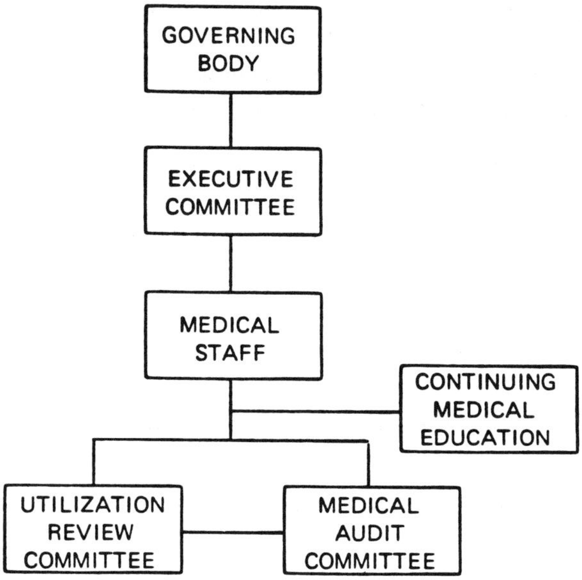

Figure 19-1. A flow chart illustrating the scope of quality assurance in the 1970s.

designates the responsibility for a quality assurance program to the governing body, with delegation of the functioning of the program to the medical staff.

The efficacy of a quality assurance program is dependent on actual performance by the administrator of the program and the cooperation of the medical staff. The quality assurance program may be administered by a group, a committee, or an individual. The overall administrative responsibility of the quality assurance program should, however, be delegated to an individual who has the authority to make decisions related to recommendations for improving patient care. Careful consideration must be given to the program's objectives. Mere compliance with the regulatory requirements will not achieve cooperation from the medical staff or other health care professionals and will usually result in a nonproductive program.[6]

The purpose of a quality assurance program is to maintain and improve, as far as possible, the quality of patient care through a problem-focused approach that examines treatment programs and activities and the hospital's therapeutic environment. The quality assurance program should integrate, coordinate, and monitor a variety of evaluative processes, administrative functions, and educational programs to assure optimal utilization of services in a cost-effective manner.

Designing a coordinated program requires a detailed assessment of the facility's existing quality assurance activities. Existing patient care review and monitoring activities should be integrated into the program. To add another monitoring mechanism to those already in place defeats the purpose of an integrated quality assurance program. Examples of existing patient-related review and monitoring activities are case conferences, utilization review, medical audit, patient satisfaction surveys, and medical staff committees. There are many existing data sources, some of which include incident reports, length of stay patterns, profile analyses, third-party payer denials or reports, PSRO feedback, and financial information. (See Fig. 19-2.)k019-2

The quality assurance program must include a mechanism for problem identification, problem analysis, problem resolution, problem monitoring, and follow-up to assess improvement.

It is important to design a flexible program that is unique to the needs of each facility. There must be a written plan that describes the functions of the quality assurance program. The written plan need not include all details and may be complemented with organizational charts and a pictorial description of the flow of information in the program.[7]

Components of a Quality Assurance Plan

Following are six components that should be included in a quality assurance plan:

1. Authority: identify the individual, group, or committee that has the ultimate authority and responsibility for the various quality assurance functions. State the relationship of the governing body to the committee.
2. Purpose: state the purpose of the quality assurance program in relation to the overall objectives of the facility.
3. Organization: identify who will have the authority to carry out the various quality assurance functions and who will be responsible for coordinating and integrating the various quality assurance activities. This may be shown in the form of an organizational chart or written into the plan.
4. Scope and responsibility: describe the overall scope of the program and define the responsibility of the individual, group, or committee in relation to the functioning of the quality assurance program.
5. Description of program implementation: include problem identification, data sources, problem assessment, priority setting for problem solving, and mechanisms for problem resolution, problem monitoring, and follow-up.
6. Annual evaluation: annually assess the effectiveness and efficacy of the quality assurance program. Describe the mechanism for the annual evaluation process in the plan.[8,9]

Each facility is unique, and the written quality assurance plan will differ accordingly. The basic components and the JCAH quality assurance standard must, however, be taken into consideration when writing the plan.

The following sample quality assurance plan was developed for a private psychiatric hospital and includes the essential components.

HOSPITAL X: QUALITY ASSURANCE PLAN

Authority

The quality assurance program has been established at Hospital X in accordance with the bylaws of the professional staff, approved by the governing body. The quality assurance committee is a standing committee of the professional staff

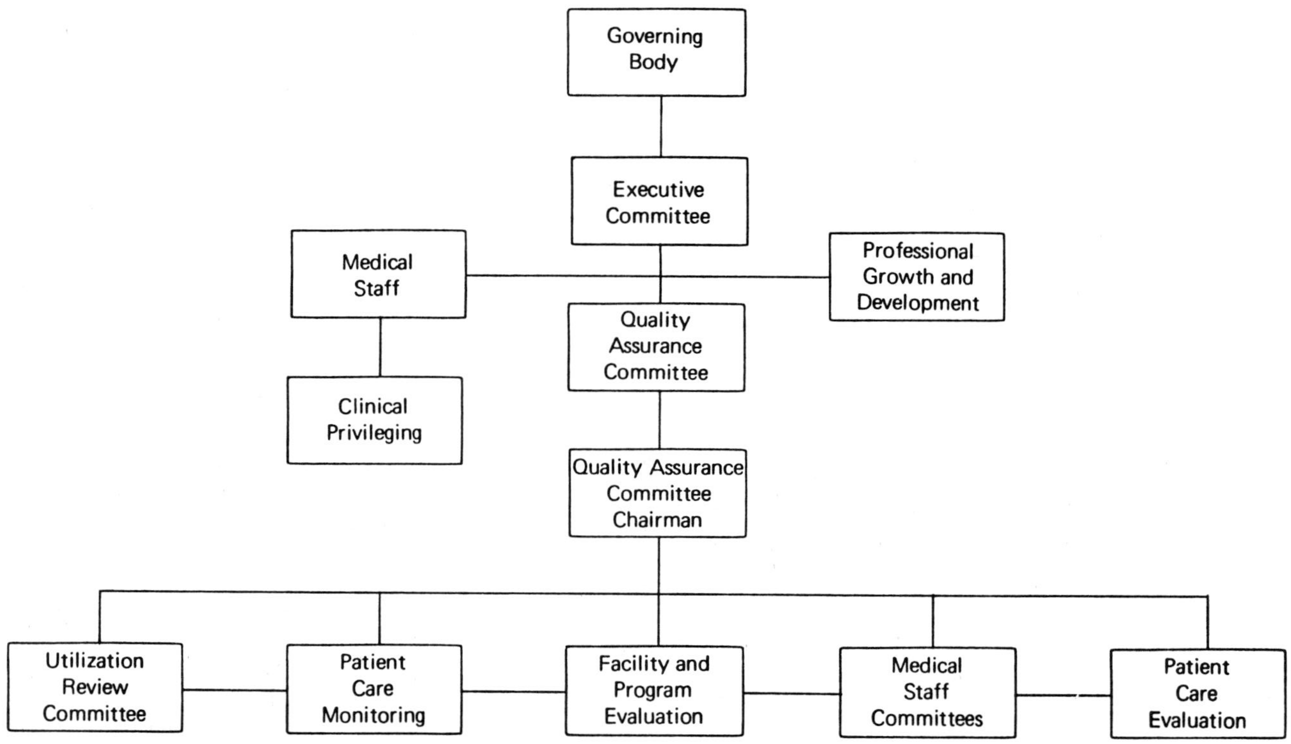

Figure 19-2. A flow chart illustrating the multidimensional quality assurance program presently required.

and is responsible for the quality assurance program. The medical director shall appoint a member of the active medical staff to serve as chairman. The chairman shall be directly responsible to the medical director, who has the ultimate authority and responsibility to assure efficient and optimum functioning of the program.

Purpose

The purpose of the quality assurance program at Hospital X is to maintain and improve, to whatever extent possible the quality of patient care through a problem-focused approach and to integrate, coordinate, and monitor evaluative processes, administrative functions, and educational programs within the hospital to assure quality patient care and optimum utilization of services.

Committee Organization

The chairman is responsible for reviewing all reported problems, for identifying and acknowledging problems that may have a significant impact on patient care, and for establishing the priority for the resolution of the problems.

The quality assurance coordinator shall provide technical assistance to the committee and be responsible for coordinating and integrating the various activities of the quality assurance program. The committee shall be multidisciplinary in membership and include members of the executive committee, the directors of the departments of nursing, rehabilitation services, psychiatric social work and pharmacy services, and the chairmen of all medical staff committees. The committee will coordinate information among hospital committees and clinical departments and identify problems relating to patient care. The committee is also responsible for assuring the maintenance of standards approved by the JCAH.

Meetings

The quality assurance committee will meet at least monthly and more frequently if deemed necessary by the chairman. The chairman will determine the time and place of the meetings.

Scope and responsibility

1. To coordinate all quality assurance activities
2. To review recommendations of other hospital committees and individuals involved in areas of quality assurance
3. To monitor the quality and patterns of patient care
4. To analyze identified or potential problems relating to patient care
5. To monitor quality assurance activities that may be performed by staff temporarily assigned by the committee to carry out such activities
6. To assure that the required patient care studies are performed and maintained and are an integral part of the hospital's quality assurance program
7. To make recommendations to the administration of the hospital for the proper resolution of the identified problem

8. To maintain an accurate record of quality assurance activities and their impact on patient care in the hospital
9. To assist as required in the evaluation of the effectiveness of the quality assurance program

Problem Identification

Problems may be identified and presented to the committee (1) during the course of a quality assurance meeting, (2) by individual hospital committees, (3) by a department or service, or (4) by a member of the hospital staff. All hospital personnel are encouraged to report any problems that affect patient care to the quality assurance coordinator. To facilitate the reporting of problems, a hospital problem report sheet may be used. Staff members may remain anonymous if they so choose. The quality assurance coordinator will present all reported problems to the chairman of the committee, who will review the problems. If it is determined that a problem can be resolved promptly, the chairman will initiate corrective action with the approval of the medical director. Other problems will be brought to the committee for deliberation and assessment.

Data Sources for Quality Assurance

The following data sources are reviewed through the quality assurance program: the patient record, incident reports, third-party payer reports, patient care monitoring summaries, financial data from insurance companies, hospital computerized clinical data reports, utilization review data, patient surveys, patient care studies, safety committee reports, clinical conference reports, and resident and staff evaluation conference summaries.

Priority Setting

The chairman and the quality assurance coordinator shall review all problems that have been reported. Priority for problem assessment and resolution shall be determined by the degree of impact on patient care and whether the problem is resolvable. If further assessment of the problem is not required, the medical director may authorize appropriate action to resolve the problem. Problems related to areas that are not the responsibility of the medical director shall be referred to the chief executive officer. Subsequent to initial assessment of an identified problem, a timetable for further assessment and resolution of the problem shall be established in the following manner:

1. Code red: this category represents problems that are felt to have a high lethality or a high injury index, affect a large number of patients, or present other serious difficulties. These problems require prompt assessment and resolution. It is the responsibility of the chairman to assure that these problems are addressed as soon as possible.
2. Code yellow: this category represents problems that because of their nature do not have the emergent nature of code red but are felt to require assessment and resolution within 6 months.
3. Code green: this category represents problems that do not have the emergent nature of code yellow or code red. Problems that are complex or difficult to

assess may also be in this category. These problems should be resolved within a year.

Problem assessment

The chairman shall assign responsibility for problem assessment to an ad hoc committee composed of staff members from the related area, a standing committee in the hospital, or to an individual. Assessment may be accomplished by observation, interviewing, or data analysis. Clinically valid criteria shall be established for objective assessment. The status of the assessment and recommendations shall be reported to the quality assurance committee monthly unless otherwise specified.

Problem Resolution

When the cause and scope of the problem are known, corrective action can be undertaken. The chairman of the quality assurance committee has the responsibility to accept the recommendations made and obtain authorization, if necessary, from the medical director, the chief executive officer, and the governing body for implementation of the recommendations. Any problem that cannot be resolved because of its complexity or because of external circumstances will be noted in the minutes of the quality assurance committee.

Problem Monitoring/Follow-up

The medical director and the quality assurance committee are responsible for determining that the problems have been resolved or reduced to an acceptable level. The quality assurance committee will request periodic monitoring of the results of any corrective action.

Reporting

The minutes of the quality assurance committee shall be reported to the medical staff at its regular monthly meeting and forwarded to the chief executive officer and to all committee members. Quality assurance status reports will be sent quarterly to the medical director, the chief executive officer, and the governing body.

Annual Evaluation

The effectiveness and efficiency of the quality assurance program shall be evaluated at least annually. The chairman of the quality assurance committee is responsible for an annual report, which includes a summary and review of the activities of the committee, the committee's assessment of the overall effectiveness of the program, and recommendations for changes in the program. The assessment will be based on maintenance and further improvement of quality patient care and treatment. The report shall be sent to the chief executive officer for his review and approval and subsequently to the governing body.

QUALITY ASSESSMENT AND CONTROL ACTIVITIES

Utilization Review

Utilization review is a valuable component of a quality assurance program and is a requirement of both the JCAH and the federal government. The purpose of utilization review is to determine if the health care services provided to the patient are medically necessary and provided in a cost-efficient manner. This review process is the responsibility of the medical staff, and the committee should be a standing committee of the medical staff. Facilities must have a written plan that describes the committee's functions. Approval of the plan by the professional staff and the governing body is necessary.

Specific areas outlined by the joint commission as well as the federal government for inclusion in a utilization review plan are as follows:

1. Committee composition, authority, and responsibility: the committee should be multidisciplinary in membership, including a representative from the hospital administration and one from the medical records department. It is the responsibility of the hospital administrative staff to provide the committee with records and pertinent material to facilitate its operation.
2. A conflict of interest policy: this policy applies to everyone involved in utilization review activities. Any person who holds financial interest in any hospital is not eligible for appointment to the committee. It is the responsibility of a reviewing member to disqualify himself if he has been professionally involved in the case being reviewed.
3. Confidentiality policy: this policy should apply to all utilization review activities, findings, and recommendations. Committee minutes and reports should not identify patients or physicians by name.
4. Description of the method used to identify utilization-related problems: medical care evaluation studies may be used for this purpose. If this function is delegated to another committee, it must be so specified in the plan.
5. Selection of cases for review: concurrent review may include all patients or be a random or focus selection. All Medicare and Medicaid patients should be included in the sample.
6. Procedure for conducting admission and extended stay reviews: criteria and length of stay norms that have been approved by the professional staff must be utilized in performing concurrent reviews. A qualified nonphysician representative of the committee, often referred to as a utilization review coordinator, may perform the review function. The coordinator does not have the authority to deny an admission or extended stay and must refer all questionable cases to a physician member of the committee. If it is determined that an admission or extended stay is not medically necessary, the patient or the responsible party and the facility must be notified in writing.
7. A mechanism for initiating discharge planning: discharge planning should be

initiated as soon as possible after admission to facilitate the patient's discharge as soon as medical services are no longer required.

8. Records and reports: the committee must keep records of its deliberations, findings, and instructions. These records are subject to review by the state agencies, the PSRO, and the fiscal intermediary in their evaluation of the facility's compliance with utilization review requirements.

Medical Audit

While medical audit was once thought to be a complete quality assurance program, it is now viewed in a more proper perspective as a quality assurance mechanism for the study of difficult patient related problems.

A medical audit is a systematic method of measuring the quality of patient care as it is reflected in the patient's record. It is a vehicle to assess clinical practices within a facility and identify patterns of care. This review method may be referred to as a medical care evaluation study, patient care study, quality assurance study, or medical audit. There are various study techniques that may be used. These include: outcome audits, which focus on the desired end results of medical intervention and treatment; process audits, which focus on the activities of the health care professionals providing direct care to patients during the ongoing treatment process; concurrent audits, which are performed while the patient is hospitalized and designed to look at both the process of care being delivered and the end result of treatment and retrospective audits, which are performed on a group of discharged patients based on the completed medical record and designed to focus either on the process or outcome of patient care.

Although the technique may vary, a study must include the following steps:

1. The topic selected for study should be related to an identified or potential problem that may affect patient care.
2. Valid measurable criteria must be established. Criteria should be developed by professionals relying on expertise and the professional literature.
3. Analysis by peers: charts that do not pass the criteria screen must be reviewed by professionals to determine if there is a clinically justifiable reason why the criteria were not met.
4. Corrective action: this should be specific to the problems identified through the study.
5. Follow-up studies: these should be performed to assess whether or not the identified problem has been eliminated. The date of the follow-up study should be based on the impact of the problem on patient care.
6. Reporting: the general findings and the specific recommendations resulting from the evaluation study must be reported to the medical director, the chief executive officer, and the governing body.[10]

The results of an evaluation study should also be reported to the quality assurance committee, the utilization review committee and the professional staff.

Although the medical audit is no longer a requirement of the JCAH, it continues to be a useful assessment tool. The findings of a medical audit should be used in continuing education programs and determining clinical privileges.

Internal Peer Review

Peer review by definition is a term signifying review by physicians of medical care. Internal peer review is a developing concept that involves the review and monitoring of patient care and treatment by the medical staff of the facility as an alternative to review by an external review agency. In this process, the treatment of all patients in a facility is reviewed at specific intervals by a panel of peers from the active medical staff. For a peer review program to be meaningful and to have a positive impact on patient care, the process must be thorough, and those involved in the peer review process must be prepared to make recommendations to correct any identified clinical problems. Cases with identified problems must be re-evaluated within a reasonable amount of time in order to assure that any deficiencies have been corrected. Absent or unclear documentation must be corrected promptly.

The advantages of an internal peer review program include the following:

1. A medical staff may develop its own peer review criteria that are consistent with national standards of care.
2. Length of stay will be determined by medical need.
3. Confidentiality of patient records will be improved.
4. Unexpected third-party denials will be eliminated, and payment of submitted claims will be timely.
5. A significant educational mechanism will be provided for the medical staff.
6. It will provide the foundation for the facility's patient care monitoring system.

The participatory peer review process may well be the best of many different programs to provide continuing education for the medical profession. An effective peer review program will be a vital component of a facility's quality assurance program. The program will have an impact on clinical privileges and reappointment. For all of the obvious advantages of an internal peer review program, there are situations that must be both recognized and considered when developing such a program. These include (1) inadequate or poor documentation, (2) physician resistance to the concept of reviewing or being reviewed, (3) professional time required for proper peer review, and (4) inprecise measurements to assess response to an outcome of treatment.[11,12]

Data Sources

Essential to quality assurance, utilization review, and peer review is a medical record that is accurate, well organized, timely, and complete. It is the clinician's responsibility to create a medical record that accurately reflects the patient's history, diagnosis, and treatment.

Another data source of the quality asurance program is risk management. A risk management program can increase efficiency and cost effectiveness in a hospital and assist in controlling liability. An efficient program should decrease the risks to the patient along with the potential for possible litigation directed toward the hospital.[13]

Facilities may use central tabulating services such as the Professional Activities Study (PAS), the Medical Audit Project in Ann Arbor Michigan, and the

Hospital Utilization Project (HUP) of the Allegheny County Medical Society to obtain data for use by the medical staff for comparison studies, analyses, and continuing education.[14]

MEDICAL REVIEW ACTIVITIES—MALPRACTICE RISK?

The question of whether or not medical review activities may expose facilities to significant legal hazards is of concern to physicians and administrators. Many states have confidentiality provisions that explicitly exempt medical review committees' proceedings from discovery or use in any civil action. Laws regarding medical review vary, however, in all states. Please refer to Chapter 26 for more detailed information.

A quality assurance program will enable hospital management to set optimal quality care standards and will provide the mechanisms to assure that these standards are met. The concept of quality assurance has been in transition over the past decade and will continue to respond to the state of the art and regulating mandates.

REFERENCES

1. The Washington, D.C. PSRO decision. Conn. Med. 43:107–109, 1979
2. Root J: PSROs in Connecticut—past, present, and future. Conn Med 39:793–795, 1975.
3. P.S.R.O. Program Manual. Rockville, Md, Department of Health, Education, and Welfare, 1974
4. Federal Register (Part 2 and 3), vol. 39. Washington, DC, US Government Printing Office, 1974, pp 41603–41649
5. Board revises audit requirements, in Perspectives on Accreditation: Chicago, Joint Commission on Accreditation of Hospitals, 1975
6. Vanagunas A, Egelston E. Hopkins J, et al: Principles of quality assurance. Quality Assurance Rev Bull (Special Edition), May 1979:4–7
7. Joseph E, Fox L, Stearns G: Management Solutions for Mental Health. Chicago, Care Communications, 1980
8. Consolidated Standards Manual for Child, Adolescent, and Adult Psychiatric, Alcoholism, and Drug Abuse Facilities. Chicago, Joint Commission on Accreditation of Hospitals, 1981
9. Quality Guide for Psychiatric and Substance Abuse Facilities. Chicago, Joint Commission on Accreditation of Hospitals, 1980
10. The Pep Primer for Psychiatry. Chicago, Joint Commission on Accreditation of Hospitals, 1975
11. Greenspan J: Accountability and Quality Assurance in Health Care. Bowie, Md, Charles Press, 1980
12. Manual for Psychiatric Peer Review. Washington, DC, American Psychiatric Association, 1981
13. Monagle J: Risk management is linked with quality of care. Hospital 54:57–59, 1980
14. Holloway D, Wiczai L, Carlson E: Evaluating an information system for medical care evaluation studies. Medical Care 13:329–340, 1975
15. New JCAH Standard: Legal Perils of Compliance. Hosp Peer Rev 5:5–12, 1980

GLOSSARY

clinical privileges. Authorization by the governing body to render patient care and treatment services in the facility within well-defined limits, based on the individual's professional qualifications, experience, competence, ability, and judgment.

concurrent review. An ongoing review of the patient's treatment while the patient is hospitalized.

criteria. Statements written by peers, setting professional standards that define optimum levels of patient care. The audit committee uses criteria as measurement tools for screening patient records.

extended stay review. A review to determine the medical necessity for continuation of hospitalization.

goal. A statement of level of functioning the patient may be expected to achieve.

governing body. The person or persons with ultimate authority and responsibility for the overall operation of the facility.

HUP. Hospital Utilization Project, 400 Penn Central Boulevard, Pittsburgh, Penn 15235.

JCAH. Joint Commission on Accreditation of Hospitals, 875 North Michigan Avenue, Chicago, Ill. 60611.

medicaid. A program of medical assistance funded by the federal government and the state for low-income individuals who are aged, blind, or disabled or members of families with dependent children.

medicare (PL 89-97). Federally funded health insurance for the aged and disabled.

Objective. A statement of desired outcome of treatment or service that is time specific and measurable and relates to one or more of the problems.

Norms. Numerical or statistical measures of usual observed performance.

PAS. Professional Activities Study, 1968 Green Road, Ann Arbor, Mich, 48105.

PEP Performance evaluational procedure for auditing and improving patient care. JCAH audit methodology.

PSRO. Professional standards review organization (Public Law 92-603).

Quality assurance program. A method of accountability to the patient, third-party payers, and outside reviewing bodies utilizing problem-focused, result-oriented methods, which should result in the maintenance and improvement of the quality of patient care and treatment.

Quality assurance studies (i.e., patient care studies, medical care evaluations, medical audits). A method of measuring the quality of patient care as it is reflected in the patient's medical record. Usually, a focused review of a potential or identified problem area.

Risk management. A program designed to increase efficiency and cost effectiveness in a facility and assist in controlling liability.

Standard. Professionally developed expression established as a measurement model to which a norm or criterion should conform.

Utilization review. A review mechanism to determine if the health care services provided to patients in a facility are medically necessary and provided in a cost-efficient manner.

William A. Hargreaves, Ph.D.
C. Clifford Attkisson, Ph.D.

20

Program Evaluation

Program evaluation is a general term for the process of making judgments about program effort, effectiveness, efficiency, and adequacy based on systematic data collection and analysis. The manager of a community mental health center, psychiatric hospital, or larger mental health organization depends on this systematic data collection and analysis to keep the organization "visible" and therefore manageable. The focus in this chapter is on the *internal* evaluation of a mental health organization. The manager calls on the program evaluator, or program evaluation unit, to provide staff support for the two general tasks faced by every manager: maintaining the effectiveness of the internal activities of the program and representing the program to the outside world. The reader should be aware that much of the literature on program evaluation refers to activities such as policy analysis, evaluation research, program audits, and citizen review and consumer advocacy, which do not represent internal program evaluation in the sense of the term used in this chapter.[1]

Policy analysis. Policy analysis is the examination of the operational and political feasibility and desirability of a proposed change in policy. While the methods can be applied at any program level, policy analyses typically serve as an aid in developing national or state legislation.

Evaluation research. The aims of evaluation research are to provide scientific evidence for the effectiveness of treatment interventions or types of programs. Evaluation research is expensive and highly technical, is typically federally funded, and often takes the form of multi-site, collaborative, randomized, or quasi-experimental clinical trials. This type of evaluation research is rarely a part of internal program evaluation except in university-affiliated clinical programs.

The program audit. Many managers in mental health programs are familiar with the program audit evaluation procedure. Usually initiated by federal or state mental health authorities or the Joint Commission on the Accreditation of Hospitals, program audits are typically brief site visits for the purpose of assuring that the program meets structural standards and measures, measures of effort and service utilization, and conformity with regulations.

Citizen review and consumer advocacy. Federal and state legislation have encouraged citizen review and consumer advocacy over the past two decades. While citizen review has not in most cases become a meaningful part of program governance, consumer advocacy has become an increasingly important force for change in the more restrictive aspects of the mental health system.

None of these activities can take the place of capable internal program evaluation. Without the "eyes and ears" of appropriate and timely information about the program, mental health managers risk struggling and stumbling from one crisis to another, experiencing increasing demands on their limited time and attention, and may progressively lose confidence in their capacity to manage effectively. It is hoped that this chapter will guide mental health managers in creating the organizational "program evaluation capability" that best will serve their needs.

THREE ASPECTS OF EVALUATION CAPABILITY

Program evaluation capability in an organization must be developed over a period of time. To make progress in this development and get a useful return on the effort it requires, managers and evaluators must plan the development process realistically. The plan must reflect (1) the organization's present level of development of evaluation activities, (2) the kinds of new information tools that will be needed, and (3) the multiple roles that are and will be expected of the evaluator. The first aspect, *level of evaluation activity,* reflects what the authors have observed as typical developmental stages in program evaluation capability. The other two aspects, *information capability* and *functional roles of the evaluator,* have important effects on the quality and utility of evaluation activities within a mental health organization.

Evolving Levels of Evaluative Activity

The authors have found it useful to think of four general levels of program evaluation activity. These levels seem to represent common developmental stages in the growth of both management capability and program evaluation capability in mental health organizations.[2]

At the first level, *systems resource management,* the focus is on the most basic internal operations of the mental health organization. The perspective broadens as management and program evaluation capacity develops, first gaining a clear picture of patient *utilization* of services provided by the program, then considering the *outcome of intervention* with program patients, and finally attending to the *community impact* of the program as a whole. Table 20-1 shows the typical management tasks and evaluation activities at each of these four levels of evaluation activity. A newly formed organization, or newly formed evaluation unit in an established organization, often must focus entirely on the first level, while well-developed evaluation units will progressively address all four levels as conditions allow.

Systems Resource Management

The functions of evaluation at this level include several activities that are critical to effective program planning and management: (1) assisting the organization in meeting minimum standards for mental health settings; (2) assisting in the formulation or revision of program objectives based on mandated services and documented needs; (3) identifying the information that will be needed for continuing review of the attainment of program objectives; (4) identifying and monitoring the allocation of the flexible resources of the program, primarily staff effort; and (5) monitoring the degree to which program priorities have been translated into appropriate intervention activities.

To enable the evaluator to function effectively at this level, the manager must be sure that the evaluator understands the organization's commitments and agreements regarding its core operations. The evaluator should be familiar with such documents as the budget, fiscal management and audit procedures, state and local reimbursement requirements, third-party billing regulations, job descriptions and staff employment contracts, hospital or mental health center accreditation requirements, and other contractual and quasi-contractual records. This understanding is needed in developing monitoring procedures to flag errors and deficiencies that threaten smooth operation and effective performance in relation to external requirements placed on the program. Analysis of these external commitments also provides a framework for exploring the further aspirations of administration and staff for improving the scope and excellence of organizational services. The manager might then ask the evaluator to formulate the organizational objectives in measurable terms, which will not only aid in sharpening the definition and priority of objectives but will prepare the evaluator for developing monitoring procedures to reveal how well program objectives are being attained.

The final set of evaluative functions at this level will aid the manager in monitoring the allocation of organizational resources. Financial records accomplish only part of this function. In the typical mental health organization, the bulk of the *flexible* resources, those easily reallocated by the manager, consist of staff. Routine information about staff effort is needed if one is to manage effectively. This is especially true in managing people who are expected to carry out a large variety of functions and positions in which the work load is not closely determined by external demand factors. For example, a clinician in a mental health clinic may primarily perform psychotherapeutic work with patients in the program. That person, however, may allocate his time between individual and group interventions and may perform consultative or outreach functions with other agencies, intake functions, and so forth. Furthermore, even staff who devote full time to clinical work rarely spend more than 50–60 percent of their time in actual patient contact. They may provide in-service training or supervise other staff and will devote some time to receiving supervision and participating in peer review, general staff meetings, paperwork, and leave time. Effective management of clinicians requires clear expectations understood by both supervisor and clinician as well as a monitoring system, usually designed and implemented by the program evaluator, that documents activities in relation to these expectations.

Such effort-monitoring systems are crucial for the middle manager, who implements programs primarily by allocating the effort of existing staff or by con-

Table 20-1
Typical Management Tasks and Evaluation Activities at Four Levels of Evaluation Activity

Level of Evaluation Activity	Typical Management Tasks	Typical Evaluation Activities
I. Systems resource management	Clarify organization objectives	Formulate objectives and indicators of attainment
	Establish lines of responsibility	Clarify roles of evaluator
	Allocate budget and staff effort	Monitor deployment of staff effort
	Establish or modify services	Develop integrated data collection and analysis
	Meet reporting and program standards	Assemble data to meet reporting requirements
	Establish fees and billing procedures	Determine unit costs of services
II. Patient	Make workload projections	Monitor number of patients, units of service, caseloads
	Assure adequate treatment planning	Install problem-oriented record, review patient needs
	Assure continuity of care	Analyze patient flow, referral rates, continuity of care
	Establish quality assurance program	Support utilization review and patient care audits
	Maintain efficiency of service delivery	Analyze cost per episode for specific groups or settings
	Assure equity of service accessibility	Compare patient demographics to census data to identify underserved groups
	Assure appropriate patient screening and treatment assignment	Study premature dropout and under-utilization of care
III. Outcome of interventions	Detect and correct grossly ineffective service activities	Compare patient change from beginning to end of service with expected change
	Select the most cost-effective approach to serving a specific patient group	Compare costs and outcomes of different existing service approaches to the same type of patient
	Establish the improved effectiveness of a proposed new type of service	Carry out a treatment experiment comparing the new type of service to the standard type of service
	Assure that services are acceptable to patients and referral sources	Study the satifaction of patients and referral sources

Level of Evaluation Activity	Typical Management Tasks	Typical Evaluation Activities
IV. Community impact	Participate in regional health planning Develop joint interagency services and administrative support systems Collaborate in integration of services for multiproblem patients Provide useful primary prevention and indirect services	Contribute to regional needs assessment activities Establish evaluation liaison with other programs, funding agencies, and community advisory groups Identify patients and patient groups using or needing services in other programs Evaluate consultation and education services

verting existing positions in order to replace existing staff with persons with different skills. Effort monitoring is also useful, but less crucial, as an aid to face-to-face supervision when effort information is partly shared informally or at higher levels of administration in which control is exerted primarily by adding or removing staff positions and assigning leadership responsibility.

Patient Utilization

When basic systems resource management issues are under control, attention can be devoted to understanding patterns of patient utilization. Program evaluation activities at this level monitor patient characteristics at entry, referral patterns, units of service rendered, lengths of service episode, and occupancy rates or degree to which service capacity is being utilized. These data are also used to analyze the factors that influence service delivery patterns, patient demand, and reimbursement. The need for such information is often first recognized because it is required to be submitted to funding agencies. This represents an aggravation for the administrator and the program evaluator, especially since the information demands from different funders or government agencies are often poorly coordinated and frequently change from year to year. Managers who experience capable patient utilization monitoring, however, quickly come to see how important it is both for internal management and for program advocacy activities such as writing funding proposals.

Examples of internal management uses of patient utilization evaluation are easy to find. An outpatient clinic finds that half of its admissions are persons with severe problems with alcohol, and special services are established for this group. A 24-hr psychiatric emergency clinic averages only four visits each day and is merged with a hospital emergency room with on-call backup by the mental health staff. Patient referrals from schools drop off dramatically, leading to the discovery that all school psychologist positions have been deleted from the public schools due to funding cutbacks, so each clinician in the child mental health services unit is assigned to spend a half day per week in outreach consultation with school faculty. Hispanic persons are seen rarely in relation to their prevalence in community census data, and a special effort is made to hire Spanish-speaking professionals. The patients who ranked in the top 5 percent in the total cost of services received in the past year received 40 percent of the service resources, and peer review attention to these cases uncovers many with inadequate treatment plans. Patient utilization evaluation, especially when combined with evaluation at the level of systems resource management, is essential for the manager who aspires to move from "brushfire management" to a style of anticipatory problem solving.

Needs assessment—the identification of populations of potential patients who should be served—can first be addressed at this level of program evaluation. The logic adopted for this task is often erroneously simple: needs are estimated by the distribution of types of patients who are already being served. The focus of modern needs assessment in mental health services is on circumstances in which service patterns are inconsistent with program objectives. Needs assessment, therefore, typically involves comparing patient utilization data to other information in order to draw conclusions about "underserved" groups. Ethnic minorities and the poor are often discovered to be underserved or served inappropriately, so all managers must be prepared to address such issues with regard to their own mental health programs. Methods for needs assessment have been summarized elsewhere.[4,5]

Service utilization analyses are best supplemented by social indicator and citizen survey approaches. The social indicators approach, based on census data and other public records, is being progressively strengthened by validation studies comparing it to the much more expensive community survey approach to psychiatric epidemiology. The manager should expect the program evaluator to keep abreast of these research developments. It should be possible to obtain summaries of census data by mental health catchment area from federal or state mental health agencies and to use these to make plausible estimates of the relative need for mental health services in one's own catchment area compared to other catchment areas in the same region or state.

The severely and chronically mentally ill are the other group that must be the focus of incisive needs identification and planning. This group will be quite visible to mental health managers in some communities where nearly all become known to the mental health system. In other communities, the chronically disabled mentally ill may migrate into areas with inexpensive housing, be supported on supplemental security income, and be known only in the welfare or criminal justice systems, so that mental health utilization statistics identify only part of this target population. There may be an argument that severely mentally ill persons who never seek services and never appear because of the complaints of others should not be sought out by the mental health system, but the issue calls for careful judgment.

In most communities, the bulk of the severely mentally ill will at some time appear in the mental health system and be recognized as needing services. The evaluation task is then not to identify those who are not served but to identify this high-risk group and ensure that appropriate continuity and integration of service are planned and implemented. Many community mental health programs are experimenting with new ways to organize community support programs for this group in order to assure adequate case management. As with any new or experimental service strategy, the manager will want to direct special program evaluation attention to examining resource allocation and patient utilization in order to "tune" the implementation of these program changes.

The final focus of activity at the *patient utilization* level of program evaluation activity is quality assurance (see also Chapter 19). Many managers will find it sensible to ask the program evaluator to provide staff support for the peer review procedures of utilization review and patient care audit. The ongoing monitoring activities developed by the program evaluator can incorporate procedures for selecting cases for review. The peer review process of selecting and structuring topics for patient care audits can be made into a reasonable planning mechanism for certain special program evaluation studies. If externally required quality assurance activities are integrated with internal program evaluation activities, the manager may find that both activities are more meaningful parts of management. On the other hand, the manager may find that the externally required activities may simply expand to consume all of the resources allocated for program evaluation, leaving management without the other information it needs for internal decision making.

Outcome of Intervention

The most common motivation for an outcome study is to aid management and clinical staff in a specific major decision about program change. Such studies must be carried out as time-limited projects rather than ongoing monitoring activities. An example would be a comparison of two different approaches to dealing with "treatment failures" in a day treatment program.[6]

Here the objective is to establish a treatment approach that maximizes the cost outcome for this specific patient population. The utility of a comparative outcome study is most obvious when a new approach is proposed to replace a current procedure and when it is unclear whether the new method will be an improvement. The steps in designing comparative outcome studies and appropriate measurement instruments for such studies have been summarized elsewhere by the authors.[7,8]

Such studies are usually not possible to carry out adequately within the budget of a treatment organization and therefore are rarely seen in mental health organizations except those with a specific research budget or those affiliated with a university.

A second approach to outcome analysis, more closely linked to day-to-day management, is routine monitoring to detect specific program strengths, weaknesses, or trouble spots. Only simple and inexpensive outcome indicators are practical to include in routine monitoring, the most common being a global rating of functioning by the clinician at the beginning and end of treatment and a measure of patient satisfaction. A more face-valid measure is information obtained from the patient by someone not involved in his treatment, both at the beginning of treatment and again after some fixed time interval when most patients will have completed their treatment. However, even the most rudimentary methods using a mailed questionnaire with telephone follow-up cost about 5 percent of the cost of the typical outpatient treatment episode per patient successfully followed up.[9] In-person follow-up interviews are considerably more expensive.[10]

There have been some proposals at federal and state levels for routine outcome monitoring of samples of patients in mental health programs. As of this writing, these activities have been restricted to pilot programs. There is as yet no consensus that routine outcome evaluation of this sort would lead to program improvements sufficient to justify the cost. In the meantime, some states have required routine global ratings by clinicians of patients at intake and discharge and sampled patient satisfaction studies. While the authors have heard a few anecdotal reports of local or state utilization of such data, certainly no consensus has developed that such program evaluation efforts come close to the management utility experienced from evaluation activities at the "systems resource management" and "patient utilization" levels.

The lack of established outcome evaluation approaches leaves the psychiatric administrator with the dilemma of managing programs where effects are largely invisible and therefore cannot directly be optimized in relation to costs. Controlled clinical trials and other clinical research, primarily funded by the federal government and by pharmaceutical companies, will continue to be the primary source of reliable and generalizable evidence about the effectiveness of mental health interventions. The psychiatric administrator must continue for the foreseeable future to rely on whatever guidance can be drived from such research, and on the generally accepted traditions of good clinical practice, in maintaining the quality and effectiveness of mental health care.

Community Impact

Program evaluation at the community impact level is the least technically developed of all, yet it is the most relevant to the *preventative* goals of mental health programs. At this level, the aims of management are to relate the mental health program to its community environment, to understand and make its interlocking actions and effects optimal in relation to other mental health programs in the community, to private practitioners, and to the larger health and human service system. The manager may ask the program evaluator to aid in coordinating comprehensive regional health and human service networks through the sharing of data and participation in planning activities. The evaluator should be asked to maintain liaison with evaluators and planners at other levels in the mental health system and at other sites at the same level, to identify opportunities for collaborative work that may benefit the program, and to anticipate changing external requirements that may impinge on the program. When evaluative work at the patient utilization level has identified a poorly served group of multiproblem patients, the manager may ask the evaluator to support advocacy for new interprogram linkages, collaborative agreements, or funding needed to meet the needs of these difficult patients. The distinguishing feature of evaluative work at this level is the shift away from an internal program focus, giving attention to the larger human service system to seek opportunities for preventative integration of services or mutual enhancement of program effectiveness.

At this level, the evaluator's attention naturally turns also to the outreach and prevention-oriented components of his own mental health program. These may include consultation services to schoools, mental health education, and the like. Approaches to evaluating such "indirect services" are discussed by others.[11–13] Having discussed the developmental levels of evaluation activities, the authors now turn to two organizational characteristics that largely determine the ultimate utility of these evaluation activities.

Informational Capability

A critical limit on program evaluation capability is the capacity of a mental health organization to capture and analyze relevant program data economically, promptly, and flexibly. In the typical mental health program, several record and data sources are created that function relatively autonomously. Examples of these are patient care records, financial records, billing systems, statistical monitoring systems, personnel records, logs, rosters of open cases, other informal records, and even the interpersonal grapevine of verbal contacts and memos. Often, these are entirely uncoordinated "natural" data systems. Each serves the immediate operational purpose for which it was created but is virtually inaccessible and totally inflexible for any other use. Even within a single record system, there may be no regular procedure for getting an overview or summarizing trends. It is essential for most mental health systems to develop some type of integrated information system that encompasses and gradually supplants these redundant natural data sources and allows the collected data to be used economically for multiple purposes.

An integrated information system does not necessarily imply computerization, although the advantages of a *successfully* computerized information system are impressive. Where a computerized system becomes necessary because of the size or complexity of the program, its development must be undertaken carefully if the many pitfalls are to be avoided. Even with the newest and fanciest equipment and excellent utility software already in place, there is no royal road for introducing automated data systems into an organization. The methods and choices one faces in considering automated data systems are discussed in detail in Chapter 22. The authors restrict themselves here to issues in planning integrated information systems that apply whether or not automated techniques are used.

If the manager determines that a major information system improvement is essential, it should be identified as the major task of the program evaluator and his support staff during the period in which the improvements are to be made. It is not at all unusual for a program evaluation staff to devote most of their effort to developing such information capability for a period of 2 or 3 years. When the new information methods are running smoothly, the same level of staff resources will be sufficient to take on a much broader program evaluation role. This gradual development of information methods under the close control of program staff, with a development budget that is not substantially larger than the ongoing resources that will be available for its maintenance and utilization, has generally yielded good results. The horror stories of wasted investments and poor performance have most often been heard when programs have attempted rapid, ambitious developments that were well beyond the capacity of program staff to control and monitor, even when the technical work was capably performed by outside contractors. Program evaluation staff need to understand the information system, be able to modify it inexpensively, and be able to maintain its effective operation in spite of the departure of a key staff member or the collapse of an outside contract.

Improving the integration of the information systems of a mental health organization involves a series of steps that require great attention to detail. The evaluator must identify which elements of system information are meaningful and needed for various planned data summaries without overloading the system with every kind of information that anyone thinks might someday be "nice to know." The availability of essential data must be assured by identifying the staff responsible for recording the information and establishing timely quality control review of data for completeness. Clear record forms must be designed that can be used reliably by staff to capture relevant data at its original source while minimizing the degree of reliance on professional staff for data collection. Redundancy of data collection must be minimized; a useful rule of thumb is to try not to introduce a new form that does not replace at least one form already in use. High priority must be given to returning useful information directly to those who collect it; for example, intake and termination forms can enable the information system to provide a current roster of active cases, eliminating the need to maintain a manual file at the reception desk. The routine reports needed by management for decision-making use must be identified and designed and production procedures must be worked out before data collection procedures are implemented so that input data are available in the form needed and useful output from new information procedures does not lag years behind the installation of new data collection procedures. Finally, centralized data files must be maintained in a form that allows unanticipated specialized analyses at reasonable cost. Information capability that incorporates these characteristics will repay itself many times over in management utility.

Functional Roles of the Evaluator

To ensure that evaluation can function usefully in program management, it is necessary to recruit talented evaluators and to underwrite the evaluator's role with sufficient authority and sanctions. Creative program evaluation depends, however, not only on the evaluator's training, experience, skill, and mandate but also on a closeness to management concerns. Evaluative capability is thus enhanced by the evaluator's access to the decision-making process. This allows the evaluator to ask relevant questions, propose appropriate studies, suggest planning strategies, and have a strong hand in implementing changes that are decided on as the result of an evaluative activity.

Integrating an evaluator into the mamagement process may seem an obvious necessity, but in the authors' experience, it is not always accomplished. Sometimes the evaluator is not a member of the management group but simply a statistical clerk who assembles data for routine reports and has neither the perspective nor the mandate to raise general policy issues. In other instances, people with research training and interests may be recruited as program evaluators with the expectation that the role allows them to pursue their own research interests in exchange for a few data analysis chores for the program, an attitude that is unlikely to result in close attention to management concerns. Alternatively, evaluators may expect themselves to be objective external critics of the program, but such a role is appropriate only for someone hired by an external finding agency or advocacy group. Trying to be the external critic of the management level by which one is exployed often leads to unresolvable role ambiguity and ineffectiveness as a program evaluator.

In large organizations, the program evaluator may be well integrated into certain levels or aspects of management and not others. Sometimes this results when a poorly integrated evaluator forms close working collaborations with specific program units that seek out program evaluation assistance. Alternatively, the evaluator may be well integrated into top management but not have the time to be involved in other components of the organization. In this case, subordinate evaluation staff members can be assigned to liaison with specific units, which may greatly improve the effectiveness of evaluation activities at these lower-management levels.

When the evaluator is effectively integrated into the management process, one often sees the following sequence of events: (1) a specific problem area is identified as requiring evaluation support; (2) relevant information is gathered and analyzed; (3) reports are generated and presented in a form compatible with the management decision process; (4) alternative solutions or actions are posed and reviewed in the light of both evaluation data and other factors; and (5) a decision is implemented, often with continued monitoring of the effect of the decision on the attainment of program objectives. While this process can be seen even at the most rudimentary level of evaluation activity, as the organization develops its evaluation capability along the dimensions we have described, this process can be applied to a wider range of problems with results that are increasingly timely and focussed on crucial management issues.

REFERENCES

1. Attkisson CC: The manager as evaluator. New directions in mental health services Middle Management in Mental Health 8:77–90, 1980
2. Hargreaves WA, Attkisson CC, McIntyre MH, et al: Current applications of evaluation, in Zusman J, Wurster C (eds): Program Evaluation: Alcohol, Drug Abuse and Mental Health Services. Lexington, Mass, Heath, 1975, p 181
3. Attkisson CC, Hargreaves WA: A conceptual model for program evaluation in health organizations, in Schulberg HC, Baker F (eds): Program Evaluation in the Health Fields, vol. 2. New York, Human Sciences Press, 1979, p 53
4. Siegel LM, Attkisson CC, Carson LG: Need indentification and program planning in the community context, in Attkisson CC, Hargreaves WA, Horowitz MJ, et al (eds): Evaluation of Human Service Programs. New York, Academic Press, 1973, p 215
5. Bell RA, Nguyen TD, Warheit GJ, et al: Service utilization, social indicator, and citizen survey approaches to human service need assessment, in Attkisson CC, Hargreaves WA, Horowitz MJ, et al (eds): Evaluation of Human Service Programs. New York, Academic Press, 1978, p 253
6. Donlon PT, Rada RT, Knight SW: A therapeutic aftercare setting for "refractory" chronic schizophrenic patients. Am J Psychiatry 130:682–684, 1973
7. Hargreaves WA, Attkisson CC: Evaluating program outcomes, in Attkisson CC, Hargreaves WA, Horowitz MJ, et al (eds): Evaluation of Human Service Programs. New York, Academic Press, 1978, p 303
8. Hargreaves WA, Attkisson CC, McIntyre MH, et al: Outcome measurement instruments for use in community mental health program evaluation, in Hargreaves WA, Attkisson CC, Sorensen JE (eds): Resource Materials for Community Mental Health Program Evaluation (ed 2). DHEW Publ. No. (ADM) 77-328. Washington, DC, 1977, p 243
9. Schainblatt AH: Monitoring the Outcomes of State Mental Health Treatment Programs: Some Initial Suggestions. Washington, DC, Urban Institute, 1977
10. Showstack JA, Hargreaves WA, Glick ID, et al: Psychiatric follow-up studies: Practical procedures and ethical concerns. J Nerv Ment Dis 166:34–43, 1978

11. Broskowski A, Driscoll J, Schulberg HC: A management information and planning system for indirect services, in Attkisson CC, Hargreaves WA, Horowitz MJ, et al (eds): Evaluation of Human Service Programs. New York, Academic Press, 1978, p 189
12. Canfield M, Kliewer D: Conference evaluation manual, in Hargreaves WA, Attkisson CC, Sorensen JE (eds): Resource Materials for Community Mental Health Program Evaluation (ed 2). DHEW Publ. No. (ADM) 77-328. Washington, DC, 1977, p 389
13. Taylor EN, Vineberg R: Evaluation of indirect services to schools, in Attkisson CC, Hargreaves WA, Horowitz MJ, et al (eds): Evaluation of Human Service Programs. New York, Academic Press, 1978, p 445

Ethel M. Bonn, M.D.

21

Accreditation and Regulation of Psychiatric Facilities

External reviews of psychiatric services are required by third-party payers and governmental agencies concerned about cost-control and quality of care. Uncoordinated demands for data tend, however, to waste resources and may undermine, rather than improve, the quality of patient care. Service-providers are therefore often justifiably skeptical about any redeeming value of the process.

The psychiatric service provider must, however, meet the requirements of accreditation bodies and reimbursement and regulatory groups in order to "do business." There is a growing recognition, by providers and by accrediting and regulatory bodies, of the need for better management of, rather than management by, the multiple surveys, inspections, and demands for data. There are ways of coping with the process that are better than mere acquiescence and cliff-hanging survival. A review of the background of accreditation and regulation is essential to coping with, and even benefitting from, the process, which does not have to be adversarial.

BACKGROUND

From 1918 to 1951 there were increasing efforts by the American College of Surgeons (ACS) to review and standardize hospitals; they undertook this work to correct the terrible conditions existing in hospitals. In 1951, the ACS joined with the American College of Physicians, the American Hospital Association, the American Medical Association, and the Canadian Medical Association to form the Joint Commission on Accreditation of Hospitals (JCAH). (The Canadian Medical Association withdrew in 1959.) The JCAH standards were applicable to general medical and surgical hospitals; these standards were also applied—often with less than satisfactory results—to psychiatric hospitals. As they have evolved, the standards of JCAH have shifted from being the "minimum essential" to the "optimal achievable."

Beginning in the 1950's, the American Psychiatric Association (APA) which has never been a "parent" of the JCAH, published standards for psychiatric hospitals and clinics. (In addition, state, county, and city departments of health have traditionally promulgated hospital and clinic standards for licensure purposes.) Having no legal jurisdiction over psychiatric facilities, the APA used its standards for teaching, advisory, and consultative purposes as a guide for administrators, legislators, and other interested citizens.

In the mid 1960's, the federal government made accreditation by JCAH a requirement for reimbursement by Medicare and Medicaid, and various states made JCAH accreditation a requirement for facility licensure. As a result of the Medicare and state health department adoption of JCAH accreditation as mandatory, the JCAH became identified with regulation. Strictly speaking, JCAH cannot regulate; only governments can regulate, through licensure and other mechanisms.

Beginning in the late 1960's, the JCAH worked with the APA and nine other psychiatric and mental health organizations to form the JCAH Accreditation Council on Psychiatric Facilities (ACPF). The council produced the *1972 Accreditation Manual for Psychiatric Facilities* (the "Green Manual"),[1] a comprehensive set of standards for psychiatric hospitals as well as mental health clinics and centers, which were also applied to programs in alcoholism and drug abuse treatment, child and adolescent psychiatric, and other facilities such as psychiatric units in general hospitals.

For many programs, hospitals and non-hospital, the "Green Manual" standards were a real advance, but they were still found unsuitable by many of the ACPF organizations. In response, the ACPF developed, and JCAH published, separate standards for child and adolescent facilities (1974), alcoholism facilities (1975), drug abuse facilities (1975), and community mental health centers (CMHC; 1977). These standards were made increasingly more specific in order to match the expressed needs of specialized facilities for standards that really fit their programs, many of which were staffed by a high proportion of non-professionals, accentuating the need for explicit standards.

Four of these manuals of standards were subsequently combined in one manual, the *1979 JCAH Consolidated Standards for Child, Adolescent and Adult Psychiatric, Alcoholism and Drug Abuse Programs*—the "Rainbow Book",[2] which did not cover CMHC's. The *1979 Consolidated Standards* suffered from some overspecificity and internal duplication, several omissions, and a few controversial standards.

As a result of the JCAH reorganization, the ACPF was dissolved in 1979, and its advisory functions were taken over by the Professional and Technical Advisory Committee for Psychiatric Facilities (PTAC). This committee assisted the staff of the Accreditation Program for Psychiatric Facilities (APPF) in revising the *Consolidated Standards.* A reorganized version, with a new standard on quality assurance, a clarified standard on professional and medical staff responsibilities, and a number of additional standards, was published in January 1981.[3]

A major issue, strongly articulated by the APA and other groups, arose from differences of interpretation of the JCAH–ACPF standards on the organization and governance of clinical staff in psychiatric facilities. The *1979 JCAH Consolidated Standards* required that there be a single organization of the clinical staff, *either* medical *or* multidisciplinary (not both), with its own rules and regulations as well as credentialing and privileging mechanisms. Some parts of the field did not accept or understand the "either/or" provision, and much confusion ensued.

The view of the APA has been that if a facility is to be labeled and operated as a *psychiatric* facility, then it must have an organized psychiatric staff (rather than an organized multidisciplinary staff) accountable and responsible for the total quality of patient care.[4] For both hospital and non-hospital psychiatric facilities, JCAH has changed the concept from "clinical" to "professional" staff in the 1981 revision of the *Consolidated Standards.*

Power and shifting of power are important elements in the accreditation and regulatory drama. The recent polarization of psychiatric and mental health organizations around JCAH issues may lead to the splitting of the accreditation process, with separate standards for psychiatric facilities and all other mental health facilities. Although accreditation by JCAH is a voluntary, confidential process (unlike governmental regulation per se), JCAH accreditation is tied to reimbursement and other funding, which are not, practically speaking, "voluntary" issues.

COPING WITH SURVEYS AND REVIEWS

Preparing an agency for review by any accrediting or licensing body has many parallels in preparing for a school examination. Working smart is better than working hard. It is smart to routinize those activities that must be or can be ongoing. Moreover, it is smart to identify those activities that can best be carried out episodically and then schedule them in advance.

Systematic use of the JCAH standards for psychiatric facilities will give comprehensive, but not total, preparation for many other surveys. It is therefore essential to ascertain one's compliance with all applicable standards and to be able to demonstrate compliance through on-site evidence and/or supportive documentation. The performance characteristics of a facility, the style of its management, and the quality of its services will determine the amount, kind, and intensity of work to be done.

Psychiatric facilities vary in their patterns of response to external reviews. At one extreme are those that characteristically have an ongoing pervasive commitment primarily to quality of care and secondarily, but clearly up front, to compliance with accepted standards, i.e., such facilities manage the process rather than the reverse. At the other extreme are those doing "business as usual," interrupted by an 11th-hour recognition of being "due for survey, " followed by a hasty search for "that letter we got from the Joint Commission or health department," correcting the "easy" deficiencies and hoping to "hide" the others, dusting off manuals of policies and procedures, exhuming files of committee minutes, doing some extraordinary cleaning and beautifying of the environment—in short, engaging in a last-ditch "cosmetic" campaign to "get ready." Most facilities are in the middle of the continuum, with at least a little of both extreme characteristics. After assessing the facility's strengths and weaknesses and setting priorities derivative from these, the prudent administrator should lay out his plans.

Goals should include setting in motion those systematic activities that will pay off simultaneously for improving quality of patient care *and* for establishing compliance. Such tactics have the best chance of achieving success and minimizing last-minute panic and disruption of programs. Procrastination will virtually guarantee that the administrator and staff will be reactive victims of their own poor management.

The administrator and staff should do the following well in advance of any survey or site visit: (1) understand the scope of the practices to be reviewed; (2) comprehend the *intent* of the applicable standards as well as their *content* by attending relevant workshops and seeking consultation; (3) change practices, if indicated, and systematically develop documentation of compliance with standards—*one's own* as well as those of the review body; (4) assign responsibility for achieving further compliance, set target dates, *and follow up*. It is indeed possible to have a reality-based grasp of the entire survey process. Sizing up the surveyors should be the last item of business.

After the survey a slump may set in, and an attitude of "business as usual" may prevail—until the next review. The alert administrator must guard against this. Essential to the process of overcoming resistance to improvement is leadership that helps the management and supervisory staff to see beyond the short-range, day-to-day priorities and to understand and accept the longer-range priorities inherent in a successful approach to all accrediting and regulatory requirements. Motivating staff and overcoming organizational and individual resistance are part of every psychiatric administrator's challenge.

THE BENEFITS OF ACCREDITATION

Sooner or later, the psychiatric administrator must face the inevitable question: Why bother with all this accreditation and regulatory madness? The psychiatric administrator and staff will ask the question and imply, if not say, "Who's crazy? We used to think it was the patients! But now . . . ?"

Part of the administrator's preparation for reducing staff resistance will come from getting sufficient information about accreditation and licensure and thinking through their real benefits and pains, weighed against nonaccreditation, loss of license, and the imagined hazards and benefits. The psychiatric administrator should strive to resolve his or her own ambivalence about these requirements and work with all management and supervisory staff toward resolving theirs. Necessary changes in these attitudes cannot be accomplished by edicts and directives. Not all staff, key or other, will "come around."

Clarity of the administrator's position does help, however. The administrator might simply state, "We will be in compliance with these standards even if the JCAH or the Medicare people or the health department were never to come here again." Whatever operational approaches are used, the psychiatric administrator and staff should give primary emphasis to quality of patient care and, in that context, to achieving and maintaining accreditation or licensure.

The psychiatric administrator is faced with the prospect of obtaining accreditation or losing the following:

1. The institution's license
2. Eligibility for third-party insurance payments, Medicare, Medicaid, and so on
3. Affiliation with training programs for mental health professionals and other practitioners

4. Certain federal grants
5. Eligibility for other awards
6. The confidence of the public

The administrator who communicates to his or her staff members the above potential consequences of not having, or losing, accreditation may yet find staff indifference to accreditation. Staff may say, "So what if we lose our accreditation? What difference will it make?" Staff members should be informed that facilities that lose accreditation experience the following consequences:

1. The governing body loses confidence in and seriously "wonders" about the capability of the psychiatric administrator and the staff.
2. The funding source withholds funding for new programs and/or pay increases for management and/or clinical staff; third-party payers withhold reimbursement.
3. The press has a field day, with headlines, about the loss of accreditation and hints at the need for an investigation.
4. The news media give the facility long-overdue visibility but at a time of embarrassment and crisis.
5. The public—including prospective patients, staff, and citizen volunteers—lose confidence in the facility, which, in turn, may lose income and have trouble recruiting staff and volunteers.
6. The morale of the staff sags; many raise questions about the competence of the administration.
7. The patients lose confidence in the quality of care.

Unfortunately, some of the consequences of losing accreditation or licensure can only be appreciated through direct experience.

QUALITY ASSURANCE AND QUALITY OF CARE

Accreditation, licensure, certification, peer review, utilization review, clinical privileging, patient care audits, staff development, program evaluation, and various other quality assurance activities measure or improve quality of care to the extent that the facility comprehensively integrates its quality assurance activities with its day-to-day operations. (See Chapter 19.) If these activities become only paper exercises, they will neither measure nor improve the quality of care.

Quality assurance can be defined with various words, but the key ingredients are (1) assessment of quality of care, followed by (2) corrective action for any problems indicated by the assessment, with (3) accountability to the "powers that be" in the supervisory and management hierarchy, up to and including the psychiatric administrator, his governing board, or central office, and eventually accountability to funding sources and reimbursing payers, patients, and the public. Assessments, corrective actions, and follow-up on the status of correcting *high-priority problems* must be documented in accessible, suitable, retrievable form for use by authorized persons and agencies. To meet JCAH standards, for example, not all problems require formal assessment, correction, and documentation, just those with high-priority.[5]

Quality of care is an elusive concept that is subject to various interpretations. Agreed-upon definitions of quality of care are dependent on a variety of subjective and objective considerations. On the one hand, there are those who say, "I can't tell you what quality of care is, but I know it when I see it." On the other hand, there are growing bodies of empirical and scientific evidence for what produces quality of care. The various accepted quality producers come from known facts, widely accepted beliefs, and requirements stemming from societal custom, economics, laws, and regulations. The standards of accrediting and regulatory bodies vary in their comprehensiveness but are based on many of the same factors. Quality of care measures leading to a rational program of quality assurance can be developed from these agreed-upon standards. Needless to say, the process is anything but perfect, but it is improving.

RESISTANCES TO ACCREDITATION AND REGULATION

Physicians and psychiatrists have long considered themselves—and the public has tended to expect them to be—guardians of the quality of patient care. If this is the case, why do physicians and psychiatrists resent and resist the intrusions of accrediting and regulatory bodies? Why the resistance if indeed quality of care is to be enhanced by the use of *professionally defined* standards that promote the continual upgrading of quality of care?

From her observations, the author believes that much resistance is derived from fear of intrusions upon professional autonomy. Another factor is the often genuine concern about burdensome quality assurance activities and paperwork. A lesser concern arises from real disagreement with the substance of standards.

The Fort Logan Mental Health Center, 1962–1976

As the clinical director (1962–1967) and the director (1967–1976) of the Fort Logan Mental Health Center (FLMHC), the author was accountable and responsible for an innovative public (state) mental hospital, with a strong community orientation. In preparing for surveys for accreditation as a hospital (JCAH), as a teaching facility (AMA, APA, NASW, and other groups), and for state licensure (state department of health), the FLMHC had the advantages of being adequately staffed with well-trained personnel and in relatively new buildings with modern furnishings, equipment, and supportive services and of having a new patient population. Our patient records were variable in quality, and we had some deficiencies in life safety. Otherwise, we met the standards well and received full accreditation during the 1960's and early 1970's.

Fort Logan nevertheless anxiously prepared (at first in the eleventh hour) for each of the surveys. The upper administrative and supportive services staff felt the anxiety and pressure rather acutely, while many of the clinical staff looked upon each site visit as another opportunity to "show and tell." Many staff at all levels of the hospital worked hard to "get ready."

The first three surveys were conducted under the JCAH standards for general hospitals (hospital accreditation program). The first surveyor was a retired urologist, and the next two were retired internists. All three concentrated on the medical records, the physical plant, the medical staff bylaws, rules, and regulations, and minutes of medical staff committees. The first surveyor recommended we keep a fire axe in our walk-in refrigerator in case someone got locked in; the second surveyor recommended we use a ball-peen hammer instead; and the third surveyor suggested we install a threaded, U-shaped bolt, equipped with wing nuts, for opening the latch from inside. Later, during long-overdue consultations with another hospital, we learned about the refrigerator safety devices on the market for a number of years, and we installed one.

The fourth survey was conducted by two surveyors, a psychiatrist and a hospital administrator, using the *1972 JCAH Accreditation Manual for Psychiatric Facilities*. At that time, we felt some special investment in these standards because Fort Logan had participated in the field trials of an early draft. Our preparations seemed less hectic than before. The surveyors spent time discussing treatment programs with staff. The staff were generally pleased with the survey, and some developed a strong interest in improving medical records.

The fifth survey was conducted by two surveyors, a psychiatrist and a hospital administrator. There were some recommendations about our records and about fire safety in the halfway houses that lacked sprinklers.

About a year later, we invited the psychiatrist–surveyor to teach a hospital-wide workshop on Problem Oriented Medical Records. In response, one team did a thorough job of successfully implementing POMR, while others made stabs at it. Over the years, the priority of "working with people instead of paper" had been institutionalized at Fort Logan. Paperwork was viewed as "compulsive" activity, and most people hated it. We found that the best records were useful, succinct and well focused, while the worst were voluminous, rambling, incoherent collections of paper. We did not completely solve these problems, not because they were insoluble but because we did not maintain the full-scale intensity of staff education, re-education, and supervisory follow-through necessary to success in this difficult area.

Multiple Facilities 1976–1978

In 1976, after leaving Fort Logan the author became a full-time surveyor for the JCAH (ACPF) and, in surveying a great variety of programs, learned much from the "other side of the fence." The professional and nonprofessional direct patient care staff's attitudes of concern about quality of patient care were impressive; by contrast, administration and upper-management staff were mainly concerned about "getting accredited." Psychiatrists and other physicians were often indifferent, even hostile, toward the accreditation process.

Veterans Administration Medical Center/Brentwood, 1978–1981

In 1978, the author became quality assurance officer and staff psychiatrist at the Veterans Administration Medical Center/Brentwood, California. The third JCAH survey under the 1972 "Green Manual" had resulted in a two-year accreditation. Two years later, in 1980, the survey under the *1979 Consolidated Standards* resulted in a one-year accreditation. Limited follow-through on the 1978 recommendations and less than enthusiastic complicance with the stricter *Consolidated Standards* in 1980 were factors in the one-year accreditation. Better follow-through on the 1980 recommendations resulted in a substantially better compliance level at the time of the 1982 survey.

CONCLUSION

From my experiences as a psychiatric administrator, as a surveyor, and as a quality assurance coordinator, I offer the suggestions discussed in the following section.

Quality Assurance Staff

Preparing at the last minute for a survey or inspection is potentially disruptive to programs, undermines quality of care, and invites disaster. It is preferable to develop and maintain an evenly paced program of compliance with standards and systematic upgrading of quality of patient care.

The administrator, all management personnel, and all supervisors should be accountable for the quality of care and for quality assurance. Achieving such a commitment depends heavily on the quality of the management of the facility. A qualified quality assurance coordinator, directly accountable to the administrator, is essential in carrying out the monitoring, follow-up document collecting, and preparation of status reports on a timely basis, at a centrally located point. The accrediting and regulatory bodies indicate in their standards and their presurvey instructions what documentation is required for demonstrating various aspects of compliance.

Example 1. Often, the chief of medical records has the "accreditation coordinator" role in addition to other duties. This arrangement may still work in some settings, but these days, a full-time, qualified person with *adequate* office and clerical assistance is the minimum. A "qualified person" is an experienced, mature professional, preferably in a mental health field with a substantial administrative background, good communication skills, and a good understanding of data analysis. Nurses and doctors of various specialties, psychologists, social workers, Registered Records Administrators, Accredited Records Technicians (RRAs)/(ARTs), and so on, are among the professional disciplines represented in quality assurance coordinator positions at psychiatric and other types of facilities.

Example 2. At the Brentwood VA Medical Center, we first had a nurse with experience in program evaluation as health systems review organization (HSRO)–systematic internal review full-time HSRO–SIR coordinator, accountable to the chief of program evaluation. Next, the author, a psychiatrist, with a background in psychiatric hospital administration and JCAH surveying, became the full-time quality assurance officer accountable to the director. While the backgrounds and styles of these respective coordinators certainly influenced their organizational effectiveness, the direct accountability of the quality assurance officer to the director and his consistent follow-through and follow-up were perhaps the most telling factors in improving the effectiveness of the quality assurance program, center-wide. Moreover, the inclusion of service and program chiefs as well as chairpersons of the quality assurance-related committees as members of the center's quality assurance committee was important in strengthening the quality assurance program and meeting the intent of the *1981 Quality Assurance Standard* of JCAH. Members of the committee have served as "internal surveyors," reviewing the various services and programs, the documentation, the physical plant, and so on, between surveys. Such reviews have positive effects transcending the value of the self-surveys per se: staff can learn about program features not necessarily evident through other channels of communication.

It is critically important for the quality assurance officer (or coordinator) to assume a "staff" role despite pressures to get involved in the line responsibilities of those who are accountable and responsible for the quality of patient care.

Internal Review Processes

Properly managed, the accreditation and regulatory process can be a useful learning experience and can improve the existing quality of care.

Over time, the repeated surveys and inspections can stimulate upgrading of the quality of care, but only if systematically followed up with the facility's own internal processes of review and quality assurance.

Example 1. Since 1972, the VA has required its facilities to be accredited by JCAH. Beginning in 1974, the VA implemented the HSRO, with its systematic internal review (SIR) and systematic external review programs (SERP), using VA standards (SCEMs) to be applied to all VA facilities. Recent improvements in SERP and in JCAH survey methods should enhance further the quality assurance programs of the VA.

Example 2. The psychiatric administrator can—in fact, should—foster the quality of patient care through legitimate use of the accreditation process, without misrepresenting the facts about which standards are being cited. Unfortunately, psychiatric (and other) administrators may invoke "accreditation" requirements in order to coerce staff into compliance with various policies, procedures, and practices, e.g., sometimes JCAH related, sometimes only "in the name of" JCAH—whether JCAH ever had such a standard or not.

Administrators may use recommendations by JCAH, Department of Health and Human Services (HHS), SERP, et al., in justifying additional moneys for staffing, furnishings, equipment, building improvements, and so on. Conversely, ritualized compliance with JCAH and other standards may be reinforced by making licensure and funding contingent upon accreditation. Understanding the intent of any applicable standards and their relationship, if any, to quality of patient care is essential to offsetting such negative effects.

Staff-Surveyor Interaction and Review Standards

Staff at a facility to be surveyed have a right and a responsibility to know by what standards and how and by whom their programs will be judged.

Recognizing this, JCAH, the VA, state departments of health, and other standard-setting groups have developed increasingly explicit objectified standards, available well in advance of the survey. Moreover, the various review bodies are now selecting their surveyors more carefully and training them more intensively. Such steps should minimize "surveyor variance" in interpreting standards. When documentation is well prepared, staff–surveyor interaction can be directed into a consultative and educational mode more effectively. Focusing staff attention (and pinning hopes) on the personal qualities of surveyors should become less of a preoccupation of facility staff as surveys become more objective. (Unfortunately, no matter what the objectivity of the survey, facility staff may still regard a survey with favorable outcome as "fair" and a survey with an unfavorable outcome as "unfair.")

Once a survey gets under way, facility staff and surveyor(s) quickly become engaged in working toward presumably common goals, at best, or become adversaries, at worst. A cooperative, if not collaborative, working relationship tends to be the rule. Staff should be encouraged by the administrator to participate actively in the process, asking questions, seeking clarification, and challenging recommendations that do not make sense. Too often a wish to "let sleeping dogs lie" and/or fear of upsetting the surveyor may inhibit facility staff and reduce chances for learning—both ways. Accepting uncritically a surveyor's recommendation or suggestion is not a good practice. (Remember the fire ax!) Of necessity, it is prudent and professional to disagree without being disagreeable.

Improving the Quality of Care

Facility staff appreciate and respond positively to having opportunities for learning and for improving the quality of care.

When conducted in a positive spirit, the survey or review can provide such opportunities in addition to serving as an inspection and thus be less of a crisis. In fact, the quality of patient care should be improved by the survey process itself. Careful notes should be taken about all findings and any recommendations. Some deficiencies can be corrected on the spot, some soon after the survey, and others still later. Staff can also learn much of relevance to improving quality of care from a skillfully conducted survey, with or without reference to deficiencies per se, and staff derive a sense of accomplishment.

It is better to respond promptly to recommendations than to wait for weeks or months until the formal report of findings and recommendations is received. By then, the attention and interest of the staff will have diminished. Ideally, the notification should give further impetus to the already "in place" process of maintaining and improving quality of care.

The Relevance of Accreditation and Regulatory Surveys

Differences of opinion persist as to the relevance of accreditation and regulatory surveys to quality of patient care.

Variations in quality between surveys and inspections contribute to some of the skepticism, as do misunderstandings about the intent of the standards. Remember: many standards are written from the patient's point of view. Constructive impact on the accreditation process can be provided by psychiatric administrators and other practitioners lending their assistance through active input into the policy-making, standard-setting, and accreditation processes of voluntary organizations such as JCAH, APA, and other groups and into the analogous processes of governmental agencies. The JCAH voluntary, confidential accreditation process responds to input from the field and is considered by many (including the federal General Accounting Office) to be preferable to governmental methods for standard-setting and reviews.[6]

Joint Surveys

Too many surveys by multiple agencies are indeed causing real hardships for many facilities in every state.

Service providers have demanded that accrediting and regulatory bodies conduct their reviews jointly and/or at least accept all or part of each other's standards, reviews, and reports as equivalent.[7–9] It is a hopeful sign that in at least 23 states, the surveys of the JCAH and of state health departments are being conducted jointly, and 17 others are considering such arrangements. These collaborations have been commended by the General Accounting Office of the U.S. Congress, as cost-containing efforts that successfully reduce some of the duplication of preparation and the overuse of scarce resources, which could better be used toward the improvement of quality of care.[6,10]

PROFESSIONAL STANDARDS REVIEW ORGANIZATIONS

Established by PL 92-603 in 1973, the professional standards review organizations (PSROs) are the regional mechanisms for monitoring the services provided by those receiving reimbursement through Medicare and Medicaid. Their purpose is to achieve cost containment by the review of utilization of resources through establishing medical necessity for admission, length of stay (LOS) and utilization of ancillary services.

Routine review of medical necessity of every admission and of every case exceeding the specified LOS is generally not productive. There has been a shift to selective, problem-focused reviews, which produce more useful information, improvement in quality of practices and quality of care, as well as more cost effectiveness. There has also been increasing use of generic screening of problem-focused medical audit topics in addition to diagnoses or procedures as topics. The *1981 Quality Assurance Standard* of JCAH emphasizes a problem-focused approach. Given the complexities of psychiatric problems and problem solving, the advice to start with the relatively simple issues in order to experience early success in utilization reviews is well taken.[11,12]

HEALTH SYSTEMS AGENCIES

Health systems agencies (HSAs) were instituted by PL 93-641, the National Health Planning and Resources Development Act of 1974. Under the Department of Health, Education, and Welfare, this powerful structure for planning and regulating health care in the United States was established to supersede all preexisting planning agencies.

At the time PL 93-641 was passed, psychiatrists were advised to familiarize themselves with the legislation and take steps to ensure adequate psychiatric representation on the governing boards of the HSA responsible for a given area. Now, some seven years later, the same advice is being repeated, from New York State in particular.[13,14]

Some HSAs (e.g., Northern Virginia) are systematically trying to exclude physicians from participating in health-planning decisions.[15] The experiences in New York and Virginia, while not necessarily duplicated in other states, should be carefully studied as examples of what psychiatric administrators and other psychiatrists and physicians can expect and might do. Meanwhile, the AMA and American Hospital Association (AHA) have continued to advocate that HSAs and PSROs be abolished and new state-level regulatory structures be developed.[16,17]

REFERENCES

1. Accreditation Manual for Psychiatric Facilities. Chicago, Joint Commission on Accreditation of Hospitals, 1972
2. Consolidated Standards for Child, Adolescent and Adult Psychiatric Facilities, Alcoholism and Drug Abuse Programs. Chicago, Joint Commission on Accreditation of Hospitals, 1979
3. Consolidated Standards Manual for Child, Adolescent, and Adult Psychiatric, Alcoholism, and Drug Abuse Facilities. Chicago, Joint Commission on Accreditation of Hospitals, 1981
4. JCAH agrees to new wording on standards. Psychiatric News 15: 1980
5. Quality Assurance. Consolidated Standards Manual for Child, Adolescent, and Adult Psychiatric, Alcoholism, and Drug Abuse Facilities. Chicago, Joint Commission on Accreditation of Hospitals, 1981, p 33–37
6. Perspectives, JCAH, July-August, 1979, 4:1–2,1979
7. Perspectives, JCAH, January-February, 1981, 1:1, 1981
8. Schlicke CP: JCAH and the federal government. Bull American College of Surgeons, 64:23–28, 1979
9. McLerran A, Grinspoon L, Gudeman J: A surfeit of surveys: escalating data demands on community mental health centers. Hosp Community Psychiatry 30:243 247, 1979
10. La Violette S: Simpler JCAH standards on drawing board. Modern Health Care, 1981, p 33–34
11. Skillikorn S: Quality and Accountability: A New Era in American Hospitals. San Francisco, Editorial Consultants, 1980
12. Bonn E, Kiriakos R, Messick J, et al: Report of the Subcommittee on Utilization Review. VAMC Brentwood, July 1979, unpublished
13. Feigelson EL: Psychiatry and health systems agencies. The Bulletin of the Area II District Branches, American Psychiatric Association, vol. 18, No. 7, March 1976
14. Keill S: The HSA and psychiatrists. The Bulletin of the Area II District Branches, American Psychiatric Association, vol. 22, No. 5, February 1980
15. Mamana J: HSA's versus physicians—health planning adversaries. Hospital Medical Staff 9:10–13, 1980
16. Editorial, 93-641: American Medical News 24:1981, p 4
17. AHA delegates urge PSRO repeal. American Medical News, 24:1981, p 1,17

Zebulon C. Taintor, M.D.

22

Automated Data Systems

There has been a recent resurgence of interest in the use of computers in psychiatry. At the 1981 American Psychiatric Association annual meeting, the course on computers was among the first to sell out in advance registration.[1] Presenters at symposia and panels have discovered they no longer outnumber the audience, and a journal on uses of computers in psychiatry is now in its fourth year.[2] Most of the new wave of interest is from psychiatrists who hope to find new uses for their home microcomputers. They are exhilarated to have so much responsive energy at their command. Some have ventured into automated psychological tests, which is almost as far as one now can go beyond small business applications with a microcomputer. While this chapter is not written for the new individual computer users, it owes a debt to them, for their complaints about the contrast between satisfaction with their own machine and their frustration in attempting to use or improve information systems at work may improve the latter. Like the rest of us, they wonder why they have to fill out so many forms to receive expensive, inaccurate, out-of-date reports.

Explanations of the contrast have to do with much more than the economics of scale, public versus private, or the need to do something oneself if it is to be done well. Answers are to be found in the study of information systems, so new a field that it is not widely recognized or taught to psychiatrists and administrators. This chapter attempts to provide a practical guide for psychiatric administrators who are involved with information systems: getting a system, using an existing system better, or—the most common situation—trying to improve an existing system.

The principal conceptual issue has had to do with appreciating the difference between a reporting system and an information system and greatly underestimating the technical and personnel requirements of the latter. A reporting system

---

This chapter was written by Zebulon Taintor, in his private capacity. No official support endorsement by the Alcohol, Drug Abuse and Mental Health Administration is intended or should be inferred. Dr. Taintor was director (1975–1979), Multi-State Information System (MSIS), Information Sciences Division, Rockland Research Institute, Orangeburg, NY 10962 (to which inquiries about systems can be directed).

merely involves providing data to others. It assumes an authoritarian relationship: some workers provide input, but only one user at the top gets reports and makes all decisions regarding the system. An information system involves creating a pool of data with the capacity for input and updating from many sources. Retrieval and reporting demands are enormous, since many are served. Inevitably, a successful information system levels authoritarian relationships. Information in the bureaucracy is currency; its sudden availability and discussion force a search for new values.

CLINICIAN RESISTANCE

Initial federal efforts, such as funding of the development of the Multi-State Information System in 1966, assumed that computers would be of use to clinicians. Printouts of admissions data, histories, mental status examinations, and so on were produced from check lists. Contrary to expectations, clinicians did not welcome these, but administrators embraced the statistical reports.

Clinicians became alienated from the use of computers in part because of their popularity with other groups, especially program evaluators, who often struck clinicians as excessively reductionistic, the quantitative type described by Talbott.[3] Clinicians complained about paperwork and the diversion of funds from patient care to the purchase of expensive computers. They noted that greater reporting and accountability had been associated with declining budgets. Computers seemed to promote administration per se. While a tool does not decide its use, the human element that was learning about information systems should have interpreted the process for others. The obvious naïveté of information systems developers in failing to distinguish among the various actors in the mental health treatment drama and the uses to which they would put computers contributed to the situation.

The question of whether computers can help clinicians is still being debated in 1981 despite favorable assessments based on the accumulation of more than a thousand published reports on the use of computers in mental health. It is only in recent years that computer applications have emerged that are clearly clinically relevant. Common interests should develop among clinicians and administrators, since the general considerations that apply to good information systems in psychiatry, beyond the individual practitioner, are roughly the same as those that apply to the achievement of good clinical care.

COMPONENTS

This section both defines the usual components of a system and describes related problems for the psychiatric administrator.

Hardware

It has been usual to speak of main frame computers, minicomputers, and microcomputers. All have a central processing unit with core memory, peripheral memory, printer(s) and input devices, cathode ray tubes (CRT), card readers, and so on. Historically, large computers had 32-bit words, minicomputers had 16, and microcomputers had mostly 8-bit words. Micros are now moving into 16-bit words, while minis are moving into 32-bit words. The internal architecture of machines has differed historically but has become increasingly similar as different computer chips have developed. Memory size used to be a distinguishing feature among machines. Minis formerly had less than 16-K bytes, but that is smaller than many of the micros of today. Ability to handle peripheral equipment and interactive transactions, price, and the number of programming languages have been differences that are now blurred. As of this writing, a microcomputer tends to be slow, has up to 32-K bytes in memory, and less of all of the above features, especially regarding data-based management systems. (see below.)

At this point, the major differences to bear in mind about machines are as follows: (1) There is an enormous turnover of manufacturers, and this year's maker of lowpriced machines may be bankrupt before next year; (2) Equipment still varies widely in terms of reliability, availability, ease of repair, and other service parameters, so cost should not be overemphasized; (3) Compatibility among machines, peripherals, and software cannot be assumed until actually tested, no matter what the specifications say. Do not purchase a machine until you have seen how well your programs run on it (benchmarking). Talk to other users before buying. Vendors will lie to be able to have low bids accepted, knowing that once the agency has been committed, it will be difficult to withdraw without seeming foolish; (4) Hardware requirements are often underestimated, since successful information systems tend to generate much more data and processing requirements than anticipated. Some equipment is so new that no one knows what it really will do.

Microcomputers are not fast or large enough and do not have a sufficiently wide range of capabilities for administrative applications within institutions, although microcomputers are improving very rapidly.

Typical mistakes in purchasing hardware include (1) having to go by competitive bids and getting an IBM competitor that did not last (GE, Westinghouse, etc.) (2) believing the manufacturer's statement that no air conditioning was required (the machines melted), (3) getting a machine on which to develop software instead of getting software that is later brought in house.

Software

Software, the programs that run on the computer, can be divided into several types:

Program Language

Program language is the language in which all other programs are written to run on a given machine. The program language converts what is written in it (e.g., admission tracking) into the machine language actually used in processing. Examples are COBOL, Basic, PL-1, Fortran, Pascal, and so on. Different programming languages become an issue in that a system generally should be written in one language. Applications are sometimes not easily transferred from one machine to another because they are either in different programming languages or the translation to a particular machine language may not work exactly: IBM PL-1 may be different from your machine's PL-1. MUMPS, a popular medical computing language, has developed several dialects.

System Control Languages

System control languages arrange to run multiple jobs submitted by multiple users on large computers. They are usually invisible, but they can become a barrier to information system software transfer between machines because a data base management system that is crafted to work under one system may not work in an otherwise identical computer with a different system control language.

Data Base Management Systems

The key to any information system, these systems describe how information is actually stored within the machine. The simplest array of data is a sequential system, which is best envisioned as having records laid end to end like the pages of a book before binding. Any word on any page may be accessed directly. The machine, however, would have to read every page before the one on which your chosen word is situated in order to get to it, so it is better to set the pages in a more compact form and have access to them through a root system, which serves the same function as the title on the spine of a bound volume. A fixed root segment with the data configured underneath it like an upside-down tree is called an hierarchical arrangement. The computer, however, can alter the ways of tapping into the data through a series of simple commands. It need not be fixed in the way books are printed or arranged in your library, since computers can rearrange data and how they function internally. Some have virtual machine capability that enables them to act as though they are much larger than they actually are. Thus computers can arrange your hypothetical library by author, title, first lines, length, and so on, altering the root segment as necessary. This sort of data base is called a relational data base. There are other data base systems, such as networks, and so on. Suffice it to say that a data base management system of some sort is an absolute requirement for gathering a variable amount of data of different types on patients or staff. Data base management systems are not easily transferred either and may pose considerable difficulty for programmers. Underestimation of problems dealing with data base management systems has accounted for the failure of many systems.

The initial time that it takes to translate even relatively simple concepts into computer applications is repeatedly underestimated. Quick and dirty jobs are often very poorly documented and difficult for successors to understand and change. Since talented people in the computer business tend to be lured away to higher-paying jobs in the private sector, administrators must ensure that documentation (both for users and programmers wanting to make changes) of systems is understandable and complete.

Statistical Packages

Statistical packages perform many statistical tests on data with minimal instructions. Examples are the Statistical Package for the Social Sciences (SPSS),[6] The Biomedical Computer Programs P series (BMDP),[7] and the Statistical Analysis System (SAS).[8] The statistical packages all run against sequential data, although SAS has a limited data base management capacity. Even statistical packages may vary in different machines: SPSS runs differently on Honeywell than on IBM.

Communication Software

Communications software is used by machines to communicate with one another, with terminals for receiving data or printing reports. It is often underrated as a cause of problems and underestimated regarding cost of revision. One state that had successfully insisted that a vendor put all of its software into a transferable form found itself locked into a long-term arrangement with the vendor because none of the contractual provisions had specified that the communication software should also be transferable. The communications language was so enmeshed in all the other programs that the vendor's terminals and core could not be separated from the operation of the system.

Operations

Processing

Processing may be interactive or batch. The first involves being continuously on line with the computer from the beginning of a job until its completion. Access to the central processing unit of the computer is instantaneous. In batch processing, jobs are read first and processed later. There is no continuous connection with the computer. Interactive processing seems desirable by definition, but batch processing is often less expensive (depending on charges for connect time) and a more efficient use of resources. Sometimes the delay is only seconds. Programs involving statistical packages are almost always submitted in batch, as are most statistical reports or anything else involving complicated input or long output. Interactive processing requires safeguards against suddenly obliterating one's records by hitting the wrong key.

Terminals

Terminals may be dumb in that they only transmit and receive data or intelligent (special purpose microcomputers with reduced flexibility and lesser cost, or micro-mini computers). Systems typically underestimate the number of terminals that will be needed or the amount of time that it takes to enter data. As they grow, the terminal becomes a bottleneck; hence the argument for batching high-volume data entry. Although public facilities tend to overbuy processing equipment, they typically underspend both on personnel (because of the public-sector pay scale) and on peripheral equipment (that would make the system work better).

Trade-offs

Different processing arrangements have different loci of costs.

Dumb remote job entry terminals on line have the advantages of simple field hardware, no field software, and easy user software development, since it is all at the host and usually cost shared by many users. Such a host is likely to be dedicated to a mental health system and will not have to interrupt mental health work to process drivers' licenses or to do other work. The disadvantages are (1) high communications costs, (2) response times that are sensitive to host load if the host is utilized to capacity, and (3) a high sensitivity to host malfunctions.

The host system with an intelligent terminal has the advantages of no host software changes, reduced communication costs, reduced host workload, local editing, and quicker responses. The disadvantages are higher field hardware cost, that form-prompting programs then to be developed in the field, and some sensitivity to host malfunction.

Minicomputers with local data bases have the advantages of (1) reduced host workload, (2) reduced communication costs, (3) interactive queries of local data bases, (4) possibly more responsivity to user demands (depending on local support), and (5) less sensitivity to main-frame down time. Heavy field investment in hardware and software is needed, however, there are problems keeping data bases current, and many management issues in field security and software development appear. Most facilities have not managed minicomputers very well.

Eventually, there may be networks linking minis at the many facilities. The advantages are low communications cost and the possibility of high redundancy of processing capability with low total hardware cost and considerable user responsivity. Sophisticated networks are required, however, and management issues having to do with security, compability, and so on, have not been solved yet. At present, there is no mininetwork in mental health that offers the range of services described here.

Generalized Retrieval

Generalized retrieval of data combined from many systems and sources should be possible. It has been argued that computer development is like the spread of electric motors. It was first thought that each household would have one large electric motor off of which numerous operations would be performed. Instead, there are many little electric motors to perform specialized tasks in each house. Should there be many little specialized computers? Electric motors no more resemble computers than muscles do brains. We have many different muscles that perform specialized functions around different joints but only one brain. The greater the capacity, the more integration that can be achieved efficiently and the better off we are. While systems can become top-heavy with data base problems, it should be possible to generate lists and tables with a wide variety of data from many systems.

What else should the administrative psychiatrist know about hardware and software? Enough to raise the issues, since computer technicians, for various reasons, will sometimes neglect one or another. The facility should avoid becoming "one of a kind," using hardware or software, since there is safety and security in numbers and user groups. It is generally better to get *computing* services rather than a *computer* because all your time may be spent struggling with the computer while other systems forge ahead. Use software you like via a remote location and then bring it in house if it is more cost effective (including costs of software update and equipment maintenance) to have your own computer than to be processing remotely. The psychiatric administrator should know how the system operates at his facility. This both demonstrates administrative support, leads to sophistication about the system and who is using it well, and generates a consensus about where to go next.

Personnel

Computer Scientists

Computer scientists have advanced theoretical knowledge of computers and their modes of operation, usually at the master's or doctoral level. Computer scientists are a necessary component of the operation of large information systems to evaluate and use the components described above; the field is changing so rapidly that solid grounding in theory is required.

Systems Analysts

Systems analysts translate obtain specifications of the applications to be written and communicate these to the *programmers*. The usual way that systems are developed involves working backward from outputs. Specify a table or list; this will reveal the data elements. Consider who should gather the data, how they are to be entered, and soon. The analyst tells the programmer how the table should look; *the programmer* tells the computer how to produce it.

Problems between mental health personnel and computer workers fall into three areas: communication gaps, cognitive styles, and resistance to understanding psychological issues. Clear communication with systems analysts, most of whom know very little about mental health, is essential. Failure to understand alternatives available or to say exactly what is really wanted is a frequent cause of failure. Mental health staff, accustomed to improvising, resist spelling out (in what they consider excessive detail) what they want or how the system will work. Some arguments justify their empirical approach. No living system is ever finished. Each answer begets two questions. No form is perfect; every one is a compromise. Direction often changes in midstream. Allow for change and expansion in budgeting all resources. Answers, however, must be found to all questions eventually, and sooner is better than later.

Cognitive styles differ between clinicians and computer workers. Computers require a dichotomous and either/or logical linking of alternatives and attract people who reason that way, while clinicians often think along spectra and dimensions in a nonquantitative and intuitive way.

Some systems analysts have great resistances to psychological phenomena and clinical settings. Systems have failed because systems analysts could not become sufficiently involved in hospitals and the milieu to understand what was really happening. One thus sees claims for systems that may not only be untrue but quite uninteresting to clinicians who have a better way of accomplishing the task. Who would be interested in a medication-ordering system that advertised itself as being a good source of what drugs had been ordered for a patient? One can look at the cardex on the unit where nurses have legibly written not only the orders but also whether the patient actually took the medication.

Those who deal with computers often do not derive much self-esteem from providing service but rather from advancing the state of the art. It is often difficult for clinicians who emphasize service to patients to understand that computer scientists find dealing with users to be confusing and disorganizing and get more professional rewards from staying in their offices planning future developments. There are, of course, wonderful exceptions to these observations, and psychiatrist-administrators must learn to look for them.

To operate, information systems need three other sorts of workers from a central source and two at the facility. Using the Multi-State Information System (MSIS) terminology:

Technical Assistance Persons

Technical assistance person(s) can be called by the terminal operator or anyone else who is having trouble running a job on the computer. There must be a friendly, sympathetic voice at the other end of the telephone who can say what should be done next. These people solve minor technical problems in the information system that would overtax the capabilities of the average user, e.g., setting up new facility data bases.

Retrieval Personnel

Provision of output is the major test of any system. A good information system will provide special help in this area in the form of helping users to get data back, circulating successful reports, working with user groups, demonstrating how to run standard reports, such as the *National Institute of Mental Health Inventory of Community Mental Health Center Services and Personnel Reports,* and so on.

Liaison Staff

Liaison staff meet users personally. They provide a structure for communicating about long-range issues and user problems with the system. How can it be made more useful? What applications should be developed next? Why does it take three weeks for the form on a new patient to go from the admitting office to the terminal room? Why is the census generated by the night switchboard operator in her idle moments more accurate than that maintained in the computer? When is a treatment episode to be terminated? Is the local data processing manager correct in saying that a frequently requested report simply cannot be produced? Advice from persons outside the facility who have broad experience with other users can be extremely helpful.

Data Processing Managers

A technician in each facility must oversee all aspects of the computer operation. Mental health skills are desirable, but warmth, genuine interest, empathy with others, initiative, and an eye for problems are absolutely essential. A good indication of the quality of a data processing manager is whether after being on the job for 18 months, he has been elevated to or is still a member of the institution's executive committee.

User Group(s)

User group(s) must be convened to develop an atmosphere of trust and cooperation, define data elements, and discuss what reports are to be produced, who is to get them, and how data are to be used. The group provides an immediate check on the data processing manager, since individual members will eventually become quite sophisticated. A well-developed system has many more functions (clinical, administrative, evaluative, research, and so on) than can be subsumed by a data processing manager's supervisor, whatever the discipline or location within the formal table of organization. Evaluate your proposed system by its attention to these factors.

CONTENTS AND USES

Most information systems have the following components, which may be separate systems in themselves, depending on the data base management system and the hardware involved. In a sophisticated system, most of the components described below feed into structured data bases on patients, personnel, and things. A good patient system will not be designed exclusively for clinicians or administrators, since the data therein will be of interest to everyone.

PATIENTS

Admissions/Census Movement

Basic demographic data on patients usually include birth date, sex, census tract, address, and so on, which are helpful for planning and billing. Basic counts document which patients are admitted to a facility, where they come from, where they are currently located, and their present clinical and legal status. Lists include an alphabetical listing of all patients currently admitted to a facility. Individual ward or unit rosters, and monthly, quarterly, and yearly admission/discharge statistics are useful as well as reports concerning length of stay and readmission rates. Most such systems also provide basic data on patient problems, referral sources, diagnoses, and so on. Cohort studies of patients are used in length-of-stay and discharge studies. Patients who stay longer than any specified period can be listed for study. The admissions data with specified census tract locations provide utilization data by area and can be used to decide the location and sorts of services to be provided within the community. Admission data can be computer merged with census tract data for other planning and projection studies.

Services

What services were provided to each patient? By whom? Where? How long did the service take? When? All services provided to each patient are documented and maintained in a data base. The frequency of specific services or categories of services can be obtained for individual patients or groups of patients through routine tabulations of all services required and stored in the system. Simple listing reports illustrate all the services and their frequencies provided by a person, unit, discipline, or the entire organization for any time period. Any of these can be compared with another. Such services can be used on an inpatient basis to produce detailed hospital bills on an outpatient basis.

Diagnosis

Especially since the advent of DSM III, there is a need to record as many psychiatric and medical diagnoses as clinicians wish, as well as to record the duration of a diagnosis when it is changed separately from the rest of the patient data base. Psychiatric administrators should verify that their information systems have this capability. Computer-assisted diagnoses can provide logical prompts interactively on a CRT,[9] suggest diagnoses from the history and mental status,[10] or suggest diagnoses through actuarial comparisons of a given case against the data base.[11] Prompting DSM III is like any other computer-assisted instruction, a useful way to learn but slower than one's mind after learning has occurred. Clinicians will use the program while it helps them to learn DSM III (no small achievement) but will then prefer the speedier method of directly entering the diagnosis. Automated diagnostic suggestions inevitably suffer from being unable to capture all the facts needed for data entry.[13]

Medication Orders

All medications ordered on a particular patient are entered much as the services are recorded, but the data entry form for services is usually completed by secretaries. If clinicians report services, it is usually on a single line. The form of data entry for medications has been, however, a battleground between the information system specialists, who favor forms, and clinicians, who prefer the usual blank order sheet. It is strange that nurses and other clinical staff have been able to decipher order sheets while data entry personnel and computer types seem unable to do so. The situation is complicated by consent decrees and regulations requiring more specificity in orders (e.g., start and stop date) and the need for frequent renewal of some orders. Ideally, this component should be invisible to clinicians (data entry to be taken from the order sheet) and will (1) maintain inventories, (2) print labels for unit doses as necessary, (3) preprint monthly orders so that a physician need only indicate changes before signing his name, and (4) assist quality control. Large computers can compare each medication order with predetermined guidelines for dosage, polypharmacy, and drug interactions. Computers can suggest cases for peer review and can serve as an up-to-date electronic textbook for indicating the need for such review. Such a system is presently being installed throughout New York State[12] and will probably represent a principal defense against class-action suits related to tardive dyskinesia. This system can be expected to work only in an atmosphere of trust and collegiality to minimize inevitable fears that Big Brother is watching. The human component must be stressed to avoid giving the impression that medical decisions are dictated by the remote group of experts who are setting the guidelines within the computer or that the computer is itself somehow making medical decisions. Suggestions of what should be prescribed have been attempted[14] but suffer from the same data entry problems as dianostic suggestions.

Patient Assessment

Patient assessment, such as detailed histories,[15–19] psychological tests,[20–23] mental status examinations,[24] and a host of other clinical forms, many of which were developed in conjunction with drug trials,[25] can enrich the data base. Gathering such data is very much in the interest of administrators, since clinicians are encouraged to reflect about their practice and all or a sample of the patient population can be described more exactly. Such descriptions help the public and other reviewers to appreciate differences in patient populations among facilities and to be more realistic regarding treatment and outcome. Detailed patient assessments before and after treatment are the only way to capture outcome. Automation promotes statistical comparisons.

Treatment planning

Recording of treatment plans is under way in many mental health information systems. Administrators are unaware of the enormous potential that this component has for documenting budgetary needs. Treatment plans should be recorded with the idea that some of the services suggested will be provided by the institution, some will be provided by community resources (which can be identified through an automated resource directory), while other needs will be unmet. The last can be automatically totaled to provide measures of community and facility need and are incontestable budgetary documentation. The component works like the service recording system except in a future mode: what should happen rather than what has.

Administrative interest in treatment planning includes program evaluation. For example, use of an information system for recording psychiatric consultations showed that psychiatric residents had a very narrow range of treatment recommendations for geriatric patients as compared to younger patients.[26]

Computer-Assisted Progress Notes and Discharge Summaries

Most major mental health information systems are working to assist clinicians in producing progress notes that meet accreditation requirements and help monitor patient problems, goals, and particular treatment programs. A printout of all relevant items in the patient data base is provided before dictation, e.g., of discharge summaries. The Institute of Living has taken the lead in this regard, including notes from nursing, social services, psychology, dietary staff, and notes regarding restrictions on mail, telephone, and/or visitors, physical examination data, and various information alerts and statistical indicators.[4] (See also Chapter 19.)

Incident Report

Even with all systems running routinely, a special system to collect and process information about patient incidents, such as injuries, accidents, or any other unusual or reportable events defined by policy, is desirable. This allows the review of incidents and ensures that a standard data set is gathered through the report, investigation, and review process. Reports can identify adverse incident trends and problem units or areas and be used to plan improvements in physical plants or program emphasis so as to reduce incidents. Reports can also identify patients who are more likely to be involved in incidents so that individual treatment plans can be modified.

Referral, Tracking, and Resources

A consortium of users can simplify patient information flow among facilities. Lucas County, Ohio, using MSIS on a regional basis, developed a discharge referral printout that transmits previously negotiated information between agencies while the system is monitored automatically to ensure that the patient has been picked up by the accepting agency. An exception report shows which patients were not; these are followed up by the referring agency.

Since most catchment areas have dozens or hundreds of agencies to which patients can be referred for housing, legal, recreational, or other services, keeping them all in mind and not settling into a referral rut can be a problem. Resource directories are usually outdated as soon as they are produced. A data base (usually simple sequential) on resources can be developed by having agencies describe themselves on a checklist (as MSIS is doing for the Diabled Children's Program, N.Y. Office of Mental Retardation). Updating occurs by circulating printouts to agencies periodically so that only corrections need be noted. Returns are good since agencies know the data are used for matching ptient needs with agency abilities and location. Facilities can maintain confidential information or prompts (e.g., "See Mrs. Perkins on South before referring to this residence") that are not circulated to agencies. Consortia will probably pool resources to maintain telephone services for agencies that have no terminals of their own.

Physical and Laboratory Data

Physical and laboratory data have not yet been integrated widely into patient data bases in mental health information systems, but many physical examination checklists and automated laboratory systems, as well as specialized electrophysiology applications exist.[28] The laboratory has been described as the melting pot for medical and information sciences.[29] The psychiatric administrator's special expertise can be applied to sifting the relevance of these.

Data Entry

The projected accumulation of a large patient data base inevitably poses problems of data entry. Everyone would like more information than anyone can take the time to enter. One solution to this problem is to have patients put in the data, as is done in the automated history taking and psychological testing. It has beeen shown repeatedly that patients are actually more truthful in reporting histories to computers than in face-to-face interviews.[15,27] The computer provides only the facts, however, and not the affect, although presumably one could assess affect through on-line physiological monitoring of galvanic skin response, pulse, and soon. Applications so far have not provided much editing help in detecting malingerers or pranksters, and a willful respondent can create chaos with such instruments. While patient entry devices should continue to be developed, the best way to build up patient entry data is to enter small amounts over time into data base management software from which all data can be retrieved easily. Clinicians are generally resistant to sitting at CRTs. Systems requiring them to do so have not survived. The paper record is here to stay; computers can be used to print and organize it but not to replace it except for long-term reference when the written record is too cumbersome (e.g., a list of medications and response, admissions, services, etc., over the past 5 years).

Prediction

Large data bases have been used for sophisticated prediction applications associated with computer diagnoses,[30] suicide,[31] psychotropic drug assessment, patient length of stay, and so on.[32] Hedlund notes that "despite strong evidence of the computer that carefully developed prediction models can do at least as well as the clinician whenever explicit criteria are available, such applications continue to meet with a good deal of clinical resistance and scepticism."[33]

ADMINISTRATIVE

Personnel

The next most common data base is kept on personnel. Personnel systems increasingly capture more and more data on workers, which include demographic and qualification data such as education, licensure, certification, language abilities, interests, promotional information, continuing education, and so on. Each worker's data base is structured like a patient's except that instead of services, systems routinely accumulate assignment data on individuals, sick leave, overtime, continuing education, payroll data, and so on.

Another personnel-related file, usually a simple sequential file rather than one of the move involved data bases used for patients or individual workers, contains all positions, including title, grade, location, current occupant, and so forth.

Personnel data are used for employee tracking, and determining staffing patterns, especially required staff-patient ratios when combined with patient locations obtained from the admissions census component. Such ratios have become important in accreditation and consent decree work. Information system data bases offer the main hope of determining how necessary a given ratio may be. The data can be very helpful in the management and allocation of personnel and are generally welcomed by personnel if they are aware that job preference data and other items of concern to them are being maintained in the computer and will be produced whenever certain questions are asked. This provides some reassurance against favoritism or being forgotten.

Inventories and Facilities

Things as well as people are tracked through inventory control systems, which enable facilities to monitor the acquisition, storage, and distribution of inventory items. Requisitions, issues, items received, adjustments, and so on, are typically recorded and stored in the computer. Requisitions and issues can generate orders automatically. Usual systems automatically calculate and flag reorder requirements, minimizing the likelihood that needs will not be met or that perishable items will accumulate. Purchasing departments receive computer-generated reports reflecting current and prior item usage, order slips to be signed, notice of overdue deliveries, and other information that aids in the procurement of supplies. The accounting department and the psychiatric administrator receive reports on costs and cost distribution for all items in the system. Comparisons between inventory amounts calculated by the computer and periodic physical inventories help detect pilferage and other inventory problems.

Inventory control systems have been extended to track furniture and less perishable items. The data base eventually can be expected to expand to include all items within the facility and some parameters of the facility itself, such as depreciation.

Billing

Billing programs merge admission/census services received and financial information to produce bills for patients and/or third-party payers or can save the delay, expense, and inaccuracy of keying data by producing tapes that are read in place of paper to produce bills directly. Desirable presently available features on which to insist include ability to bill multiple payers, automatic rebilling and concern when no payment is received, increasing a localized admission/census module that suggests patient eligibility for coverage, and some ability to develop service cost systems.

Budget

Agencies frequently produce several budgets that represent a range of possible expenditures (e.g. − 5 percent, + 5 percent, + 10 percent). MSIS developed an interactive system for the New York Department of Mental Hygiene that recalculates tables and related variables when one figure or set of figures is changed. Budget simulation applications can relieve drudgery and assist in projections.

Cost Finding, Rate Setting, and General Ledger

While several cost-finding and rate-setting programs are available (MSIS, New York State, Missouri, etc.), their usefulness depends on being able to use a variety of cost-finding methods simultaneously[34] and the degree to which data can be fed in automatically from other components of the patient, personnel, and financial data bases. The last is least well developed, although some agencies have specialized applications (e.g., Tennessee). While there are many general ledger and billing systems available commercially, success in transferring these systems is small and expert financial consultation is to be recommended rather than any one package.

OTHER USES

Program Evaluation

The use of computers has radically altered the task of the program evaluator. The problem is no longer how to get data but how to cope with what may be too much data. Hundreds of studies have dealt with process evaluation, measures of who is doing what for whom and why, since all of these elements can be brought from the computer very easily.[35,36] Outcome evaluation, while less well reported, is eased by systems that routinely record patient status before, during, and after treatment.[37,38] If cost and resources information can be linked to service and outcome data, cost effectiveness studies can be undertaken.[40] Computer applications have been reported for needs assessment for peer review systems.[41,42] The program evaluator's concern with the reliability and validity of the data must be supported by the psychiatric administrator. Administrators must emphasize that the computer system is regarded as speaking the truth and that the data reported must be scrutinized as carefully as one would scrutinize a bank statement. The administrator must ensure that program evaluators have appropriate skills for dealing with computers and an appetite for printouts. The administrator must ensure that all key staff to be involved in program evaluation define the variables to be measured and frequency of measure and discuss action to be taken on the reports. Computerized information systems can produce so much data that facilities may find themselves in more of a goldfish bowl setting than they had anticipated. It is the administrator's task to guide the facility through this process and to draw appropriate lines of communication.

Quality Assurance

Reviewing items from the data bases described against guidelines yield cases or situations for review such as excessive length of stay or amount of service, and so on. Computerized systems also have important capabilities in determining norms that professional standards review organizations can use to detect variant cases.[43] While measures of congruence between plans and treatment are being developed, review against guidelines for a particular area can occur in a setting that promotes continuing education, as is done with medication ordering by MSIS.[12]

Accountability

Funding and regulatory agencies typically enjoy the products of information systems. Facility staff, having gone from poverty to plenty as data are reaped, are properly concerned when output from information systems is misused and they are judged arbitrarily. It is most important that communication of results be accompanied by face-to-face discussion. An effective format for this sort of discussion is a regional or a state-wide user group. Some regulatory agencies have asked for tapes of patient data bases from which all identification has been removed so that their own analyses can be undertaken. There is no legal requirement that these data be provided. Individual facility directors must strike the appropriate balance of communication.

Staff Training and Evaluation

Among the many reasons that information systems fail is inattention to the fact that all information systems require human contact to prosper and survive. Particularly important is a good data processing manager and an active user group at the facility level that functions in an atmosphere of collegiality and trust. The data processing manager typically is most effective when reporting to program evaluation. He is not infrequently also head of medical records, as the record becomes increasingly automated and procedures for checking completeness and storage of manual records are also automated. The principal staff burden, data entry, is typically underestimated, and systems analyses and frequent evaluations of staff are required to ensure that the data entered are complete and reliable.

Validity checks involving the filling out of selected rating instruments by others should be carried out periodically. Most information systems require some seasoning before proper editing and security measures are installed. The administrator should insist on reviewing these procedures. Confidentiality requires special vigilance regarding privacy; user groups must stay alive to the question that each report produced raises questions of access. Although automated data bases represent an exponentially greater risk in terms of being tapped and exploited, the measures taken so far have resulted in no recorded incident of a major infringement of confidentiality in any of the major mental health information systems. This record is a striking contrast to the sometimes lax security that obtains in individual facility record rooms.

PROTECTING AGAINST FAILURES

Since the advantages of systems are so obvious, while achievements are mixed, it is important to be aware of the many reasons for failures other than those already mentioned.

1. Lack of administrative support: the administrator must recognize that the installment of a system will require a great deal of visible support as the system is set up. All voices must be heard and technical advice checked repeatedly. Systems usually die when staff become aware that the administration is ignoring the system. Administrators must participate in user groups. Installation steps must be carefully understood. The National Institute of Mental Health has provided a useful guide,[44] as do many systems. The general medical experience is also relevant.[45,46]
2. Starting with too much: it is best to start with one or two components and work up to a full system, starting on a unit where success is assured so that those who would resist cannot argue with the local success.
3. Lack of user involvement: while avoiding reinvention of the wheel is heartily recommended, it is also true that cooperation with an information system is greatly enhanced if clinicians feel they have played a role in developing or adapting a system. Participants should have a sense of ownership in the system; clinicians must be rewarded for their efforts by getting back useful data. They do not like to feed researchers who may try to transfer a system that works well in the research setting with committed staff. Stereotyped reports, e.g., printouts of the history from checklists, must be understood as collecting only core data so that clinicians have free time in which to add individual data of their choosing. If the computer-generated report is taken to be all there is, there will be an inevitable rebellion.

Since clinicians distrust impersonal information, it must be repeatedly reemphasized that the data at hand are no different from those which the clinicians have contributed initially. Clinicians should be encouraged to carry on their own research projects and to look at their own patterns of practice. Most importantly, the psychiatric administrator must provide a positive role model of using the data for what it is worth while projecting an awareness of the limitations of data and information systems.

REFERENCES

1. Taintor Z: Working with computers, Course, Annual Meeting, American Psychiatric Association, New Orleans, May 1981.
2. Computers in Psychiatry/Psychology. Available from Marc Schwartz, MD, Editor, 23 Trumbull St, New Haven, Conn 06511. In general medicine, there are several learned journals. New technical developments can often be found in the Medical Computer Journal (and Newsletter), 42 E High St, East Hampton, Conn 06424. The AMA publishes Computers and Medicine
3. Talbott J: The death of the asylum. New York, Grune & Stratton, 1978
4. Conklin T, Boren CW, Zeman PM, et al: Computers: A benefit to the hospital clinician? Issue Workshop, Annual Meeting, American Psychiatric Association, New Orleans, May 1981
5. Hedlund JL, Zieweg VW, Wood JB, et al: Computers in Mental Health: A Review and Annotated Bibliography. NIMH Series FN #7 DHHS Pub. No. (ADM) 81–190, Washington, DC, Sup of Docs, USGPO, 1981
6. Nie N, Hull C, Jenkins J, et al: Statistical Package for the Social Sciences (ed 2). New York, McGraw-Hill, 1981
7. Dixon WJ, Brown MB (eds): Biomedical Computer Programs P Series (BMDP). Berkeley, University of California Press, 1979
8. Statistical analysis system user's guide 1979. Raleigh, NC, SAS Institute, 1979
9. Gottfredson DK, Schmidt LJ, Christensen PW, et al: Computers in mental health treatment: The Salt Lake VA Medical Center experience. Computers in Psychology/Psychiatry 3:6–8, 1980
10. Spitzer RL, Endicott J, Cohen J, et al: Constraints on the validity of computer diagnosis. 31:197–203, 1974
11. Sletten IW, Ulett GA, Altman H, et al: The Missouri standard system of psychiatry (SSOP): Computer generated diagnosis. Arch Gen Psychiatry 23:73–79, 1970
12. Laska E, Siegel C, Simpson G: An automated review system for psychotropic drug orders. Arch Gen Psych 37:824–827, 1980
13. Taintor Z: Computers and diagnosis, Am J Psychiatry 137:62–63, 1980
14. Heiser JF, Brooks RE: Design considerations for a clinical psychopharmacology advisor, in Orthner FH (ed): Proceedings of the Second Annual Symposium on Computer Applications in Medical Care. New York, Institute of Electrical and Electronics Engineers, 1978
15. Angle HV, Ellinwood EH, Carroll J: Computer interview problem assessment of psychiatric patients, in Orthner FH (ed): Proceedings of the Second Annual Symposium on Computer Applications in Medical Care. New York, Institute of Electrical and Electronics Engineers, 1978; Hay W, Hay L, Angle H, et al: Computerized behavioral assessment and the problem-oriented record. Int J Ment Health 6:49–63, 1977
16. Greist JH, Klein MH: Computer programs for patients, clinicians, and researchers, Sidowski JB, Johnson JH, Williams TA (ed): Technology in Mental Health Care Delivery Systems. Norwood NJ, Ablex, 1980
17. Lucas RW, Mullin PJ, Luna CBX et al: Psychiatrists and a computer as interrogators of patients with alcohol-related illnesses: A comparison. Brit J Psychiatry 131:160–167, 1977
18. Metz JR, Allen CM, Barr G, et al: A pediatric screening examination for psychosocial problems. Pediatrics 58:595–606, 1976
19. Johnson JH, Williams TA: Using on-line computer technology to improve service response and decision-making effectiveness in a mental health admitting system, in Sidowski JB, Johnson, JH, Williams, TA (ed): Technology in Mental Health Care Delivery Systems. Norwood, NJ, Ablex, 1980
20. Elwood DL, Clark CL: Computer administration of the Peabody Picture Vocabulary Test to young children. Behavior Research Methods and Instrumentation 10:43–46, 1978
21. Elwood DL, Griffin HR: Individual intelligence testing without the examiner: Reliability of an automated method. J Consul Clin Psychol 38:9–14, 1972
22. Fowler RD: Automated MMPI, in Sidowski JB, Johnson JH, Williams TA (ed):Technology in Mental Health Care Delivery Systems. Norwood, NJ, Ablex, 1980
23. Johnson JH, Williams TA: The use of on-line computer technology in a mental health admitting system. Am Psychol 30:388–390, 1975
24. Endicott J, Spitzer R, Fleiss J: Mental status examination record (MSER): reliability and validity. Comp Psychiatry 16:285–301, 1973
25. Guy W: ECDEU Assessment Manual for Psychopharmacology DHEW Publication

No (ADM) 76-338. Rockville, MD, Department of Health and Human Services, 1976
26. Taintor Z, Strain J, Gise L, et al: Recording psychiatric consultations: a preliminary report. Gen Hosp Psychiatry 1:139–149, 1979
27. Lucas R, Mullin F, Luna C, et al: Psychiatrists and a computer as interrogators of patients with alcohol-related illnesses: a comparison. B J Psychiatry 131:160–167, 1977
28. Remond A (ed): EEG Informatics: A Didactic Review of Methods and Application of EEG Data Processing. New York, Elsevier, 1977
29. Lincoln T, Korpman R: Computers, health care and medical information science. Science 210:257–263, 1980
30. Morsicato RS: A Staff Allocation Model Applied in a Multimodel Alcoholism Rehabilitation Facility. Bufallo, NY, Research Institute on Alcoholism, 1980
31. Glueck BC, Stroebel CF: The computer and the clinical decision process. Am J Psychiatry 125:2–7, 1969
32. Altman H, Evenson R, Hedlund J, et al: Missouri actuarial report system (MARS). Comp Psychiatry 19:185–192, 1978
33. Hedlund JH, Evenson RC, Sletten IW, Cho DW: The computer and clinical prediction, in Sidowski JB, Johnson, JH, Williams TA (eds): Technology in Mental Health Care Delivery Systems. Norwood, NJ, Ablex, 1980
34. Sorenson J, Phipps D: Cost-finding and Rate Setting for Community Mental Health Centers. DHEW Publication No. (ADM) 78-291, Rockville, MD, Department of Health and Human Services, 1978
35. Siegel C, Goodman A: Evaluating the attainment of process objectives of community health centers using MSIS, In Laska EM, Bank R (eds): Safeguarding psychiatric privacy: computer systems and their uses. New York, Wiley, 1975
36. Siegel C, Goodman A: An evaluative paradigm for community mental health centers using an automated data system. Community Ment Health J 12:215–227, 1976
37. Evenson RC: Program evaluation using an automated data base. Hosp Community Psychiatry 25:80–83, 1974
38. Evenson RC: Community adjustment changes after treatment for 1,851 psychiatric patients. Newsletter for research in mental health and behavioral sciences. 18:12–14, 1976
39. Evenson RC, Sletten IW, Hedlund JL, et al: CCAPS: An automated evaluation system. Am J Psychiatry 131:531–534, 1974
40. Fishman DB: A computerized, cost-effectiveness methodology for community mental health centers, in Sidowski BJ, Johnson JH, Williams TA (ed): Technology in Mental Health Care Delivery Systems. Norwood NJ, Ablex 1980
41. Goodman AB, Siegel C: Differences in white-nonwhite community mental health center service utilization patterns. J Eval Program Planning 1:51–63, 1978
42. Miller RR, Black GC, Ertel PY, et al: Psychiatric peer review: the Ohio system. Am J Psychiatry, 131:1367–1370, 1974
43. Siegel C, Laska EM, Griffis A, et al: Quantitative care norms for a psychiatric ambulatory population in a county medical assistance program. Am J Public Health 68:352–358, 1978
44. Laska EM, Bank R (eds): Safeguarding Psychiatric Privacy: Computer Systems and Their Uses. New York, Wiley, 1975
45. Paton J. Dhuvvetter P: Automated Management Information Systems for Mental Health Agencies: A Planning and Acquisition Guide. Mental Health Service System Reports, FN #1, DHHS Publication No. (ADM) 80-797. Rockville, Md, National Institute of Mental Health, 1980
46. Covvey H, McAlister N: Computers in the practice of medicine. Reading, Mass, Addison-Wesley, 1980

PART V

Facility Management, Budget, and Finance

Frederick D, Raine, M.B.A.

23

Facility Management

There are many ways to organize the nonclinical management of a psychiatric hospital, but certain tasks, common to all hospitals, must be accomplished. Discrete departments or contractual arrangements handle each of these tasks, which include personnel, accounting, purchasing, food service, plant and maintenance, housekeeping, data processing, payroll, laundry, and security. Such functions can be handled in house or purchased from an outside source. In either case, they must be accomplished, and the hospital administrator must have some means of determining whether jobs are done efficiently, effectively, and professionally.

This chapter will review each of the administrative departments in order to examine the usual tasks required and to suggest some common-sense guidelines on how to judge if a department is operating effectively.

One factor is common to all administrative departments; indeed, the entire hospital—the people. Each department must be managed by the most competent and knowledgeable people available to perform the required functions. Department heads must regard themselves as part of the hospital's management team, whose primary goal is to do the best possible job for the hospital. They must each be delegated sufficient administrative responsibility to accomplish the tasks they are required to perform. A hospital is made up of the people who work for it, and one of the main tasks of an administrator is to recruit and retain the best possible staff. Once this is accomplished, most of the other problems tend to solve themselves.

PERSONNEL

The personnel department is listed first with good reason. A psychiatric hospital is a labor-intensive institution that requires an efficient personnel operation responsive to the needs of employees and the hospital.

A hospital with more than 100 employees needs to have a separate personnel department led by a professional personnel manager. Smaller organizations need to have some method for accomplishing all of the personnel functions and a knowledgeable person to direct the personnel activities of the hospital, although not necessarily full time.

Personnel administration is a highly technical field requiring a specific knowledge of federal, state, and local laws and regulations. The personnel manager must have a working knowledge of labor relations, recruitment policies and techniques, position classification systems, wage and salary administration, benefits, unemployment compensation regulations, and grievance procedures. The director of personnel is frequently the in-house expert on techniques of supervision and provides guidance to other department heads on how to handle difficult supervisory problems. The larger the facility, the more people will be required to manage the personnel operation. A useful rule suggests the utilization of one person in the personnel department for every 150 employees.

There are numerous ways for an administrator to judge the effectiveness of personnel department management:

1. Keep track of employee grievances. How many are handled by supervisors before they get to personnel, and how many are handled by personnel before they get to the administrator? Make sure that the hospital's position is fair, defensible, and legal. Too many grievances are a sign of employee unrest or unfair policies. There may also be a problem if a hospital receives no grievances because it may be a sign of employee distrust. If a hospital wins all employee grievances, then someone may not be listening to the needs of employees.
2. Keep track of employee turnover. Are too many employees resigning compared to other hospitals and related organizations? Are employees giving specific reasons for their resignations? The cause of high employee turnover may lie within a department or may be due to low salaries or noncompetitive benefits. The reasons need to be explored and remedies suggested when warranted. An annual turnover rate in excess of 20 percent can be a sign of trouble.
3. Keep track of wages and benefits. Periodic reports must be prepared to make certain that compensation plans and benefit packages are realistic and competitive.
4. Monitor benefit administration. Spot checks should be made to ensure that employees do not have to wait an inordinate amount of time to collect on their benefits.
5. Monitor vacant positions. A system of position control is essential to make sure that departments stay within their budgets and to spot areas that pose recruitment problems.

The personnel administrator should be included in the hospital's central administrative team. It is important for the personnel administrator to be called on to make the technical recommendations about the viability of job descriptions, the advisability of promotions, the setting of job rates, and the appropriateness of disciplinary actions. The personnel administrator should be on the front line to ensure that all employees are treated fairly and honestly, and his demeanor will have an effect on everyone who works in the institution.

ACCOUNTING

Budget and finance will be covered in Chapters 24 and 25, but it is important to recognize how the accounting department relates to the central administration of a facility. There is usually a close tie between the accounting department and the administrator of a hospital—usually closer than the tie to any other department. For that reason, it is somewhat easier for the administrator to judge if the accounting department is meeting the needs of the institution by providing the reports and services that are required and desired.

Most accounting departments are responsible for the general ledger, accounts payable, accounts receivable, and the budget. Accounting is also usually responsible for payroll and credit and collections, although it is also common to find these functions set up separately. For example, payroll is sometimes the responsibility of the director of personnel; credit and collections are sometimes set up as a separate department or become the direct responsibility of the administrator. In a long-term psychiatric hospital that has fewer than 50 admissions a year, the administrator may want to review each admission to ensure that proper financing is available. In a hospital with hundreds of admissions, this function must be delegated.

As is the case with all of the administrative departments, the accounting department is providing a service—money management and financial information management. The administration needs to be given that information in a form that is understandable and allows ready identification of potential problems and trends. This usually means more than a simple income statement and balance sheet. Information needs to be compared with past years' figures as well as the current budget. Significant variances with the budget or the prior year's expenditures need to be explained. Information must be made available in a timely and regular fashion, and bills need to be paid according to the hospital's plan.

Special reports are an ongoing requirement that usually falls to the accounting department. Filling out financial questionnaires, preparing annual cost reports, dealing with auditors, and handling other special requirements would seem to be ad hoc tasks, but these tasks can keep someone busy throughout the entire year. It is important to have the staff available to handle these special assignments as they occur.

PLANT AND MAINTENANCE

The third major arm of administration is usually the plant and maintenance department. In many ways, this is the "action" arm of the central administration; it is the group that gets things done. The nature of the hospital's physical plant will dictate the type of plant and maintenance department required, e.g., a new physical plant will primarily require ongoing maintenance programs, while older plants will require both maintenance and construction services.

The effectiveness of plant and maintenance departments is hard to judge in the short run because their activities are so spread out. Perhaps the best way to judge the effectiveness of routine maintenance activities is to take a walk through the hospital to observe conditions objectively. Check to see that walls are painted, doors work easily, water fountains work properly, and sinks do not drip. Fire extinguishers should have a current inspection tag. If there are too many such problems, there is something wrong with the hospital's preventive maintenance programs.

Hospital maintenance needs to be a combined effort to keep abreast of all the items requiring attention. Plant and maintenance staff need to tour the hospital on a routine basis to identify items that need repair or to replace items on a preventive maintenance schedule. Nursing and housekeeping staffs must be alert and notice items that need attention, reporting them to the plant and maintenance department for appropriate action. Something as simple as a lightbulb will never be replaced if there is no system in place to handle it.

Construction projects and new work requests require a more complex monitoring system. Goals need to be set to identify which projects will be addressed during a given period. This is frequently done as part of the capital budget process. Reasonable timetables need to be set for each project, and variances with the timetable need to be explained.

A plant and maintenance department needs to have good lines of communication with other departments both to inform them when work will be scheduled and to find out what needs to be done. All requests coming to the plant and maintenance department require a response, even when the response is negative.

Appropriate feedback should be sent to the requisitioner if a work order goes on hold. The requisitioner should be notified, for example, of delay in the arrival of parts or equipment or of any other reason for delay. The best method to keep track of work orders is to assign someone in plant and maintenance to expedite all requests, which includes setting priorities and informing the requisitioner when the work will be accomplished.

Plant and maintenance usually has the responsibility for the institution's fire safety program, which includes making sure that the institution is operating in accordance with all applicable fire codes. Fire safety in a psychiatric hospital is a serious business because some psychiatric patients set fires. It is important to make sure that there are written fire plans that cover what each employee should do in the event of fire. Fire procedures need to be drilled and rehearsed, and employees need to be quizzed to make sure they understand their responsibilities when a fire occurs.

Finally, a plant and maintenance department needs to maintain good records, plans, and drawings of the institution. The filing system needs to be straight forward so that future generations can find out where service lines are buried or how to turn off the fire alarm. In this respect, plant and maintenance provides the archives for the physical plant that will become increasingly important as the building ages.

FOOD SERVICE

Everyone has an opinion about an institutional food service; usually, the less institutional the food service, the better people like it. One of the easiest ways to check on the food service is to eat the hospital's food. The administrator needs to go to the hospital cafeteria from time to time; if something does not seem right, he should discuss it with the director of food service.

The most important planning document the food service prepares is the menu. The menu reflects the budget, staffing, inventory levels, and food acceptance. If the administrator does not feel that the menu is appealing, chances are that the patients and the rest of the staff will agree. A food acceptance survey to check on what the patients and staff like best and least about the menu can be a valuable tool.

A food service needs to be managed by someone who understands food production to ensure that the end product is prepared, cooked, and served as well as possible. A dietitian is essential to a hospital's food service to plan and prepare menus and to handle all of the special diet requirements, but it is not advisable to put the dietitian in charge of production unless the dietitian is experienced in that specific area. Similarly, an executive director of food service who never goes near the kitchen will not be in a position to guarantee the final product. While there are exceptions to every rule, the best restaurants are run by people who understand food and know how to cook, and hospitals could learn from this example.

A food service needs to be cost conscious and have suitable procedures and systems in place to control inventory and to minimize the opportunities for pilferage. Periodic reports should be prepared on the number of meals served and the cost of a meal, and the costs ought to be compared to other similar hospitals. If there are large variations, they need to be explained.

A hospital is a social institution, and special functions that require food service support happen all the time. A food service that can handle a special luncheon or dinner can be a tremendous asset to an institution, and it is important to have the staff and equipment available to handle such occasions when they occur.

HOUSEKEEPING

Everyone can judge the cleanliness of an institution by simply walking around. A hospital must be kept clean or else it develops a poor image that will take years of hard work to overcome.

To accomplish a clean institution, there must be a sufficient number of people and equipment to do the job and a sufficient number of supervisors to manage the work. A reasonable ratio is one housekeeping employee for every 12,000 sq. ft. to be cleaned, depending on the age of the institution, and how it is furnished. There must also be a well-thought-out cleaning plan that can be easily followed by the staff.

There are numerous common-sense steps that can be taken to help the hospital's housekeeping department.

1. Make sure that the director of housekeeping is involved in furniture and decorating acquisitions to ensure that items purchased are easy to keep clean.
2. Make sure that policies are in place and enforced to keep storage items off the floors so that the housekeepers can keep the floors clean.
3. Carpet is easier to clean and looks richer than hard floors and can be used

extensively in psychiatric hospitals as long as the fire-spread ratings are within code limits.

An important adjunct to a housekeeping department is a group of people who can provide moving services. In larger hospitals, this can become a full-time job because there are always heavy moving jobs to be done.

A well-managed housekeeping department that keeps the institution immaculately clean helps foster a sense of pride in the institution that everyone appreciates.

LAUNDRY

The laundry service is closely related to the housekeeping department. Sometimes the laundry is administatively part of the housekeeping department, and sometimes it is a free-standing department.

Standards of the Joint Commission on Accreditation of Hospitals require that patients have access to a washing machine so that they may wash their personal laundry. As a result, hospital laundries are mainly required to handle towels and linens, and most personal laundry is done elsewhere. Many institutions have made economic decisions to close their laundries and use outside or cooperative services. But whether the laundry is located in the hospital or off site, the administrator should visit it periodically to make sure the facility is clean, following routine infection control procedures, and has adequate equipment and staff to do the required work.

An institution needs to have an adequate supply of linens and towels on hand and a distribution system in place that makes sense for the physical plant and avaiable manpower. If the staff has confidence in the linen distribution system, they will not need to hoard sheets and towels, and the entire system will work better.

SECURITY

Most hospitals have a security department. Security is usually asked to patrol the hospital and the grounds, control parking and visitor access, recommend measures to minimize thefts and pilferage, help with eloped patients, and investigate unusual occurrences related to the security of the hospital

Security officers are frequently asked to handle unusual situations on their own, and it is important that they have sufficient training to anticipate the categories of incidents that may occur and know how to handle them.

A well-trained security department will instill confidence, and that is extremely important to the staff, especially to those who work on the evening and night shifts when the hospital feels more isolated. There needs to be someone available at all times who can handle any problem that may arise in a professional manner.

The administrator needs to read the daily security reports to find out what incidents occurred and how they were handled. If there is disagreement on how to handle a specific situation, the problem needs to be discussed and the relevant policy or procedure clarified.

A security department is not a police department, and a hospital training program for security officers is usually not as comprehensive as the training for police officers. Hospital security officers need to be aware of their own limitations and should know when to call on the local police for assistance. A good working relationship with the local police is essential.

PURCHASING

The purchasing function of a hospital must be handled expeditously and according to clearly understood written policies and procedures. The director of purchasing must be delegated the primary responsibility to determine which companies will be invited to bid on hospital requirements and which products meet approved specifications. The director of purchasing, rather than the department head who requisitions an item, is the primary source for issuing all purchase orders and is the person primarily responsible for obligating the hospital to a contract to purchase any product or service. Exceptions to such rules can be made for certain products such as pharmaceuticals or petty-cash purchases, but the exceptions need to be fully delineated in the purchasing department's policies and procedures.

All significant hospital purchases should be subject to competitive bidding procedures. These procedures should be under the control of the director of purchasing, and the bidding should be open to the scrutiny of both department heads and bidders. Department heads may ask the director of purchasing to disregard a low bid, but the reasons need to be convincing and stated in writing.

Food, medical supplies, and all other items the hospital requires must be purchased, and if there is a bottleneck in the purchasing department, the effects can be devastating. For that reason, the purchasing department should be monitored closely. The administrator should be sure that:

1. The time delay between when a requisition is received and a purchase order issued is not excessive.
2. Products are always equal to or surpass hospital specifications.
3. A competitive sampling of vendors is invited to bid on requirements. If the same vendor is always the low bidder, the reasons should be investigated.
4. Department heads report excessive delays in obtaining needed supplies and materials. If this occurs frequently, the reason needs to be determined and the problem corrected.

DATA PROCESSING

Hospital billing and accounting procedures are so complex that almost every hospital requires data processing assistance to cope with the paperwork. Smaller institutions are purchasing small computers as the price of such equipment becomes more reasonable. An industry average would suggest that 1.5–2 percent of an institution's operating budget should be spent for data processing services.

Institutional requirements may vary, but most organizations seek to automate payroll, general ledger, accounts payable, billing, personnel data systems, budget controls, departmental expenditure reports, medical information, daily census reports, and so forth. The possibilities are limitless, and good data processing services can save thousands of dollars each year in reduced labor costs. For a complete description of computer services, see Chapter 22.

Administration has to decide whether to develop an in-house data processing facility or to purchase the service through one of the many time-sharing services. That decision may be significantly influenced by the hospital's ability to recruit the technical staff required to run a data processing department.

Regardless of whether the data processing is handled inside or outside the institution, it must meet the needs of the institution. The administrator must make sure that every system is backed up with duplicate copies of the data, and there must be written procedures explaining all systems and how to use them.

Computer services, data processing, word processors, and the like have proven their value, and it is clear that the most efficient organizations will rely on these technologies in ever-increasing ways.

SPECIAL SERVICES

There are a series of miscellaneous tasks that are an essential part of facility management although not carried out by a separate department. Examples include space management, outside survey supervision, and coordinating special meetings and functions. In most hospitals, the administrator is responsible for coordinating those ad hoc activities that do not clearly fall within the usual assignments of any single department. It is important to have a system in place to handle such matters in an organized fashion.

CONCLUSION

This chapter highlights the administrative departments most closely associated with facility management. It was stated earlier that a hospital is made up of people, but it is also organized into a series of departments. Each of the departments must be properly managed and have its own set of working policies and procedures to describe its activities and to set the parameters for its operations. The administrator's main task in managing the facility is to coordinate the movements, communications, and interrelationships of all the hospital's departments so that they work toward the single goal of quality patient care.

Haroutun M. Babigian, M.D.

24

Budgeting

Funding limitations of public and private mental health facilities make fiscal efficiency a critical dimension of organizational effectiveness and survival. Since mental health administrators tend to have extensive professional training but little administrative background, budgeting is an area that has received little emphasis in psychiatric administration.

DEFINITION

Berman and Weeks[1] appropriately describe a budget as "a comprehensive financial plan, based upon anticipated outputs and predetermined hospital goals and policies for future operations which is expressed in dollars of expense and corresponding dollars of revenue." This definition captures the concept of a budget as the culmination of a sequence of activities aimed at bringing the organization into synchrony with its context or, in a mental health setting, providing the quantity, type, and quality of services to meet optimally the mental health needs of the community at the least possible expense. Significant effort should be expended in areas of planning, priority setting, and goal development before a budget is derived. (See Chapters 17 and 18.) The power of the budget as a statement of organizational policy can be seen in the approach taken by President Reagan's administration toward governmental change. In an effort to reduce the size of the federal government, the budget was consistently viewed as the major tool for change. Administration policies and goals were often initially expressed through the budget.

COMMON PROBLEMS IN MENTAL HEALTH BUDGETING

Inappropriate use of the budget is relatively common in mental health agencies and may often result in organizational mismanagement. It would be a mistake, however, to place all blame for fiscal and budgeting problems on inept

The author would like to thank Sylvia K. Reed, Ph.D., for her invaluable help in the preparation of this chapter.

administration. In fact, mental health financial management may present a challenge even for professional administrative personnel due to several complications in funding and accounting practices. Despite increasing adeptness of mental health personnel in budgeting, the following types of problems persist:

Annual Budget

It is not unusual to find mental health agencies whose budgets have not changed in 10 years. For most mental health directors, budgeting financial resources is a nuisance, so the tendency is to rely totally on reviving the previous year's budget. They thereby avoid a stepwise budgeting procedure that would permit them and their management personnel to improve the organization's responsiveness or efficiency. This practice freezes the organization into a mode that is relatively unresponsive to changes in delivery systems and treatment modalities as well as changes in community needs. Meanwhile, the organization has learned nothing about operating efficiently and is less able to cope with reductions in available funding. Often, this practice reflects a general lack of attentiveness to basic management and planning, which may result from appointment of clinical staff into administrative positions for which they are not properly prepared. Mental health professionals tend to resist the view that their organizations are businesses, preferring to concentrate on the image of an organization designed to perform a needed and beneficial clinical service. With an executive director of a mental health facility who is also a clinician, a conflict of roles may develop that is difficult to surmount. Levinson and Klerman[2,3] state the conflict as follows:

> A person can remain in an executive position and find his work reasonably satisfying, useful, and fulfilling, only if he can come to terms with the fact that his primary functions are executive. He may have other functions such as teaching or research, but these are of necessity secondary. His chief responsibility is to further the growth of the organization toward the realization of goals and values to which he is committed. If this work is congenial to him, he will find ways to engage in it creatively and to go on learning; if the work is not congenial, his remaining in it is a disservice to himself and to society.*

From the perspective of good management, this role conflict is exacerbated by the fact that medical schools and psychiatric residency programs rarely focus on administrative problems and practices. Even the recent tendency to include some training along these lines (see Chapter 14) has not yet brought clinical staff to a point of being able to communicate and work effectively with professional administrators. Increasingly, professional administrators have been hired to manage mental health institutions. Whether to enhance their ability to communicate with administrators or to prepare them for their own executive roles, mental health personnel would benefit from some training in administration and management.

---

*From Levinson DJ, Klerman GL: The clinician-executive revisited. Adm Ment Health 1:52–67, 1972. With permission.

Reimbursement

The kaleidoscopic array of reimbursement plans available to the mental health field has something of the quality of an Escher design. These reimbursement plans, which provide payment for patient services, involve such agencies as Medicaid, Medicare, Blue Cross and Blue Shield, health maintenance organizations, and an assortment of other third-party payers. A single patient visit may require billing and receipt of revenues from three different reimbursement sources, each basing the amount paid on different criteria. One payer may reimburse 50 percent of the charge, up to a maximum charge of $45. Another payer may cover a flat fee of $32 for each hour of individual therapy. After the first transaction has taken place, the remaining portion of the original charge is assessed for a second billing. When all third-party payers have been duly billed in a specified order, the unpaid portion of the charge is billed to the patient, possibly on a sliding scale based on ability to pay. Charges remaining after the patient has been billed are recorded as losses. This obscure procedure requires the development of an incredible monolithic billing mechanism of great complexity and creates untold headaches for accounting and billing personnel. To further complicate matters, the billing procedures must be flexible enough to accommodate changes introduced by political processes, since reimbursement depends heavily on public funds and legislative limitations. There are undoubtedly mental health centers that have been unable to collect some revenues simply because their billing and accounting systems could not keep pace with the complexity introduced by assorted reimbursement plans.

Financing Systems

Due to chronic inability of many psychiatric patients to pay for long periods of intensive service and the reluctance of third-party payers to provide extensive mental health coverage, a heavy percentage of such care is financed through public funds. A typical community mental health center (CMHC) receives as much as 50 percent of its total budget from local, state, or federal funding. This dependence on the vagaries of federal and state funding formulae can be frustrating for the mental health administrator and sometimes destructive to the organization.

Deficit Funding

Current practices in financing mental health agencies do not provide incentives for management efficiency. Much federal and state funding is based on what is called "deficit funding." In New York State, 25 percent of the revenue-to-cost deficit (typically around 50 percent of budget) is sought from local funding agencies like United Way. The county then matches this with another 25 percent derived from local tax dollars. Finally, 50 percent matching funds are provided by the state mental health department. If an organization sacrifices to improve efficiency, it simply receives less money, while the less efficient organization receives more money. Indeed, efforts to improve efficiency can even be suicidal. For example, one CMHC created severe budgetary deficits in an effort to decrease hospitalization. Since the center relied on partial hospitalization and ambulatory services to decrease bed utilization, it set itself up for fiscal disaster because the local insurance plans covered inpatient care fully but not partial hospitilization or ambulatory care. Simultaneously, budgeted personnel costs associated with unused beds could not be greatly reduced, so the resultant loss of revenue was not offset by reductions in expense. The result was a deficit of $50,000 for each percentage point reduction in occupancy. This provided a challenging test for the limits of the deficit funding system, which proved unwilling to cover a deficit that was unexpectedly larger than in previous years.

There is also no incentive to seek funding elsewhere, since the effort required is not rewarded. The deficit funds received are simply reduced by the amount received from other sources. If mental health agencies are to have the organizational health required to function optimally, changes have to be made in the financing systems, and incentives must be built into funding programs to reward good management and discourage inefficient practices. Along these lines, an experimental program has been developed in the Rochester, New York, area that provides for local control of funds used in operating area hospitals. Planning occurs on a community-wide basis, and incentives are included to enhance efficiency. This concept is dealt with in more detail in the section on community planning.

Long-Range Planning

Almost every mental health agency reaches the point where a large amount of money is needed in a relatively short period of time to develop a new system or a new program to address a new need. For example, many organizations could benefit greatly over time from the installation of a good management information computer system (see Chapter 22) but such a system invariably requires a large investment. Funding agencies and superordinate hospital complexes do not generally allocate funds for these needs and thus frustrate efforts at long-range planning and program development. Such investments must often be funded through foundation grants or other discretionary monies. Another example of the problem is the frustration of clinical program development. A single chronic patient, who uses frequent and intensive psychiatric services over a lifetime, costs the mental health system a great deal. It makes sense that early intensive involvement in providing a thorough biopsychosocial evaluation and developing an appropriate treatment plan, which can cover a period of many years, would result in considerable savings over time. In order to save funds over a long run, however, program development funds must be spent in the beginning to acquire the type of talent and procedures necessary. It is difficult to spare these funds from existing programs or to procure extra monies from financing agencies. As a result, the normal practices in funding mental health services tend to discourage effective conversion of clinical needs and plans into budgets.

Budget Periods

Most financing agencies required that annual budgets be submitted based on the agency's fiscal year period. The hospital's fiscal year may be from July to June; United Way's from April to March; state and county cycle's from January to December; and the school district's from September to August. It is difficult to project total budgetary transactions with overlapping budget periods, since some agencies have not yet committed funds for portions of the budget period.

Fragmentation

Mental health facilities are usually part of larger organizations, such as hospitals. In these larger organizations, many of the real costs of service delivery are neither under the control of the mental health administrator nor, in many cases, even available to administrators for use in computing real costs. The hospital provides independent services such as utilities, security, engineering, laundry, personnel management and selection, janitorial services, and various other necessary support services. (See Chapter 23.) The mental health segment of this larger organization is responsible for submitting a budget that consists primarily of personnel costs, as this is the principal area for which they have management responsibility. The mental health administrator is unable to effect efficiencies in any of the areas of support provided by the larger institution until such time as he or she is able to negotiate with the hospital administration for these indirect costs and develop some mechanism to participate in and influence decisions made in central administration. To be able to proceed with authority in running his shop, the mental health administrator needs to have a budget for the responsibility center he directs, with all of the costs and income clearly included. It is common practice for mental health executives at the top and middle-management levels to think only in terms of personnel budgets and ignore all other costs. When a program director tries to enlarge a program, he usually attempts to justify the need by showing the increased revenue that an additional professional will produce that will cover his salary. He is usually unable to comprehend that covering salary alone will not be enough because the individual will require indirect costs for space, support services, malpractice insurance, and so on. It behooves all executives to train their personnel to think in terms of total costs. To be able to do so, mental health programs need to have full responsibility for their budget for both direct and indirect costs.

PREPARATION FOR BUDGETING

An exceptionally fine treatment of budgeting and other aspects of fiscal management can be found in Berman and Weeks[1], from which many of the concepts utilized in the following pages are derived. Although this text is oriented toward hospital financial management, much of the material has general applicability. Annotated bibliographies that include information relevant to budgeting are also available in Feldman[4] as well as Berman and Weeks[1]. Other perspectives on budgeting and related functions can be found in Feldman[5], Barton[6], Sorenson and Phipps[7], Silvers and Prahalad[8], Cooper[9], and Smith and Sorenson[10].

Prerequisites for Budgeting

In order to carry out properly the processes involved in budgeting and cost analysis, certain characteristics and capabilities must be adopted by the organization. Berman and Weeks[1] list these as follows:

1. A well-designed organization structure that eliminates overlapping responsibility and clearly defines all accountabilities

2. A chart of accounts that both corresponds to the organization structure and allows for the accumulation of actual cost data by cost and responsibility center
3. An accurate accounting system capable of accumulating and appropriately assigning all financial data
4. A comprehensive management information system capable of collecting nonfinancial data relative to total volume of services demanded and cost center workloads

The preceding list of budgetary requisites overlaps with requisites for cost analysis. Berman and Weeks[1] also listed three budgetary requisites that are unique to budgeting. These consist of the following:

1. Historical and current actual performance data for use in projecting future volumes and costs
2. A formal feedback reporting mechanism
3. A high level of management staff capability and sophistication

As organizational staff participate in a formal budgeting procedure over time, they will develop their abilities in budgeting and in understanding the intricacies of the mental health economic picture. Some of the prerequisites of sound budgeting may be out of the question for a specific organization at a given time. For instance, the organization simply does not have the necessary data. In this instance, the process should be conducted with best estimates and a serious effort given to developing the necessary capability in the future.

Budget Functions

Essentially, the budget is the most compelling statement of policy that an organization has, as it controls the flow of resources to the various parts and functions of the whole. Properly understood and applied, the budget process is a powerful management tool. It provides an opportunity and a structure for planning, which, in turn, forces the organization to review and define its policies. Periodic review of plans result in elimination of overlap and assures more complete coverage of organizational objectives. Lines of cost responsibility (programs) within the organization become well defined, and program costs are assessed against community benefits. The budget also performs the standard control function of assuring that fiscal performance is consonant with expectations. Although motivational effects of the budget frequently take the negative form of avoidance of excess, budgeting can be used as a positive motivational tool by constructively involving employees in the budget process. In summary, management functions potentially achieved through budgeting are extensive and include planning, developing policy, organizing cost-responsibility programs, coordinating organizational functions, motivating employees, and controlling the flow of resources.

Types of Budgets

How well the various management functions of the budget process are served depends heavily on the frequency and form of the budget.

Line Budgets

The traditional annual *object* or *line budget* provides detailed accounting of specific items of expense for the entire organization. This approach tends to diminish the policy planning and management functions of the budget, though the controlling function remains strong.

Zero Base Budgeting

As the economy has become leaner, emphasis on accountability of public funds has required more complete justification of programs. One of the popular forms this justification has spawned is the *zero base budget.* Whereas the traditional budget approach required only justification of requested increases from year to year, zero base budgeting requires justification in each budget period of all programs and expenditures as though they were entirely new. A thorough discussion of zero base budget procedures is presented in Pyhrr[11] and Berman and Weeks.[1] While the primary purpose of introducing zero base budgeting was to halt the inherently inflationary practices associated with traditional budgeting methods, it has had the corollary effect of forcing an increase in planning and management involvement in the budget process. The basic process of zero base budgeting consists of development and ranking of alternative decision packages designed to satisfy organizational objectives. Each decision package consists of a description of the program or activity in terms of its objectives, anticipated result, or benefit, as well as manpower and other operating resources. Alternative levels of activity are also projected for costs and benefits, as are alternative methods of achieving the same result. Alternative levels presented should include the current level, requested level, and a minimum feasible level. In using zero base budgeting, the program becomes the unit of cost responsibility in the decision package. This development makes zero base budgeting a logical complement to *program budgeting.*

Program Budgeting

The primary purpose of program budgeting is to allocate funds to the various programs in accordance with general management emphasis and policies. Zero base budgeting goes beyond program budgeting in that it lays the basic guideline for specific expenditures between and within areas of cost responsibility. The chief benefit afforded by program budgeting is a format for making decisions regarding allocations to the various cost responsibility centers. Beyond that point, program budgeting is limited in its usefulness in that it does not provide guidance for allocations within cost responsibility centers.

Discrete Versus Continuous Budgets

Traditionally, budgets have been updated on an annual basis. Where public funds are involved, annual budgets are still often required. Under this common form of discrete budget, preparing the budget tends to become an unpleasant chore performed once a year under time pressure, and management never becomes really adept at budgeting. With the typical annual *discrete budget,* the budget is prepared for the following 12-month period. At the end of the 12-month period, a new budget is prepared for the next 12-month period. A *continuous budget* is characterized by routine preparation of a new budget each month or quarter for the following 12-month period. The continuous budget has a number of advantages over the discrete budget, including increased sensitivity to changing trends in workload, increased budget and management ability of organizational leadership, and continuous availability of a 12-month plan. Monthly activities in continuous budgeting do not involve the full budgetary process. Typically, standard budget-monitoring reports are generated on a monthly basis, and budget and volume projections are extended to cover a full 12-month period. Comprehensive planning is carried out on an annual or semi annual basis, while fine tuning occurs on a monthly basis.

Fixed Versus Flexible Budgets

Much of the budget hinges on forecasting volume for the budget period. If this forecast is inaccurate, the budget can become contrary, controlling expenditures at an inappropriate level. Either there are insufficient funds to provide services at actual volume levels, or more funds are allocated than can be covered through revenues. If the budget period is long, as with an annual budget, a fixed budget based on inaccurate volume projections can be seriously problematic. Improved forecasting methods and use of continuous budgeting may help to resolve this problem. An alternative solution is the *flexible budget,* which is particularly attractive when annual budgeting is employed. A flexible budget actually consists of a series of fixed budgets for different volume projection levels. The original volume estimate plus or minus 10–20 percent represents a reasonable range of volume that flexible budgeting may address. Typically, a separate budget is prepared for each 5 percent increment or decrement from the original forecast volume. This technique provides a ready budget for unpredictable variations in workload. While flexible budgeting is clearly the procedure of choice, the technique requires some sophistication with regard to knowledge of fixed, variable, semifixed, and semivariable cost structure within each cost responsibility area.

BUDGET PROCESS

While a variety of budgeting options are available to the mental health administrator, understanding and appropriate application of the budget process are a primary requisite. Each organization must evolve a budgetary method that is optimal for it, since forcing an organization into an inappropriate process can be frustrating and wasteful. The process selected should provide the administrator with a feedback loop, allowing the organization to be dynamic and responsive to the pressures and needs of the community. The following comprehensive review of the budget process is designed to provide a general guideline for administrators in development of their own optimal process. A schematic of the budget process is shown in Table 24-1. Note that many of these steps are similar or identical with those presented in Chapter 18 regarding the planning process.

Development of an Environmental Assessment

Since mental health services should be responsive to community demands, the first step in the budget review process is to define the community needs and the unique position of the organization within the total mental health service

Table 24-1
Summary of the Budget Process

Step of Budget Process	Participants
1. Development of environmental assessment	Administrative and clinical leadership
2. Development of organizational objectives and policies	Governing board
3. Development of operating policies and objectives	Administrative and clinical leadership
4. Development of budget preparation package	Budget team (administrative)
5. Budget meetings	Budget team (administrative) Program directors
6. Preparation of decision packages	Program directors Line staff
7. Rank order decision packages	Budget team (administrative)
8. Detailing by line personnel	Line Staff
9. Tentative budget development	Budget Team (administrative)
10. Review and revision	Administrative and clinical leadership
11. Approval of the governing body	Governing board
12. Implementation	Program directors Line staff

delivery system. An environmental assessment summarizes the characteristics of the population, previous patterns of service, strengths and weaknesses of the organization, and any factors that might be expected to have an impact on population needs. Trends reviewed should include local, state, and national economic and political conditions affecting the system. For example, reductions in block grants to states, changes in levels of Medicaid reimbursement, or changes in legislation have potential ripple effects in the mental health delivery system and climate. The environmental assessment is presented to the governing board of the organization for use in determining general organizational objectives and policies.

Development of Organizational Objectives and Policies

General objectives and policies include only the very broadest statements of organizational purpose, such as the provision of quality mental health care at minimal cost. The board should address issues relating to the potential patients' ability to pay for services, referral policies, and scope of services to be considered, as well as any assumptions regarding future developments that might have an impact on the planning process.

Development of Operating Policies and Objectives

Armed with the guidelines of the governing board, the administrator assesses the possible directions the organization can take as well as limits to available funding for the budget period. The purpose of this step in the budget process is to define the limits and directions to be considered in order to avoid unnecessary expenditure of time preparing packages for programs that have no real chance of serious consideration. This is the stage at which the program budget is prepared, determining not only what funds are available but which programs will receive what proportions of available funds. Operating objectives are then defined in terms of measurable goals, which essentially define the magnitude of the effort to be conducted in each program area. The operating objective might state the number of inpatient days or the number of clinic visits anticipated for the budget period.

Development of the Budget Preparation Package

An administrative budget team is formed, which serves as a steering committee for the budget development process. This group is often comprised of the clinical director, administrator, financial officer, approximately two at-large program directors, the director of nursing, if apropos, and an individual designated to provide staff services (take minutes, assemble materials, etc.). The initial effort of the administrative budget team is to design and assemble the budget preparation package. The budget preparation package consists of a summary of the first three steps, a review of historical volume information, a calendar for budget development, current personnel salary information, projections of forecast volume for the budget period, blank budget detail forms with instructions for completion, and blank forms for development of decision packages. The budget preparation package is provided to each manager of a cost responsibility center. For example, the director of inpatient services, all clinic directors, and the director of the alcoholism treatment program would each receive a budget preparation package.

Budget Meetings

Next, a series of meetings is conducted to familiarize the line administrators (program directors) with the budget preparation package and the role they are to play in budget preparation. Line administrators should be informed as to the degree to which the budget process is subject to alteration, what types of assistance are available, and how to prepare their input. At this point, the budget process moves to the line level.

Preparation of the Decision Packages

Each line manager involves his staff in whatever way he sees fit to develop alternative proposals as to how to achieve the operational objectives defined for the specific program area. For each proposed activity, descriptive information, anticipated levels of benefit, personnel and supply resource requirements, and alternative methods of accomplishing the same objective are provided. The line manager and team then rank the proposed packages in terms of optimum ratios of benefit to cost and other relevant considerations.

Rank Ordering of Decision Packages

The decision packages and ranks recommended by the line personnel are received by the administrative budget team. Again, the decision packages are assessed and rank ordered in terms of available funding and cost benefit analyses.

A final ranking is derived, preferably in collaboration with each cost responsibility center.

Detailing by Line Personnel

Once rank ordering is finalized, selected program proposals are returned to the line personnel for further details. Specific and detailed information are provided regarding numbers and levels of required personnel, supply requirements, space requirements, and other program resource information. If flexible budgeting is used, several levels of detailed program resource information may be required for each program proposal. If so, fixed and variable cost information should be provided to line personnel.

Tentative Budget Development

Once specific resource requirements have been identified for each program, it is possible to develop a tentative budget for each selected program proposal. The budget team applies known cost information for specified line items and personnel wage and benefit requirements, and thereby derives a specific cost estimate to perform the activity. At this point, ranked programs are selected in the order of their ranking for each cost responsibility center until available funding for that center is exhausted. Then a complete budget can be developed combining the selected packages within each cost responsibility center into a single set of budget documents.

Review and Revision

The administrator receives the budget package prepared by the budget team. This is the fine-tuning stage of the budget preparation. Since the selected program packages are unlikely to produce an exact replication of the projected resources available for each responsibility center, decisions must be made regarding adjustments in levels of activities and possibly regarding the balance of the program mixture. The administrator identifies the impact of each of these decisions on each program for the budget team, and a revised budget is produced.

Approval of the Governing Body

The completed budget is ready to submit to the board of directors or other governing body for approval. The process that was used to develop the budget should be explained, and the materials should be presented in a simple and understandable fashion. If approval is not granted, the process is returned to whatever stage is required to remedy the difficulties cited by the board, and the budget is prepared again and resubmitted at a later date.

Implementation

The budget preparation process is now complete, and the budget may go into effect at the start of the budget period. The budget ceases at this point to be a planning and management tool and takes a primary role as a mechanism to control resource flow. It also plays a major role in monitoring the organizational activity, identifying areas of cost overrun and shortfall and allowing adjustments to be made during the budget period.

Application of this process will vary with the size and complexity of the organization.

INFORMATION GENERATION AND STORAGE

As indicated earlier, extensive information capability is requisite to budget decision making. An accurate accounting system, complete budget performance summaries, analysis of costs per unit of service for each cost center, projections of service levels for specified future periods, and historical information regarding service volumes serve as inputs to the budget process. (See Chapter 22.) Organizations which rely on hand-generated data for these purposes commit a surprisingly large number of clerical hours to keeping records of service and accounting information and monitoring billing and personnel functions. A well-designed and properly utilized computerized management information system provides vastly greater accuracy and flexibility at a potential savings to the organization. It allows for monthly budgeting without tying up untold hours of personnel time in preparing charts and tables, as these can be routinely generated by the computer at little cost.

A real-time data base system provides the greatest flexibility for records management, accounting, and billing systems. A real-time data system is characterized by the fact that it is kept up-to-date on a constant or daily basis. A data base is a filing structure that allows for random access to any bit of information without having to search through an entire file until the requested information is found. A variety of such computerized packages have been designed specifically for mental health applications. There is wide variation, however, in what reports can be generated and what functions can be performed (e.g., personnel payroll, schedule maintenance, billing, general ledger, statistical reports, cost reports, and others). The purchaser should be armed with accurate knowledge of his or her organization's administrative needs in order to evaluate properly the offerings of each software firm's package. For example, should the package use accrual accounting or another method? Should it report cost per unit of service? It would also be wise to have the assistance of an individual versed in computer capabilities and efficiencies. A complete package to satisfy mental health needs, including hardware and software to perform most desirable functions, costs approximately \$80,000–\$100,000 in the 1982 market. Less expensive contractual services are available from several locations throughout the United States to provide statistical reporting and other limited services, using either batch processing methods or telecommunications. Many of the standard software packages will accomodate time sharing with several agencies, which allows for considerable cost savings by all concerned if collaboration is feasible.

Smaller organizations or those in private practice would probably not realize any savings through computerization and thus would be wise to maintain manual accounting and information procedures.

FACTORS IN FISCAL EFFICIENCY

Although budgeting is critical to effective management of an organization, the effectiveness of a mental health facility does not depend solely on sound budgeting. A discussion of other areas that enhance efficiency in utilization of resources follows.

Quality Staff Selection

Since mental health agencies are essentially marketing a human service, the quality of their product is directly related to the quality of personnel. It is extremely difficult to make a productive employee out of an unproductive one, so the importance of careful staff selection cannot be overemphasized.

Careful Record Keeping

Accounting ledgers should be kept up to date as receipts and payments come in. This cannot be emphasized too much. Negligent failure to bill patients due to sloppy record keeping can be very destructive to the organization's finances.

Economy in Purchasing

Emergency purchases should be avoided, as they usually result in higher costs for supplies. If stock levels of necessary items are determined through experience and someone is made responsible for maintaining those levels on a regular basis, the individual responsible for purchasing will have the opportunity to make wise purchases and keep costs down. if the entire staff is reasonably cost conscious, it is much easier to maintain economy in purchasing.

FORECASTING

Since the budget is prepared for a period that has not yet occurred, the extent to which a manager can accurately estimate volume and expenditures becomes a primary dimension of successful budgeting.

Estimating Volume

It is assumed that the unit of revenue (office visit, group therapy session, inpatient day) has already been determined. The two most common procedures for forecasting volume are averaging and exponential smoothing. *Averaging* involves simply summing the previous three or more months of volume experience and dividing the result by the number of months. The purpose of this method is to obtain a relatively stable summary of recent volume experience. *Exponential smoothing* is a somewhat more complex method that utilizes the previous estimate (P estimate) and the previous actual volume (actual) to estimate current volume, using a weighting factor to determine the desired impact of recent trends. The weight is based on experience, ranging from 0 to 1, with a high weight (0.9) being very responsive to recent trends and a low weight (0.1) being relatively unresponsive to recent trends.

Exponential Smoothing Formula

Current estimate = P estimate + (weight) (actual − P estimate)

If seasonal patterns are not pronounced and volume is relatively stable or grows at a predictable rate, the averaging technique is simplest. Neither method will anticipate a new trend (e.g., a new factory in the area results in increased volume), but once a trend presents itself, the exponential smoothing method with a high weight will provide the best estimate until the trend has stabilized. Other methods of estimating volumes are available (such as regression analysis) but will not be treated here.

COST BREAKDOWNS AND INDICATORS

There are several ways of breaking out costs that are useful in understanding and adjusting the flow of resources.

Direct Versus Indirect Costs

When program budgeting is used, it is advisable to break out direct and indirect costs for each program area. *Direct costs* include all costs directly incurred in operating a program, such as salaries of program staff, supplies, and contracted support. On the other hand, administrative salaries, utilities, and rent are costs not immediately involved in operating one of the programs and are termed *indirect costs.* If several programs are involved, the typical practice is to compute direct costs and to divide indirect costs between programs on the basis of some logical dimension such as total salaries in each program or total floor space utilized.

Fixed Versus Variable Costs

For purposes of forecasting expenses for anticipated changes in volume, it is necessary to know the fixed and variable costs of the program. *Fixed costs* include all those costs that would be incurred independent of the number of patients or units of service provided. *Variable costs* identify those expenses that are directly related to volume, including such items as supplies and program personnel salaries. Building utilities, management costs, and rentals are usually considered fixed costs. Actually, costs tend to cluster into aggregate increases, based on such things as the requirement to open a new building or the need to add administrative personnel as the volume increases. These do not increase as each individual unit of volume increases and are sometimes referred to as semifixed or semivariable costs. To estimate the impact of changes in volume, it is necessary to identify the expansion points (volume levels that would require significant additional resources). Total costs are then computed as fixed costs, plus the variable cost per unit, times the expected change in volume units. If the change in volume crosses an expansion point, a new variable cost per unit of volume should be computed.

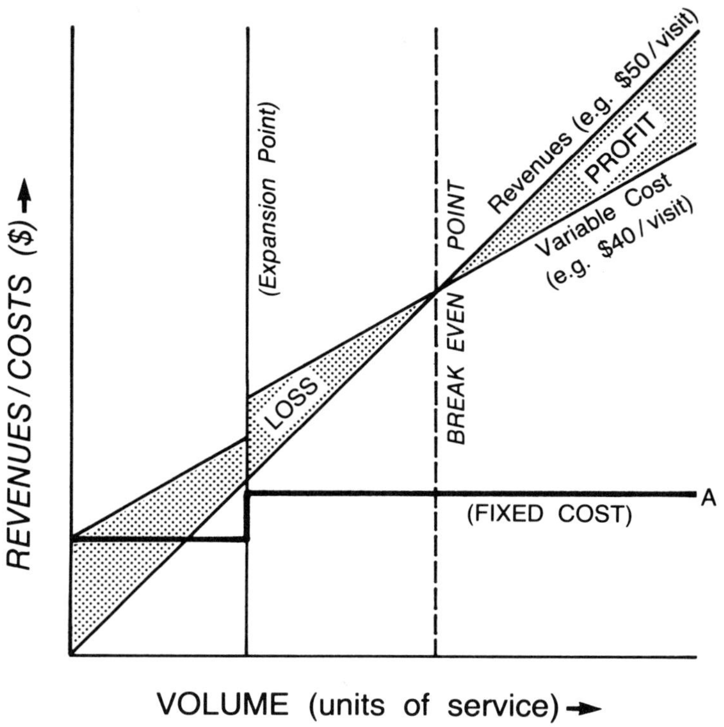

Figure 24-1. Computation of the break-even point.

Break-Even Volume

Once the fixed and variable costs have been determined, it is possible to compute the volume required to break even, as shown in Figure 24-1. Line A represents the level of fixed cost, which jumps with increased resource allocation at an expansion point. Note that the variable cost line begins at the level of the fixed cost, since total cost consists of fixed cost plus variable cost, but only variable cost increases with increases in volume. The revenues line begins at zero unless the agency is partially funded from other sources, such as grant monies. If other funding is available, the revenues line begins at that level of funding for the computation period. The point at which the cost line and the revenues line cross is the break-even volume point. Below that level of volume, the agency will suffer loss, and above that level of volume, a profit will accrue. If the projected volume level results in a loss by this computation, then it will be necessary to raise the fee for each unit of service in order to break even.

Inventory

Another indicator that can be of assistance in monitoring the organization's resource utilization is the proportion of the annual supply expenditure that is tied up in inventory on hand. If this ratio exceeds one-sixth, or a 2-month supply, inventories may be excessive, though each item's stock level should be determined by consequencies of interruption, time required to order, opportunities for economizing, and other relevant factors.

Collection Period

The ratio of outstanding or unpaid accounts to total annual revenues provides a mechanism for computing the delay factor when revenues will be received. For example, if the outstanding accounts represent 20 percent of total annual revenues, this ratio, times 365 days, yields a collection period of 73 days. Emphasis should be placed on keeping the collection period at the minimum attainable level, which may require active follow-up of delinquent accounts.

PLANNING AS A COMMUNITY

By 1978, rigorous cost-containment policies, frequent reimbursement rule changes, and diminishing dollars available for health care created an environment in which the solvency of many hospitals was in serious jeopardy. In the Rochester, New York, area, an alternative was developed to counteract these conditions and to create a mechanism for planning at the local level. The Hospital Experimental Payments Program (HEP) was developed and administered under the guidance of the Rochester Area Hospitals Corporation (RAHC), a nonprofit organization. "RAHC's initial task was to develop a payment alternative to test the assumption that a community could simultaneously enhance its hospital system's excellence and control its rate of cost increase." RAHC's mission, is, therefore, as follows:

1. To maintain and enhance the community's hospital system
2. To control the rate of cost increase of hospital services, ensuring the availability of needed hospital services in an era of increasing constraints on resources
3. To facilitate local decision making through enhanced communication and coordination
4. To maximize the cost effectiveness and benefit to the community of hospital services provided and planned[12]

In order to achieve the goals set forth in the HEP experiment, comprehensive community planning was introduced, such that overlapping services were reduced, and incentives were built into the funding formulations to improve efficiency and reduce unnecessary or inappropriate services. In the HEP program, funds allocated to each hospital for the initial five-year period were based on the 1978 allowable costs, with adjustments each year. Any efficiencies the hospital was able to achieve through reduced hospitalization or other measures resulted in residual monies for development of new or innovative programs. Since funds were allocated independently of occupancy levels, efforts at reducing hospitalization, as in the example provided earlier, resulted in savings rather than losses for the facility. After three years of developing and implementing the HEP experiment the initial results are very positive. Individual hospitals have benefited from knowing what their funding levels will be and having access to more complete cost and statistical information than ever before. An effort is now under way to develop such an experimental program for the mental health services in the Rochester area, including all public and private facilities. Since this approach to community planning represents a relatively radical departure from traditional approaches to funding and planning, it is a course fraught with difficulties and resistance, but the potential rewards are significant.

REFERENCES

1. Berman HJ, Weeks LE: The Financial Management of Hospitals. Ann Arbor Mich, Health Administration Press, 1976
2. Levinson DJ, Klerman GL: The clinician-executive. Psychiatry 30:3–15, 1967
3. Levinson DJ, Klerman GL: The clinician—executive revisited. Adm Ment Health 1:52–67, 1972
4. Feldman S, Goldstein C, Offutt J: Mental Health Administration: An Annotated Bibliography. Rockville, MD, DHEW NO. (ADM) 77-548, 1978
5. Feldman S: The Administration of Mental Health Services, Springfield, Ill, Thomas, 1978
6. Barton WE: Administration in Psychiatry, Springfield, Ill, Thomas, 1962
7. Sorenson JE, Phipps DW: Cost-Finding and Rate-Setting for Community Mental Health Centers. Rockville, MD, DHEW No. (HSM) 72-9138, 1972
8. Silvers JB, Prahalad CK: Financial Management of Health Institutions. New York, City University of New York Press, 1974
9. Cooper, EM: Guidelines for a Minimum Statistical and Accounting System for Community Mental Health Centers. Rockville, MD, DHEW No. (ADM) 74-14, 1973
10. Smith TS, Sorenson JE: Integrated Management Information Systems for Community Mental Health Centers. DHEW No. (ADM) 75-165, 1974
11. Pyhrr PP: Zero-Base Budgeting. New York, Wiley, 1973
12. Block JA, Regenstreif DI, Shute LJ: Experimental payments program: It's working for Rochester Area Hospitals. Hosp Financial Management 35:10–20, 1981

Robert C. Brice, M.S.

25

Financing of Psychiatric Services

As custodian, regulator, benefactor or scapegoat, the state has been the dominant force in mental health for 150 years. Unlike general health care, which has historically drawn its sustenance from private financing in the past, an estimated three-fourths of mental health services have been provided through public funds. Society has traditionally treated its mentally ill as an embarrassment to be removed, too costly to maintain in other than custodial settings and almost certain to be a chronic claimant on our resources and collective conscience. Accordingly, the management and funding mechanisms that evolved were quite distinct from those of general health care.

The early initiative of the states in providing a structure for mental health services was further stimulated by legislation and financial support. The New York State Care Act of 1890 mandated that "all insane persons . . . who shall become public charges shall be transferred to the respective state asylums without unnecessary delay, there to be regarded and known as wards of the State and to be wholly supported by the State"[1] It was not until the century faded that the construction of new state facilities slowed, but those being built were now enormous in comparison.

As the Great Depression of the 1930s blanketed weak and strong alike, the now giant state mental health systems entered their "saddest period." Society, caught up in its own concerns, first with the Depression and then with World War II, could effectively ignore the mentally ill to concentrate on more pressing problems. That two-decade period, however, found state governments increasingly mandating that their institutions accept ever-greater numbers of admissions, including the retarded and committed, whether or not they had the requisite funds, staff, or facilities. State hospitals that had provided admittedly low levels of custodial care were now, by the end of the war, acknowledged to be no more than "warehouses" or "dumping grounds."

In the mid-1950s, four new factors began to stem the tide of relentless state expansion. True, the nation's "resident population" had reached a record total of 560,000 inpatients, but much as a ship will coast forward after its engines have stopped, the state's lonely voyage was to take a new, less ambitious course.

A benign by-product of war is thought to be the quantum breakthroughs that often occur in the field of medicine. This appears to have been the case with the return of the psychiatrist–veteran and his patients. The optimism they generated gave positive hope that mental illness could be treated successfully. Support for this premise came from the dramatic results in patient management achieved through the use of psychotropic medication and from a new wave of "social awareness" that was to sweep the nation, an awareness that had its first stirrings in disclosure of the intolerable state hospital conditions and then gathered momentum from the plight of the elderly, those incarcerated in inner cities, and on through every cohort of the disadvantaged, underserviced, overlooked, and abused. New funds and new funding partners began to appear almost at will.

Quitely ignored in this great outpouring of new resources was perhaps the single most powerful agent for change in the history of mental health financing: the acceptance of the concept that the mentally ill could be treated in an acute-care general hospital under routine insurance mechanisms.

The states reacted relatively quickly to this change by expanding their budgets to provide for both improved plant and enriched staffing and by enacting legislation, such as the New York State Community Services Act of 1954, that provided for treatment at the local rather than state level. The former "wards of the State" were now becoming "active, functioning members of society" at a dizzying pace. By the early 1970s, the state's hospital inpatient census had declined by nearly 50 percent from its 1955 levels, with some states reporting reductions as high as 75 percent. An examination of New York's executive budget for the fiscal year 1977–1978 reveals that "although it housed some 93,000 inpatients in the mid-fifties, by November 1976, the State system served an institutional population of 28,400, less than one-third as many." The median length of stay had also "decreased from 75 days in 1966 to 34 days in 1976. In 1955, by way of contrast, it was eight months."[2]

This is not to imply that the states had, at long last, lifted this financial burden from their backs. Far from it. In the same fiscal period, New York State's projected gross program spending level called for an appropriation of $1.7 billion to treat an estimated 420,000 patients. After subtracting funds for the mentally retarded, alcoholics, and substance abusers, the balance for mental illness was an estimated $887 million.

THE LOCALITY

To support this great migration from state facilities, additional funds were diverted to community care. In states such as New York, this created dual funding streams, one for state purposes and one for local assistance. Local assistance or state-aid reimbursement, when combined with local tax levy funds, philanthrophy, Medicaid, Medicare, insurance, and agency contributions, supports a surprising number of providers, offering services such as inpatient and outpatient care, aftercare, partial hospitalization, sheltered workshops, crisis intervention, and so on.

Out of a total approaching $1 billion in the New York State "system," typically about 40 percent is budgeted for community care, and 60 percent is spent in support of state facilities. Of the portion allocated to community care, about 50 percent is provided by the state, but only about half of this in "hard dollars," the

Table 25-1.
Community Care Funding Sources—New York City

Source	$ in millions
Third-pary revenue	$35.0
State funds	29.3
Agency contributions	15.0
City tax levy	6.4
Federal sources	5.3
Total	91.0

balance being the provision of local services by state facilities and staff. Of the funding allocated for state facilities, about 65 percent comes directly from state funds and 35 percent from federal, private, and third-party support. As to be expected in such a labor-intensive industry, the greatest proportion of these monies is spent to support some 40,000 staff positions.

One locality, New York City, made available $91 million for its voluntary providers in 1980 through a shared contract mechanism. These funds came from the sources cited in Table 25-1.

Looking backward at the long and checkered era of the state, it is difficult to comprehend the vast network of services and financing now in place. This is the complex world of Medicare and Medicaid, trending factors, step-downs, and inpatient reimbursement rates approaching $400 per day. Eighty-four percent of the psychiatric inpatients in New York State still live in state facilities, but 65 percent of all admissions come through psychiatric units of general hospitals and 80 percent of the 9 million outpatient visits are provided by community clinics and agencies.[3]

THE FEDERAL GOVERNMENT

Just as the states determined the course of the first 150 years of our mental health history, so has the brief modern era been heavily influenced by the federal government. Its long, direct involvement in administering mental health services has, for the most part, been through the Veterans Administration (VA). This substantial and progressive program has been fairly static when viewed from a fundamental perspective. It is worth noting, however, that in the early 1980s, approximately 10 percent of all psychiatric beds were under the auspices of the VA.[4]

In 1946, the National Mental Health Act "authorized research related to the cause, diagnosis, and treatment of psychiatric disorders, as well as pilot and demonstration programs aimed at their prevention and treatment." This program was incorporated under the newly established National Institute of Mental Health. A summary of the awards granted gives a sense of the rapid growth of this program.[5]

In 1963, the Community Mental Health Centers Act and its subsequent amendments placed the federal government squarely at the locus of the changing mental health delivery system. The stated purpose of the program was to assist in the delivery of comprehensive mental health services at the local level by first

Table 25-2.
Grants Awarded by the National Institute of Mental Health

Year	Number of Grants	Amount Awarded ($)
1948	38	373,221
1949	45	578,695
1950	57	829,519
1955	206	3,609,166
1960	1,062	22,822,397
1965	1,623	57,227,040
1970	1,471	60,559,073

providing construction awards and, later, staffing grants. As Sharfstein notes, "The scope of its mission was deliberately writ large—a minimum of five essential services to be made readily accessible to all in need, regardless of ability to pay."[6] The underlying funding concept was one of declining "seed money," enabling the centers, in time, to become self-sufficient. Early evaluations were positive, and additional funding was made available.

Since its inception, 718 Community Mental Health Centers (CMHCs) have been funded; 97 with construction grants, 241 with staffing/operations grants, and 380 with combined grants. For the period through 1978, $2.369 billion had been appropriated.[7]

The high expectations held for the centers, however, have not been realized. Budgeted funds have been appropriated at levels lower than authorized; more importantly, the medical mode originally envisioned has evolved into that of a social agency. This has made it increasingly difficult for the centers to qualify for routine reimbursement, and a downward funding spiral threatens the continued viability of the program. Its future has become even more problematic given the growth and patient acceptance of hospital-based clinics.

PROSPECTIVE REIMBURSEMENT

The surest way to gain some understanding of the great funding engines of modern-day health care, Blue Cross–Blue Shield, Medicare, and Medicaid, is to examine the basic formula common to this form of reimbursement. It must be remembered, however, that this is a technical area, subject to constant change, and one should always assume there will be exceptions and "special situations" lurking behind every calculation.

The concepts of cost finding and prospective reimbursement underlie all modern reimbursement. Prospective reimbursement differs from earlier forms in that providers are paid unit rates, set in advance, for a fixed period. These rates are established by an external authority, and while tied to the provider's historical costs, are not based on the actual expenses incurred over the payment period. Prospective reimbursement evolved from a desire to control hospital costs by shifting the risk of their rapid escalation from the third-party payers to the provider.

A typical algorithm starts with the encirclement of a 3-year span. The middle year is used as a buffer period in which to make the calculations, typically performed during the fourth quarter. The rate year, next year, from our perspective, is the fixed period over which the rates will apply.

The base year, last year in our context, is the period for which the data on actual expenditures and service have been collected. It forms the basis on which all calculations are made. In essence, a prospective formula takes these base years costs, molds them into a common format, trims off the nonallowable items, and then projects them into the rate year's per diem payments by utilizing various economic and marketplace trending adjustments.

To determine which costs are attributable to direct patient care and, therefore, allowable, one of several step-down methods may be employed. Picture, if you will, a large, multitiered fountain. This fountain, with its empty pods, represents the provider's cost accounting system. Each pod is a defined cost center. Those nearest the base are closely identified with direct patient care services: an emergency room or an intensive care unit. Those farther up the treelike fountain—housekeeping, finance, administration, and general—are less direct. If we take a large pail of water as representative of the provider's total costs for the base year and measure it into each of the pods in the ratio of that cost center's direct contribution to the total cost, we will have the provider's expense breakdown as it appears at the end of the base-year fiscal period.

Each pod has water in it, some much more than others. Before starting the step-down process, we add yellow coloring to the water in one of the pods located about mid-level in the fountain. This pod is labeled "housekeeping" and has more water in it than most because of its large, labor-intensive structure. As the step-down pump starts, the pods at the uppermost level tilt and spill their water, or costs, downward to the pods below—not randomly or in equal measure, but by a predetermined, functional measure of the relationship each pod has to the one above it. The measure used is normally some routinely available statistic considered reasonably appropriate to the activity, It may be patient days, pounds of laundry, or actual procedures performed.

As the yellow water in the housekeeping pool begins to swell, catching more and more water from the pools above it, we see that the provider's true housekeeping costs are not merely that department's direct salaries and expenses but also include the cost of services provided to the housekeeping department by other departments, such as personnel, maintenance, and so on.

It is now time for the housekeeping costs to be allocated, and the surrogate measure chosen is square footage. As the yellow water cascades down, some falls into the intermediate pools below, but some also goes directly to the lower patient care reservoirs. One intermediate stop is the pharmacy. To its already expanding pool of costs is added the housekeeping allocation. As the pharmacy pod, in turn, is tilted, the water spills downward in yet a new allocation flow. This may now be the ratio of prescriptions or medication orders filled. Some of these costs ultimately come to rest in direct patient care pools, reservoirs greatly expanded from the initial combination of direct salaries and expense to those including stepped-down overhead costs that have themselves been increased by other stepped-down costs.

This is only one of several cost-finding techniques. While it is more reflective of the true cost relationship between departments than a direct allocation method, it is not as accurate as the double apportionment or algebraic methods that give better definition to the exchange of services between nonrevenue producing departments. In these more complex algorithms, the water in our fountain would continue to flow up and down again as long as the pods below provided some service to the ones above.

Once the institution's costs have been segregated by function, certain nonreimbursable expenses such as private-duty nursing, research, and the use of blood products are deleted. The remaining reimbursable balance is then divided by the provider's service units to arrive at a unit cost. At this point, certain underutilization penalties may be imposed. If, for example, occupancy levels in maternity were to fall below the minimum level of 60 percent, the institution must increase the denominator of their base year fraction by the amount of this shortfall just as if these services had actually been provided. This, of course, decreases unit costs and lowers future rates.

Two additional steps must be taken before the base year's calculations can be trended forward. The first is to take those costs that are expressed in fixed dollars, interest, depreciation, and so on, and merely move them ahead unchanged. Finally, the institution's adjusted unit costs are compared to those of comparable institutions in an assigned group. The base year rate then becomes either the one calculated or some percentage above the group's average cost, whichever is lower. These groupings are important, as they determine the ceilings and floors for trending purposes. An institution that is able to hold its costs below the group average may gain an immediate advantage that it subsequently loses when the rate year becomes a base year.

The trending process attempts to convert the adjusted actual base year unit costs into a current rate that approximates the change in externalities. It rests on the recommendations of consulting economists, who, by the use of a "shopping bag" of weighted cost factors, seek to incorporate into the unit cost those price increases and market conditions that have taken place over the interim period. The proposed rate may be appealed and often is.

This, in abridged form, is the prospective reimbursement rate methodology, at least as practiced in New York State. The psychiatrist–administrator should have a working knowledge of this concept. It is the method by which the institution receives the major portion of its operating income and will, in all probability, be used even more extremely in the future.

General hospital psychiatry is in a unique position. It generates the same income per patient day as other services, but at a lower cost, due both to the nature of its treatment modality and longer length of stay. It is axiomatic that the most expensive days, from the hospital's point of view, are those that occur at the beginning of the term of hospitalization. The longer the stay, the more "profitable" it becomes at the margin. This position of relative intrainstitutional strength could become one of critical vulnerability within a few years. Experimental methodologies, now being piloted, base reimbursement on "diagnostically related groups." In this model, the institution is paid a set "fee" for each admission diagnosis regardless of length of stay, the "fee" to be based on some average cost for this treatment. The inherently lower costs of psychiatric treatment could well mean lower future reimbursement to the institution under this concept.

INSURANCE

It is generally agreed that Blue Cross, or at least a prepayment plan having many of its essential characteristics, had its founding in Dallas in 1929. At the same time that the Baylor University Hospital, Dallas, was saved from a precarious financial situation, 1000 or so local schoolteachers were able to ease their medical expense burden. This synergistic relationship proved to be so effective that by 1978 Blue Cross membership had grown to 72,718,604, and 2,052,657 of these members had received coverage for 12,871,413 inpatient days and 5,616,911 outpatient visits.[8]

In evaluating the impact that Blue Cross–Blue Shield insurance has had on the delivery of health care, it is important to realize the following:

1. There are more than 70 autonomous plans.
2. Roughly 85 percent of the membership is enrolled through group plans.
3. Enrollment varies widely by region, from a high of 32 percent of the population in the South to a low of 18 percent in the West.

Coverage for inpatient psychiatric care may vary not only by plan but also among group, individual, and family contracts within each plan as well. Inpatient care coverage typically ranges from 30 to 730 days, with most plans offering the lower amount.

As the importance of general hospital psychiatry has increased, the significance of Blue Cross funding has grown accordingly, although coverage has, for the most part, not been as comprehensive as that offered by commercial insurance carriers. Table 25-3 shows the breakdown, by enrollment, in private health insurance plans as of December 31, 1970.[9]

Given their disastrous experience with psychoanalytic coverage during the early 1950s, the carrier's prior wariness concerning mental illness is understandable. Studies of the utilization rates of federal employees under their Blue Cross–Blue Shield plan, however, have shown no more than a 7.5 percent usage for mental health as compared to general health despite very liberal psychiatric benefits.[10] Additional data from a Canadian provincial study "indicate that the proportion of psychiatric care to total medical payments is between 1.4 percent and 5.4 percent in various provinces, depending on the availability of psychiatrists."[10] It has now become generally more accepted that insurance, as a means of paying for mental health services, is growing rapidly and that the range of coverage provided is also increasing.

The emergence of Medicare and Medicaid (see Chapter 3) has had an enormous and unforeseen impact on the delivery of all health care services. Enacted in 1965 as Title XVIII of the Social Security Act, Medicare is essentially two programs in one. Under part A, payments are made for hospital care, extended care, and home health services for those enrolled persons, 65 years of age or older, after the deduction of a coinsurance payment. Coverage for psychiatric patients is initially the same as for those of other patients in the hospital: up to 90 days of inpatient care with each term of hospitalization to be broken by intervals of at least 60 days between benefit periods. There is also a 60-day "lifetime reserve" that can be used to extend any benefit period. Comparable benefits are available

Table 25-3.
Breakdown, by Enrollment, in Private Health Insurance Plans as of December 31, 1970

	Blue Cross–Blue Shield (%)	Insurance Companies (%)	Indenpendent Plans (%)
Hospital care	36.0	60.1	3.9
Physician hospital visit	40.5	53.4	6.1
Office visits	20.3	70.2	9.5

for patients in a psychiatric institution but are limited to 190 days of care in the patient's lifetime and may not be extended by the reserve.

Part B is designed to help pay for physician and outpatient services. Coverage for psychiatric patients in a hospital setting is comparable to that for general health care.

Medicare is a federally funded program administered by the Social Security Administration primarily through the use of intermediaries such as Blue Cross. Unlike Blue Cross and Medicaid, however, Medicare reimbursement is actually retrospective. Periodic interim payments are made to an institution in advance based on a prospective rate target. These are later adjusted to reflect the provider's actual experience.

Medicaid, Title XIX of the Social Security Act, is a federal matching plan. The state's share of the total funding may vary anywhere between 17 percent and 50 percent. The state-administered plans also vary as to benefit coverage, but all must provide health care financing for public assistance recipients in at least four categories: those receiving aid for dependent children, the blind, the totally and permanently disabled, and low-income persons 65 years of age or older. To qualify for the program, the state plan may not exclude patients on the basis of diagnosis. Eligible psychiatric patients, therefore, are entitled to the same benefits as other recipients, with the important exception that *no federal funds may be used to support the care of persons between 21 and 64 years of age in a psychiatric institution.*

Medicare has given the psychiatric units of general hospitals the financial ability to expand their treatment of the elderly. Medicaid, on the other hand, has become a major funding resource in many states for both the care of children and the elderly in all mental hospitals. In 1974, 10 percent of total Medicaid expenditures for hospital care were for those patients in psychiatric hospitals. By 1976, over 23 million people were receiving some form of Medicaid assistance.

While these programs have thus proved to be a tremendous boon to the delivery of all health care services, they have strayed dramatically from the initial estimates of what their impact would be. Medicaid, in particular, has become a trememdous financial and administrative burden to those states offering comprehensive coverage. In addition, its image in the minds of many as the successor of earlier welfare programs raises the specter of fraud, abuse, and "freeloading" among many of the inner-city poor.

We are now well into an era in which we have the tiger firmly by the tail. Health care costs consume almost 10 percent of the gross national product; public assistance programs have fallen out of favor, politically and economically, yet both the health care industry and the needy are highly dependent on them for survival. With no alternative available, the situation becomes one of a holding action, with constant, relatively ineffectual attempts to slow the incremental growth rate as all concerned wait to see what will unfold.

NEW REIMBURSEMENT STRATEGIES

Over the past two decades, the psychiatric patient has been "medicalized" to a great extent. This status has opened the channel to substantial reimbursement sources but has also brought with it a new set of problems. Health care expenditures now represent more than 9 percent of the gross national product, with more than 40 percent provided by public sources. Hospital care is the dominant component of this cost base, and most of the new reimbursement strategies are focused on controlling the rapid rise in this area.

A "targeted days" concept is being tested in New York State. This methodology utilizes the familiar per diem rate built up by prospective rate setting. Each institution, however, has a targeted number of annual patient days, which may be the institution's actual inpatient experience in the base year as defined in our prospective reimbursement discussion. In the rate year, for each marginal day in excess of the target, the institution receives only 20 percent of its per diem revenue. For each day under the target, the institution still receives 80 percent of its daily rate even though the bed is empty. As we have seen, the rate year soon becomes the base year, and those institutions that permit underutilization will soon find themselves being "ratcheted down" through this mechanism.

Another strategy and one that has potentially serious consequences for inpatient psychiatry is the classification system called "diagnosis-related groups" or DRGs. This system, developed by Yale University, is being used experimentally in New Jersey, where hospitals are reimbursed by disease category rather than by costs or charges. In this model, each disease category is assigned a specific "price," that presumably will average out over the years, although individual cases may vary widely. Recalling our earlier discussions on rate setting, we have seen that psychiatry is the least costly per day of all the hospital's services. Because of its long length of stay, however, the fixed DRG "price tag" might still be quite high. The short-run incentive, then, will be to increase census and maximize revenue by shortening the length of stay. This will inevitably lead to a lower "price tag," which will require even greater velocity, and the downward spiral will grow.

In the final analysis, however, the utlimate arbitrator of mental health financing continues to be society's view of this problem. Not long ago, at a university Grand Rounds, a noted physician–economist spoke of a patient of his who would die within the next few days. The patient was a young man who had suffered massive trauma in a water skiing accident. The initial prognosis among the staff was unanimously negative, at only 1 chance in 100 of survival, yet life had been sustained for several months. The end was now at hand, and it was calculated that approximately $100,000 had been spent on this case. The question posed was that at an expected cost of $10 million per life saved, could society afford this treatment or should patients with this prognosis be permitted to die?

These questions are being asked with greater frequency, and one cannot help wondering how mental health will fare in this new world. Are we, perhaps, not unlike the universe, still expanding from the recent "big bang" of social awareness, only to slow in our finite world of priority constraints and then to contract back to the world of the almshouses and jails once again. Or are we forever cast in the role so eloquently expressed by the fox when he said farewell to the Little Prince:

> "Goodbye," said the fox. "And now here is my secret, a very simple secret: It is only with the heart that one can see rightly; what is essential is invisible to the eye."
> "Men have forgotten this truth," said the fox.
> "But you must not forget it. You become responsible, forever, for what you have tamed. You are responsible for your rose . . ."*

REFERENCES

1. Cahill KM: Health in New York State. Albany, Health Education Service, 1977, p 99
2. State of New York Executive Budget for the Fiscal Year, April 1, 1977, to March 31, 1978
3. Two-Year Comprehensive Plan for Services to Mentally Ill Persons in New York State. New York State 1979, vol. 2, Appendix 2, 1978, New York State Health Planning Commission, 1979
4. Financing Mental Health Care in the United States. 1973, DHEW publication No. (HSM) 73-9117.
5. Mental Health Research Grant Awards, Fiscal 1970. Washington, DC, NIMH, 1971
6. Sharfstein SS: Will community mental health survive in the 1980's? Am J Psychiatry 135:1363–1365, 1978
7. 1979 Directory of Federally Funded Community Mental Health Centers. Division of Mental Health Service Programs, DHEW publication
8. Berman H, Weeks L: The Financial Management of Hospitals (ed 4). Ann Arbor, Health Administration Press, 1979, p 139
9. Mueller MS: Private health insurance in 1970: population coverage, enrollment and financial experience. Soc Secur Bull 35:4–7, 1972
10. Sharfstein SS: Third-party payers: to pay or not to pay. Am J Psychiatry 135:1185–1187, 1978

*de Saint Exupery A: The Little Prince. New York and London, Harcourt Brace Jovanovich, 1971, p 88. With permission.

PART VI

The Law and Psychiatry

Peter M. Crain, M.D.

26

Civil Law

During the past 20 years, a great deal of litigation has created a complex interplay between civil law and clinical psychiatry. Underlying this litigation appears to be a recurrent question: how far should legal regulation be allowed to intrude into clinical practice or, conversely, should medical authority be granted free rein? The decision as to where one draws the line belongs with social policy, expressed through legislative action and judicial verdicts. Because social policy varies both geographically and historically, the ground rules established at different times or from one jurisdiction to another will change somewhat. It is essential that psychiatric administrators have available to them the services of good legal counsel. This chapter provides administrators with a basic understanding of significant trends in mental health litigation, enabling them to ask pertinent questions of counsel and plan realistic programs within the present legal climate.

SOME PRINCIPLES OF LAW COMMON TO ALL MENTAL HEALTH LITIGATION

Due Process

The Fourteenth Amendment to the Constitution of the United States guarantees that an individual will not be deprived of life, liberty, or property without safeguards to ensure fairness of the procedure. The panoply of safeguards include the following: a statement of the reason for the procedure, adequate notice, a right to representation by legal counsel, a hearing on the matter, presided over by a neutral decision maker, a right to confront and cross-examine witnesses, a written transcript of the hearing available for review and appeal, as well as a standard of evidence. The scope of such safeguards applied to clinical matters varies significantly.

Standard of Evidence

Standard of evidence refers to the level of certainty that a judge or jury must attain in order to arrive at a legal decision. The standard "beyond a reasonable doubt" applies to the determination of criminal guilt. The evidence for conviction must be 90 percent sure; in other words, social policy prefers nine guilty people to go free rather than convict one innocent person. The standard "preponderance of the evidence" means greater than 50 percent certainty. In civil suits, only a scintilla over 50 percent is necessary to establish liability. "Clear and convincing evidence" defines an in-between standard, approximately 75 percent sure. All three standards have been applied to issues involving clinical decision making.

Legal Precedence

Enactments by legislatures are called *statutory law.* When courts adjudicate or make determinations about the application of these enactments to special instances, such decisions constitute *case law.* In the absence of applicable statutes and previous adjudications, the judiciary may also refer to *common law,* a body of legal formulations inherited historically from Anglo-Saxon roots. Federal laws tend to take precedence over those of states unless ruled otherwise by the courts. Within the judiciary, supreme or appeal courts have authority over lower, district courts; hence, depending on the position of legal standards within this hierarchy, the impact on clinical practice in a given jurisdiction varies significantly. In addition, a legal standard formulated by some higher decision-making body, either legislative or judicial, though referring to an unrelated matter, may be applied in principle and taken as "precedence" in order to justify legal regulation of clinical practice.

COMPETENCY

The legal consideration of a person's competency includes the following categories: competency to stand trial, testamentary capacity, contractual capacity, marital capacity, and the related issues of guardianship.

In general, the following components apply to all categories of competency: (1) *cognitive component*—a person is capable of reasonable, rational understanding of issues; (2) *volitional component*—a person is capable of making a choice freely and independently, without undue influence or coercion; (3) *mental disorder, disease, or defect*—the diagnosed condition causes impairment of the preceding cognitive/volitional components. Although the determination of incompetency is a judicial rather than clinical matter, social policy may influence whether or not the legalistic cognitive/volitional components or clinical diagnosis are emphasized in the subsequent disposition of cases. Affective factors in mental status tend to be significant only so far as they impair the cognitive/volitional components.

Competency to stand trial is discussed fully in Chapter 27.

Testamentary Capacity

This capacity, as another example of competency, requires three abilities: (1) to understand the nature of making a will, to know that this is what he or she is doing, (2) to know the nature and extent of the property (bounty), and (3) to know the "natural" objects of the bounty. "Natural" refers to marital partners and relatives to whom a person would leave his property. If a person does have a mental disorder, including the presence of bizarre delusions, but the disorder does not affect these three abilities specifically, then the person will probably be deemed competent to make a will by a probate court.

Besides the cognitive aspects discussed above, the volitional factor must also be considered. If a person has made a will but acted under the undue influence of others, this might be construed in court as coercive—grounds to overturn the will.

It is, however, in the interest of social policy to preserve wills. Rather persuasive evidence of mental disorder is required in order to raise a significant doubt as to whether the narrowly defined abilities are fulfilled and the act occurred under undue influence. Clinical issues thus tend to be minimized.

Contractual Capacity

A third example of competency is contractual capacity. There are two types of legal tests that traditionally have been used in different jurisdictions, although the wording of the tests can vary from place to place. They tend to be called the *Understanding Test* and the *Insane Delusion Test.*[1] In regard to the Understanding Test, a contract is void if, at the time, the buyer does not understand, on account of mental illness or defect, the "nature and consequences of the transactions." According to the Insane Delusion Test, when a buyer's motivation to enter a contract is based on a belief in the reality of facts that do not exist (e.g., that no rational man would possibly believe), then the contract may be invalid. For example, that an individual makes out a promisory note based on the false belief that only this action can prevent his family from getting killed may qualify as an insane delusion. It may not necessarily correspond to a clinically defined delusion. Note that both cognitive and volitional features are included in the test.

In practice, the law does not usually rely on clinical data to resolve questions about contractual capacity. Simply having the buyer restore the property to the seller may suffice. Moreover, the buyer may not be held to the contract if the seller knew of the former's mental disturbance and took unfair advantage.

When the property cannot be restored, the buyer remains obligated regardless of contractual capacity. This places responsibility on those charged with caring for the mentally disabled person to fulfill the contract. The tests for contractual capacity tend to be applied only after the property has been restored; only then is medical authority given much weight.

Marital Capacity

In this type of competency, as in other areas, cognitive aspects are considered. For example, does the person understand the nature and objects of marriage—"bearing and rearing children, economic goals, the status attached to being husband or wife, sexual fulfillment, mutual kindness, affection and respect, emotional support"?[2] The volitional component refers to whether the person entered a marital contract without coercion.

Also involved are social policy interests. In a case in which two teenagers elope, "soft" psychiatric testimony to the effect that both lacked mature understanding of the nature and objects of matrimony may sometimes suffice as a basis for annulment. On the other hand, if during a marriage, a spouse develops a major mental disorder, the marital duties of the healthier spouse remain in force generally. In some states, in order for divorce to be granted on psychiatric grounds, "incurable insanity" must be established, not just by the demonstrated severity of the mental disturbance—how it impairs marital duties and fails to respond to various ameliorating treatments—but also by a certain number of continuous years that the disabled spouse spends confined in an institution.[3] It would appear that social policy tends to favor preservation of marital obligations, downplaying medical authority.

Guardianship

Guardianship refers to the capacity to manage one's own affairs. A typical statute taken from one state defines an incompetent any person who, because of insanity, mental illness, mental retardation, old age, physical incapacity, imperfection, or deterioration of mentality, is incapable of managing his own person or estate. The vague condition of imperfection, or deterioration of mentality, as a basis for adjudicated incompetency was contested in an appeals court, which upheld such a determination. What mattered most to the court was the petitioner's demonstrated incapability in managing the estate, not the cause of the incapability.[4] Even in the absence of clinical findings indicative of a mental disorder, social policy concerns prevailed in preserving the estate.

Conservator or Committee

A guardian refers to a person or persons who are appointed by courts to care for the estate and/or person of a declared incompetent. Although the terms *conservator* and *committee* are used synonymously in some states, in others, a conservator is appointed by the court to manage a specific area or areas of one's estate. The conservatee must have a substantial impairment demonstrated by "clear and convincing evidence." Such an individual is not considered incompetent; that is, he can manage his own affairs outside the area of adjudicated impairment. The court is very careful to define the specific area of impairment for which a conservator has responsibility to administer. A person who is declared to be a conservatee has the right to repeal this adjudication at any time and can request appointment of another conservator. In contrast, a determination of incompetency means that the individual is regarded as an infant in the eyes of the law, totally unable to manage his property or person. A trial period, perhaps a conservatorship, may be required before the drastic action of incompetency can be proposed or established. When established, a committee is appointed that then manages all of the incompetent person's affairs.

HOSPITAL COMMITMENT

Involuntary Civil Commitment—Legal Rationales

The focus of recent interest has been on involuntary civil commitments rather than on informal or voluntary admissions. There are basically two legal rationales that justify involuntary psychiatric hospitalizations. The first is *parens patriae,* which refers to the state's interest in caring for people who are mentally disabled and unable to care for themselves. Statutory criteria based on *parens patriae* may apply to the following individuals: (1) a person in need of care and treatment, (2) a person in need of hospitalization, (3) a person lacking judgment with respect to his needs. The other legal rationale is *police power*—that the state has a legitimate interest in committing mentally disturbed persons who pose a danger to self or others. At this time, all of the states except New York require a finding of dangerousness before a mentally disturbed person can be certified to a long-term facility. Short-term or emergency commitments are also based on police power. Although dangerousness is currently the rule of law with respect to civil commitment, the approach in one jurisdiction, Wisconsin, has not proved consistent. For example, 50 percent of judges in the state interpreted "substantial harm" as property damage or psychological or financial hardship to the family of a mentally ill person.[5] Such a practice suggests some blurring between the two legal rationales.

Developments in Case Law

The widespread adoption of police power as the sole rationale for civil commitment was facilitated by a particular legal percpetion; committing people involuntarily to mental hospitals resulted in serious deprivations that outweighed intended benefits. Hospitals appears to offer treatment not much better than custodial care. While confined, patients became institutionalized, exposed to a higher morbidity/death rate compared to the general population, rendered incompetent to manage their own affairs, and stigmatized upon return to the community.[6] Indeed, one court regarded the risk of committing a person not mentally ill or dangerous as "cruelty beyond comprehension," analogous to convicting an innocent man of a crime and sentencing him to prison. Consistent with this viewpoint, the court granted citizens the full panoply of due process safeguards, insisting on proof "beyond a reasonable doubt" before ordering involuntary hospitalzation.[7]

In 1979, two cases came to the U.S. Supreme Court concerned with the imposition of due process safeguards upon civil commitment. In *Addington* v. *Texas,* the court set the minimum standard of proof at "clear and convincing evidence." It recognized that an individual does have an "interest of such weight and gravity" not to be erroneously committed and concluded that the risk should be less than fifty-fifty, the "preponderance of evidence standard." On the other hand, unlike criminal proceedings, the decision to commit is based on the interpretation given to facts by expert clinicians, not the facts themselves. The subtleties and nuances of psychiatric diagnosis would not be amenable to proof "beyond a reasonable doubt." In other respects, due process safeguards would remain.[8]

In *Parham* v. *J.R.,* a different approach was taken. Here the court stated that "a neutral factfinder" should decide whether or not a child met "medical standards for admission." Due process does not require the fact finder to be "law-trained. . . . Neither judges nor administrative hearing officers are better qualified than psychiatrists to render psychiatric judgments." Apparently, children did not require the full panoply of due process safeguards because parents sought hospitalization in their best interests, while the risk of erroneous admission was reduced by careful psychiatric screening—first, by community mental health centers, and, second, by hospital physicians.[9]

While it could be argued that adults and children who need involuntary hospitalization probably have much in common, the U.S. Supreme Court would permit more medical authority and fewer due process safeguards for children in determining suitability for civil commitment.

Involuntary Commitment and Competency

In some states, civil commitment and competency to manage one's affairs are considered together in the same hearing. At the time of discharge, the hospital superintendent files a statement to the court that the individual is no longer mentally ill. The judge then decides whether or not to enter an order to restore competency.

In other states, civil commitment and a finding of incompetency are regarded as separate issues. This separation would suggest that there exists no assumed relationship between a person's need to be cared for in a mental hospital and his capacity to handle his own affairs. Usually, however, administrative regulations, issued by state mental health boards, limit the extent to which patients can, in fact, manage their affairs, even though a finding of incompetency has not been made at the time of commitment. For example, a mentally ill person may be prohibited from making a will, executing a contract, or signing any evidence of indebtedness except upon the order of a commissioner or judge, who is advised of the patient's commitment in a mental hospital. Such regulations, if enforced, would seem to treat patients as if they were adjudicated incompentent.

In practice, patients do execute wills, contracts, and deeds whether or not they are found competent. Superintendents generally enforce limitations on competency, filing a petition for guardianship only when encountering a specific problem over a patient's behavior. Even though statutory law or administrative procedure may, in effect, render an involuntary patient incompetent, such limitations are usually not enforced.[10]

"The Least Restrictive Alternative"

Under circumstances in which citizens are legally compelled to accept limitations on their freedom, such restrictions ought not exceed the minimum amount necessary to achieve socially desirable goals. In 1960, the U.S. Supreme Court ruled in one case, concerned with a state mandate that teachers make unlimited disclosure of all organizational affiliations before their contracts could be renewed, that such a mandate constituted "too wide a scope for a state to investigate competence of teachers." Judge Frankfurter suggested recourse to less restrictive methods, an availability of alternatives, to achieve the same justifiable goal.[11]

By analogy, such an approach was applied to the management of psychiatric patients. In 1966, the U.S. Court of Appeals, District of Columbia, considered the habeas corpus petition of a 60-year-old woman, alleging that St. Elizabeth's Hospital detained her illegally. A psychiatrist on the hospital staff testified that the patient "suffered from chronic brain syndrome, with cerebral arteriosclerosis. She was forgetful, became confused, and wandered the streets. If she were released . . . her only problem would be exposure to difficulty if left unattended without the benefit of supervision." Judge David Bazelon, the chief justice of the U.S. Court of Appeals, District of Columbia, insisted that the district court should explore alternatives less restrictive than total confinement in St. Elizabeth's that would "provide care reasonably suited to her needs." Such care could range from giving her an identification card (like a diabetic) in case she wandered to arranging day programs or home health visiting services. Upon reconsidering the case, the lower court found, in fact, that no suitable alternatives existed, and Mrs. Lake remained in the hospital subsequently.[12] The U.S. Court of Appeals, District of Columbia, extended the least restrictive alternative rationale from civil commitment decisions to conditions of confinement within hospitals—from maximum security to outpatient care.[13] In *Jones* v. *Robinson,* due process safeguards were introduced. Mr. Jones, a patient hospitalized at St. Elizabeth's, was accused of raping a female patient on his ward; consequently, he was transferred to the more secure John Howard Pavilion. The court questioned whether the transfer had been permissible and reasonable. On what basis had it been decided that the patient committed the alleged act? To resolve the issue, did the hospital utilize the least drastic means possible? To answer these questions, the court suggested that the hospital appoint a neutral officer or psychiatrist to interview all witnesses, conduct a hearing in which the patient with a chosen advocate could confront the witnesses, and have the proceedings written down—available to the patient or advocate. The decision and supporting reasons would then need to be affirmed by the superintendent.[14] In effect, "administrative due process" would enter into routine hospital procedure, reinforcing the least restrictive alternative rationale.

The "Right to Treatment"

In 1960, Morton Birnbaum, an attorney–physician, published a legal rationale for this right. He suggested that when individuals are involuntarily hospitalized, failure to provide ameliorating treatments not only deprived them of an opportunity to recover from mental illness but also to regain freedom from confinement. Without treatment, such persons would become virtual prisoners. From a due process standpoint, treatment must be made available, enabling committed patients to regain their freedom.[16] This rationale was read widely by the legal profession.

Judge Bazelon developed further rationales. In *Rouse* v. *Cameron* (1966), a habeas corpus case, the appellant challenged his confinement in St. Elizabeth's Hospital, which followed acquittal of a misdemeanor offense by reason of insantiy. Mr. Rouse claimed that he had not received suitable treatment. He regarded himself as not mentally ill and ready for release. Months before, he had rejected group therapy. Judge Bazelon suggested that the following factors ought to be considered: "the suitability of group therapy for his particular illness, whether his rejection of this therapy was a . . . symptom of his mental illness . . . whether reasonable efforts were made either to deal with such rejection or to provide other suitable treatment." The hospital must make a "bona fide effort" to offer the patient "adequate treatment," "suitable to his particular needs." Authority for this ruling was based on the D.C. statutory provisions, which stated that "any person hospitalized . . . shall be entitled to medical and psychiatric care and treatment." Besides referring to the due process rationale, Judge Bazelon reasoned that hospital confinement in the absence of adequate treatment constituted "cruel and unusual punishment," violating the Eighth Amendment to the Constitution: "the purpose of involuntary hospitalization (was) treatment, not punishment."[17] *Rouse* v. *Cameron* exerted slight impact on subsequent practices but encouraced civil libertarian groups to advance the right further.

In *Wyatt* v. *Stickney* (1962), such groups brought a class-action suit into a U.S. District Court against the Alabama State Mental Health Board, representing all mental and mentally retarded patients involuntarily confined to state institutions. This case continued as *Wyatt* v. *Aderholdt* (1974) and *Wyatt* v. *Harden* (1976). Referring to the rationales developed in *Rouse* v. *Cameron,* Judge Johnson declared a "constitutional right to treatment." He invited various national organizations in the mental health field to submit *amicus* briefs that would define minimum standards for care and treatment in mental institutions. When the mental health board claimed inability to meet the defined standards due to a lack of resources, the court asserted a higher constitutional authority that mandated compliance regardless of state regulations and statutes.

Judge Johnson eventually ordered the state to go into receivership, ordering certain assets to be sold off so that money could be made available to the mental hygiene system. No other federal court had gone so far in the implementation of the right to treatment. Judge Johnson mandated the following minimum standards: (1) maintenance of a humane psychological and physical environment, (2) provision of qualified staff in sufficient numbers, and (3) provision of individualized treatment plans. One of the elements in the humane psychological and physical environment was a proscription against putting patients into involuntary servitude, an allusion to the Thirteenth Amendment. If patients were to work, this should be voluntary and compensated with adequate pay. Furthermore, work should be incorporated into the treatment plan and supervised by staff. Many other details concerning "minimum constitutional standards for adequate treatment of the mentally ill" are too lengthy to discuss further here. Administrators in the mental health field would be well advised to review the itemization of standards elsewhere.[18,19]

In *Donaldson* v. *O'Conner* (1974), the plaintiff, an involuntary patient at a Florida state hospital, accused Dr. O'Conner, the defendent, of violating his civil rights and sued for monetary damages. Specifically, the psychiatrist was accused of willfully and maliciously withholding treatment from Donaldson, violating an alleged, constitutionally based right to treatment. On appeal, the U.S. Court of Appeals Fifth Circuit ruled in favor of the plaintiff, proposing a due process rationale for the right to treatment—the *quid pro quo* theory. In other words, loss of liberty incurred through hospital confinement could be justified only with the availability of treatment.[20]

Dr. O'Conner then appealed the case up to the U.S. Supreme Court in 1975. It appeared to a majority of the justices that Donaldson was a nondangerous individual, capable of surviving safely by himself or with the help of willing and responsible family members or friends. The court declared that a person who meets this criteria constitutionally cannot be hospitalized against his will even if he has been found mentally ill and able to benefit from treatment. The decision of the lower U.S. Court of Appeals was vacated.[21]

In effect, the court sidestepped the right-to-treatment issue, stressing rather minimal constitutional restrictions on the state's authority to confine individuals against their will. The court did not say who may be involuntarily confined, only who may not be. In addition, Chief Justice Berger rejected any legal rationale that would establish a tie between civil commitment and a right to treatment. He pointed out that patients such as Donaldson, with a diagnosis of paranoid schizophrenia, may indeed by untreatable due to a lack of cooperation and/or motivation. Treatments in themselves may be ineffective, leaving available only custodial care.

Yet commitment would still be justified for such a person because he continues to meet statutory criteria, established through a proceeding with the usual due process safeguards. When the reasons for confinement no longer exist, then would he have to be released.

With the exception of Judge Johnson's continuing authority in Alabama under *Wyatt,* the judicial impetus for a right to treatment appeared to come to a dead end. Alternative approaches might be considered. For example, deplorable living conditions in mental institutions could be construed as violating the Eighth Amendment—the ban on cruel and unusual punishment. Unavailability of services for the mentally disabled, which ordinary citizens obtain routinely, might suggest a lack of "equal protection." Financial considerations, such as those related to accreditation by the Joint Commission on Accrediation of Hospitals, would probably exert greater influence on standards for hospital care and treatment than judicial review. Legislative acts could make provision of services a condition of eligibility for funding.

INFORMED CONSENT

Treatment cannot be provided to an individual without obtaining informed consent. The latter consists of three components: (1) competency, (2) knowledge, and (3) voluntariness. Competency refers to the cognitive capacity needed for a person to understand and evaluate information about recommended treatment. Knowledge includes the type of information that must be presented, enabling one to reach an informed decision such as the following: (1) What is the nature of the treatment and why is it being recommended? (2) What benefit could be expected? (3) What alternative treatments are available? (4) What risks are there to treatment? Voluntariness means that the individual is not forced into a decision and recognizes that at any time he can withdraw his consent.

Whether or not social policy deems as sufficient an individual's capacity to give informed consent depends on the nature of treatment recommended and under what circumstances it is offerred. In *Kaimowitz* v. *the Department of Mental Health for the State of Michigan,* 1973, the court considered this issue regarding a prisoner who volunteered for psychosurgery designed to alleviate violent tendencies. His informed consent was declared invalid, based on the following; (1) the treatment was experimental, with uncertain benefits, significant irreversible risks, and no validation of specific medical indications or studies comparing alternative approaches, (2) the incarceration was inherently coercive in that the prisoner consented in the hope of gaining release, (3) his competency to reach an independent judgment was compromised by prison life.[22]

In contrast, one state does not require informed consent as a precondition of administering electroconvulsive therapy (ECT) to hospitalized patients because ECT "is an accepted therapy beyond the stage of experimentation".[23] The same treatment in other states necessitates the obtaining of informed consent apart from hospitalization. It would appear that society's perception of the risk-benefit ratio of a given treatment determines the threshold of competency judged sufficient, enabling a patient to give valid informed consent.[24]

The Right to Refuse Treatment

Repeated litigation has demonstrated that hospitalized patients who are nondangerous and mentally competent to give informed consent have an absolute right to refuse treatment. The thrust of recent cases has been to decide under what circumstances this right may be overriden. In *Rogers* v. *Okin* (1979), the district court in Massachusetts ruled that antipsychotic medication could be involuntarily administered during an emergency in which there existed a "substantial likelihood of physical harm." Psychiatric indications did not suffice. In nonemergency situations, only an adjudication of incompetency with appointment of a guardian to provide informed consent would permit the patient to be involuntarily medicated.[25] A year later, the higher court of appeals reconsidered the case in a manner consistent with the U.S. Supreme Court's approach in *Parham* v. *J.R.* (1979) that "neither judges nor administrative hearing officers are better qualified than psychiatrists to render psychiatric judgments." Specifically, a qualified physician could determine when an emergency demanded chemotherapy on the basis of the following estimations: (1) "the possibility and type of violence," (2) "the likely effects of particular drugs on a particular individual," and (3) "an appraisal of alternatives, less restrictive courses of action." In addition, "where any delay could result in significant deterioration of the patient's mental health," alternative means of determining cometency should be considered. In nonemergency situations, a judicial finding of incompetency was still required, but the appointed guardian would not have to give permission for "all treatment decisions involving the use of antipsychotic drugs." The lower district court was directed to devise procedures to monitor situations calling for involuntary chemotherapy.[26]

In *Rennie* v. *Klein* (1978), the district court in New Jersey had already instituted procedures applicable to such situations. In an emergency, where "life and limb" were in danger, the physician could medicate involuntarily up to 72 hours. Past this time, certification by the medical director would be required. Outside of emergencies, patients would sign forms indicating informed consent. If the physician determined the patient to be "functionally incompetent," then chemotherapy could commence without informed consent. A patient advocate, provided by the hospital, would examine the decision to medicate, deciding whether or not to refer the matter for further hospital review or request the opinion of an outside, independent psychiatrist.[27]

The type of monitoring system chosen, administrative due process or court review, would depend on society's perception of the risk-benefit ratio involved in a given treatment. For example, in some jurisdictions, involuntary chemotherapy might be monitored by procedures of administrative due process, while only adjudications of incompetency would permit giving ECT in the absence of informed consent. Occasionally, a legislature might limit, through statute, the amount of treatment given or forbid a particular treatment altogether. In the *Rennie* case, the court took notice of tardive dyskinesia, an irreversible disability associated with neuroleptic agents, and questioned whether "the cure might be worse than the illness"; such a risk would justify the instituting of due process procedures designed to give proper consideration to patients' refusals of medication. In nonemergency situations in which the objective is based on religious grounds, case law would suggest that only a court could make the overriding decision to treat.

CONFIDENTIALITY, PRIVACY, AND PRIVILEGE

Confidentiality

Among members of the legal profession, Professor Wigmore's four criteria have generally been accepted as the definition of a confidential relationship.[28]

1. Communications must originate in the understanding that they will not be disclosed.
2. This nondisclosure is an ingredient essential to satisfactory maintenance of the relationship.
3. Such a relationship is one that serves a valid social purpose and ought to be fostered.
4. The harm done to the relationship by disclosure of the communication must be greater than the benefit gained from correct disposal of litigation.

The authority for confidentiality is derived ultimately from the Hippocratic oath, an ethical code for the medical profession.

Privacy

Individuals have a right to shield themselves from public view and legal intrusion. For example, a person is entitled not to have his or her photograph shown in newspapers. No public disclosure of one's involvement in treatment or hospitalization is authorized. The U.S. Supreme Court found state statutes forbidding sales of contraceptives or abortion unconstitutional because issues concerning sexual relations and bodily privacy did not warrant legal intrusions. This fundamental right to privacy was derived from various constitutional amendments.

Privilege

The right to privilege is established by statutes in each state that protect an individual from disclosing confidential and private communications in a courtroom. Psychiatrists are included in the physician–patient relationship protected by privilege statutes. Professionals in allied mental health fields are also covered through their association with psychiatrists, or else statutory privelege may apply to psychotherapist–client relationships. In most states, however, there are specified exceptions to the right, which can be subsumed under three broad categories: (1) proceedings for involuntary hospitalization, (2) court-ordered psychiatric examinations, and (3) proceedings in which an individual's mental condition is raised as an element of a claim or a defense.

In *Re Lifschutz* (1970), the psychiatrist was held in contempt of court because he refused to disclosed any information about a former patient who had filed a suit against another individual. The California Supreme Court ruled that no absolute privilege existed for psychotherapeutic confidentiality.

In this case, the former patient's mental condition had a bearing on the suit, which waved his privilege. The benefit gained through correct litigation outweighed any injury to the psychotherapeutic relationship resulting from disclosure of information.

In a similar case, *Caesar* v. *Mountanos* (1976), Dr. Caesar acknowledged treating a patient for injuries sustained in accidents and revealed that she had been depressed; however, he refused to answer questions pertaining to the relationship between her emotional condition and the accidents. The U.S. Court of Appeals Ninth Circuit reached the same conclusion as the California Supreme Court. One dissenting justice, Judge Hufsteder, did not consider this a closed issue. In her opinion, if the psychiatrist had indicated that sensitive matters such as personal marital difficulties or sexual intimacies were at stake, then the constitutional right to privacy might compel nondisclosure, outweighing the need to correctly dispose of litigation.[30] Application of this approach would await future cases.

PROFESSIONAL LIABILITY

Negligence is conduct that falls below legally established standards that protect others against an unreasonable risk of harm. Four elements are required.[31]

1. A defined duty
2. A dereliction of that duty
3. A direct causation between dereliction of duty
4. Damage to the patient

Standards established by one's own profession, or even common sense, may constitute a duty. Dereliction can occur either by acts of commission or omission. Direct causation means that the act contributes in some way, proximate in time, to the unfavorable outcome. Violation of a legally protected interest constitutes damage. For example, alienation of affections between spouses, though associated with mental distress, is not ordinarily considered a legally protected interest. In order to prove negligence, the plaintiff must demonstrate the elements by the "preponderance of the evidence" standard; thus, a mere 51 percent certainty, just enough to tip the scales of justice, suffices.

Five themes may be discerned in professional negligence cases. First, is the service provided in conformity to professional standards? Various task force reports or other statements from the American Psychiatric Association, as well as qualified professionals, who testify as to prevailing practices, may supply standards. Second, is reasonable care exerted in providing the service? Taking prudent steps to avoid mishaps or acting in a conscientious manner are matters understandable to laymen, apart from professional standards. Third, does the service involve an acceptable risk-benefit ratio? When the benefits are dubious and/or the risk appears significant, then the question arises as to whether informed consent was obtained. Even if validly obtained, such an approach to the patient may be regarded as experimental, and the practitioner may be held liable for any adverse outcome. Fourth, *res ipsiloquitor*—the thing speaks for itself—refers to a harmful consequence, occuring around the time of treatment, which is patently obvious and qualifying for both causation and damage. In such a case, the burden shifts to the practitioner to disprove negligence. Fifth, "respondent superior" means that the professional is held accountable for the actions of ancillary staff. For example, receptionists or secretaries should be trained to avoid exerting detrimental effects on patient care.

Selected Case Developments

Release of Dangerous Patients

In 1967, a Veterans Administration hospital in South Dakota released a patient on work leave who subsequently killed his wife in North Dakota. The latter's estate successfully sued the U.S. government. The court found that the doctors had been notified repeatedly about the patient's threats. No one investigated the basis for these allegations, and no reference to the matter was made in the medical chart. At the time of work release, the employer was not informed of the patient's recent hospitalization, current hospital supervision, and inadvisability of returning to North Dakota. This constituted a dereliction of reasonable or "due care."[31] (See also the discussion of dangerousness in Chapter 27)

In *Tarasoff* v. *Regents of the University of California* (1976), a university psychologist learned that his patient intended to kill a former girl friend. He instructed the campus police to take the patient to a hospital for evaluation, but the latter was released and did not return to therapy. Two months later, the patient killed his former girl friend. The California Supreme Court ruled that "when a psychotherapist, pursuant to the standards of his profession, determines that his patient presents a serious danger of violence to others, he is obliged to exert reasonable care to protect the intended victim." Such reasonable care would include "warning the victim, others likely to appraise the victim, notifying police, or other steps." In a similar 1979 case, valid grounds for negligence could arise from a jury determination about whether a psychotherapist did or did not respond prudently enough to dangerous comments made by a patient. Furthermore, since psychiatrists routinely evaluated civil commitment according to a dangerousness standard, it was assumed that they would posses greater experience and skill in this area than layman.[33] The judges, however, did not consider the possibility that there are different types of dangerousness; the type involved in a liability suit cannot be equated with that evaluated for civil commitment.[34]

In response to such a trend, institutions appear to be developing administrative due process procedures prior to releasing allegedly dangerous individuals. One procedural approach might involve a committee of professionals to assess the pros and cons of release, preparing a recommendation for final approval to the suerintendent. This process could be monitored by a patient advocate. If such a patient after release were to commit a serious assult, then a potential court review would probably find that reasonable care had been exerted.

Liability for Suicide

Extensive litigation has demonstrated that negligence can arise from deficiencies in a number of areas.[35–37] First, an adequate number of caretaking staff need to be educated in identifying suicidal cues among hospitalized patients. Second, once such patients are identified, the attention of the psychiatrist is required. Third, the psychiatrist has to evaluate the patient's suicide risk and indicate this assessment in the medical record. Fourth, with severe or moderate risk assessment, the psychiatrist must write specific orders for suicide precautions. Fifth, caretaking staff are obliged to carry out the orders according to standards for suicide precaution established by by the hospital. If deficiencies exist in any of these areas, a completed suicide can potentialy lead to a successful liability suit.

Failure to Treat

Although the U.S. Supreme Court disallowed monetary damages in *O'Conner* v. *Donaldson and transformed the right to treatment into a narrow issue of liberty, in Whitree* v. *State* (1968), the New York court took another approach. The majority opinion stated that "Whitree" was not treated with any of the modern tranquilizing drugs . . . during his entire stay in the hospital. . . . The reason for not using such drugs was that Whitree refused them. We consider such reason to be illogical, unprofessional and not consonant with prevailing medical standards." This negligence resulted in a 12 year hospital confinement, avoidable had the patient been medicated.[38] Professionals had a duty to pursue procedures toward overcoming an incompetent refusal.

REFERENCES

1. Slovenko R: Psychiatry and Law. Boston, Little, Brown, 1973, p 317
2. Slovenko R: Psychiatry and Law, p 359
3. Sadoff R: Forensic Psychiatry: A Practical Guide For Lawyers and Psychiatrists. Springfield, Ill, Thomas, 1975, p 205–206
4. In Re Estate of Stevenson, 44 Ill 2d 525, 256, NE 2d 766 (1970)
5. Zander: Civil Commitment in Wisconsin: The Impact of Lessard v. Schmidt. Wisconsin Law Review 503–526 (1976)
6. Lessard v. Schmidt, 349 F Supp 1078 (ED Wis 1972)
7. In Re Ballay, 482 f 2d 648 (DC Cir 1973); 157 US App DC 59
8. Addington v. Texas, 99 S Ct 1804 (1979)
9. Parham v. J.R., 99 S Ct 2493 (1979)
10. Allen RC, Ferster EZ, Weihofen H: Mental Impariment and Legal Incompetency. Englewood Cliffs, NJ, Prentice-Hall, 1968
11. Shelton v. Tucker, 364 US 479; Bl S Ct 247 (1960)
12. Lake v. Cameron, 364 F 2d 657 (DC Cir 1966)
13. Covington v. Harris, 419 F 2d 617 (DC Cir 1969)
14. Jones v. Robinson, 440 F 2d 249 (DC Cir 1971)
15. Baxstrom v. Herold, 383 US 107; 86 S Ct 760 (1966)
16. Birnbaum M: The right to treatment. American Bar Association Journal 46:499 1960
17. Rouse v. Cameron, 373 F 2d 451 (DC Cir 1966); 125 US App DC 366

18. Wyatt v. Stickney, 325 F Supp 781 (MD Ala 1971); 344 F Supp 373 (MD Ala 1972)
19. Brooks AD: Law, Psychiatry and the Mental Health System. Boston, Little, Brown, 1974, pp 857–870
20. Donaldson v. O'Connor, 493 F 2d 507 (5th Cir 1974)
21. O'Connor v. Donaldson, 42 US 563; 95 S Ct 2486 (1975)
22. Kaimowitz v. Michigan Department of Mental Health, No 73–19434-AW Mich. Cir. Ct., Wayne Co. July 10, 1973. See 1 Mental Disability Law Reporter 147 (1976)
23. Stone AA: Mental Health and Law: A System in Transition. New York, Jason Aronson, 1976, p 100
24. Roth LH, Meisel A, Lidz CW: Tests of competency to consent to treatment. Am J Psychiatry 134:279–284, 1977
25. Rogers v. Okin, 478 F Supp 1342 (1979)
26. Rogers v. Okin, (1st Cir Nov 25, 1980)
27. Rennie v. Klein, 462 F Supp 1131 (DNJ 1978)
28. Wigmore JH: Evidence in Trials at Common Law, vol 8. Boston, Little, Brown, 1961
29. In Re Lifschutz, 2 Cal 3d 415; 467 P 2d 557 (1970)
30. Cawsar v. Mountanous, 542 F 2d 1064 (9th Cir 1976)
31. Merchants National Bank and Trust Co. v. United States, 272 F Supp 409 (DND 1967)
32. Tarasoff v. Board of Regents of the University of California, 17 Cal 3d 425, 551 P 2d 334 (1976)
33. McIntosh v. Milano, 168 NJ Super 466 (June 12, 1979)
34. Crain PM: Assessing dangerousness, in Rosner R (ed): Critical Issues in American Psychiatry and the Law. Springfield, Ill, Thomas (in press)
35. Lucy Webb Hayes National Training School v. Perotti, 419 F 2d 704 (DC Cir 1969)
36. Peer I: Suicide Responsibility of Hospital and Psychiatrist, 9 Clev—Mar Law Review 427 (1960)
37. Slawson P: Psychiatric malpractice, in Professional Liability Insurance and Psychiatric Malpractice, Task Force Report 13. American Psychiatric Association, February 1978
38. Whitree v. State, 56 Misc 2d 693, 290 NYS 2d 486 (1968)

Harvey Bluestone, M.D.
John T. Melella, M.S.W

27

Criminal Law

There has been an increasingly important overlap between psychiatry and criminal law in recent years. Many psychiatric patients have entered and remained in psychiatric hospitals as a result of criminal proceedings. We have been informed, for instance, that approximately 15 percent of patients currently being treated at Bronx Psychiatric Center in New York have been committed under New York State criminal procedure law. With relatively large numbers of patients entering hospitals via the criminal justice system, it behooves mental health administrators to have a fundamental understanding of the legal issues that are intertwined with patient care and treatment. This chapter intends to introduce to the mental health administrator those medicolegal issues likely to be encountered in everyday practice.

The issues to be discussed in this chapter are (1) the role of the psychiatrist as expert witness, (2) competency to stand trial, (3) insanity as a defense, (4) special categories of offenders, including alcoholics, drug addicts, sex offenders, "defective delinquents," (5) dangerousness, (6) transfer from prison to hospital, and (7) the release of criminally committed offenders. Throughout the chapter, we will use relevant court decisions to illustrate the issues at hand. Finally, perhaps the best way to illustrate what happens to a mentally ill criminal offender is to use an actual case to demonstrate what happens in each of these various parts of criminal procedure, particularly regarding the psychiatrist's role.

THE ROLE OF THE PSYCHIATRIST AS AN EXPERT WITNESS AND HIS RELATIONSHIPS WITH LAWYERS

A role of the psychiatrist in criminal proceedings is that of "expert witness" when the allegation of mental illness plays a significant part in the proceedings. Most commonly, psychiatrists are asked to give their expert medical opinions with regard to the patient's (1) competency to stand trial, (2) criminal responsibility, (3) transfer from prison to a hospital, (4) treatment, and (5) release. The psychiatrist is asked to examine the individual and submit a written report to the court answering a specific question. Sometimes the psychiatrist–expert is asked to testify in open court as to his findings. In either case, the information provided to the court by the psychiatrist is introduced as evidence in a criminal procedure.

For the uninitiated psychiatrist, courtroom testimony can be a harrowing experience. A major reason for discomfort is a lack of understanding by both psychiatrists and lawyers of the other's profession. Both parties fail to realize that each field represents a conflicting philosophical view of human behavior.

Virtually all modern psychological theories are in some way deterministic. Criminal law, on the other hand, has as its philosophical basis the concept of free will, the idea of a man as a free agent, who is free to make a moral decision as to right or wrong. These differences often emerge in a criminal trial. The criminal law focuses primarily on the crime. The psychiatrist remains concerned with the criminal rather than the crime.

Another reason for discomfort is that psychiatrists generally are not familiar with law as an adversary system, just as lawyers are not usually comfortable with the lack of certainty in psychiatric findings.

The adversary system allows the lawyer to portray the psychiatrist as a partisan for his patient rather than the presenter of objective information. In this system, the psychiatrist may find himself disagreeing with his colleagues in a battle of experts. If an attorney has little else to go on, he may attack the credentials of the psychiatrist or even attack him personally in an attempt to discredit him as a witness. Psychiatrists are used to being treated with a certain amount of deference and may resent this kind of treatment, which accounts for much of the reluctance of psychiatrists to testify when called into court.

Attorneys and courts in general do not understand the nature of psychiatric findings. They become frustrated when reports and testimony do not lend themselves to hard facts. Some do not understand the nature of mental illness and attempt to equate psychiatric diagnosis with incompetency or insanity.

The Case of Mr. Nathan

Mr. Nathan, a 55-year-old World War II veteran has been a patient in a New York State Hospital for the past 15 years. In 1964, he was accused of murdering his wife. He had met his wife while working nights as a bartender. She was a regular customer of his. They married, and while on their honeymoon, Mr. Nathan heard voices that he believed then and still believes were the devil talking to him. His wife, frightened that he was crazy, convinced him to go to a state hospital near where they lived. While on a weekend pass from the hospital, he allegedly strangled his wife to death while they were in bed. Mr. Nathan was vague about the circumstances but remembered calling the police. He was arrested and charged with murder. Since Mr. Nathan was a mental patient at the time of his arrest, the court was first interested in protecting his constitutional rights to a fair trial by establishing whether or not Nathan was competent to stand trial of the crime for which he was being accused.

COMPETENCY TO STAND TRIAL

The concept of competency to stand trial evolved out of English common law.[1] This concept grew out of the concern that the defendant should be able to protect himself in the context of a trial system in which he is involved with the prosecution in a adversary struggle.

The standard for incompetency emerged out of a series of 18th- and 19th-century trials.[2–4] These standards emphasized the cognitive capacity of the defendant to understand the procedures and to collaborate with his attorney. These standards of competency were brought to the United States, where they have been used in our court system.

Current Legal Standards for Competency

The current legal standard for competency to stand trial came out of the 1960 Supreme Court decision in *Dusky* v. *United States.* "The test must be whether the (defendant) has sufficient present ability to consult with his lawyer with a reasonable degree of rational understanding, and whether he has a rational as well as factual understanding of the proceedings against him."[5] This ruling sets forth the criteria to which all state jurisdictions must conform.

There has been a great deal of confusion, however, because the Supreme Court in Dusky did not define what a "reasonable degree of rational understanding" is. Therefore, it is left up to each state to decide its meaning. A defendant who may be found competent for a particular crime in one state might thus be found incompetent in another. Although the judge or jury ultimately makes the legal decision as to a defendant's competency, the court relies heavily on the clinical judgment of psychiatric examiners to decide if the defendant does possess the rational understanding required.

Because of the vagueness of laws regarding competency, the court's decision may be a difficult one. The American Psychiatric Association recommends that the psychiatrist can best perform his function if he presents relevant information about the patient to the court without himself attempting to make a legal determination. This is not his responsibility.[6]

When Is the Competency Issue Raised?

According to the rules set down by the U.S. Supreme Court in *Pate* v. *Robinson* (1966), prosecutors, defense attorneys, and judges are required to raise the issue of competency whenever they believe that a defendant may be ill and that such an illness may interfere with his capacity to participate in a trial.[7] Examiners can only speculate about the reason used by officers of the court that might lead them to ask for a competency determination. In the case of Mr. Nathan, a patient in a psychiatric hospital, the reason is obvious. But in most cases psychiatric examiners can only make assumptions about why a competency proceeding is being initiated by the criminal court.

The issue of competency might be raised because of prior mental hospitalizations or known history of psychiatric illness; the bizarre nature of the crime itself (sexual crimes often fit into this category); the person's strange appearance or actions in the courtroom or upon arrest; and reports from the defense attorney that he is unable to communicate with his client and is therefore unable to prepare a defense. Halpern points out that the competency procedure is often misused. He suggests that judges, prosecutors, and defense attorneys use this procedure to serve their own individual purpose. While granting their laudable motive to "keep the criminal off the streets," Halpern contends that officers of the court may use the issue of competency in order to effect continued detention of the defendant by denying bail while awaiting psychiatric examination.[8] The use of the competency procedure as preventive detention is clearly a misuse of the purpose for which it was intended.

Competency used as preventive detention is of particular importance when one realizes that before the Supreme Court ruling in 1972, which set time limits on competency laws, (*Jackson* v. *Indiana*), a person facing criminal charges on a relatively minor crime could have spent his whole life incarcerated without ever having been tried or convicted of a crime.

Mr. Nathan was repeatedly examined for competency. After 8 years in the state hospital, he was finally found competent to stand trial. Mr. Nathan pleaded not guilty by reason of insanity and was acquitted. His continued treatment in the hospital was ordered.

The Finding of Incompetence

Persons found incompetent to stand trial are sent to hospitals for treatment until competency is restored. Upon restoration of competency, the accused is returned to court. The legal proceeding then continues as it would for any other case. This presupposes that the incompetency finding is based on a treatable mental illness and that the illness can be treated within a reasonable period of time. This is often not the case. The landmark Supreme Court decision handed down in *Jackson* v. *Indiana*[9] illustrates the problem of how the state of Indiana's competency statute violated one person's civil rights.

> Theon Jackson was a mentally retarded deaf mute with the intelligence of a preschool child. He could not read or write but could communicate in sign language. In 1968, at age 27, he was charged in Indiana with two robberies. The first involved a purse and its contents, valued at four dollars. The second concerned five dollars in cash. The trial court, under Indiana Law, found Jackson incompetent to stand trial.
>
> The psychiatric testimony regarding Jackson's condition established that his mental deficiency was so severe that it would be highly unlikely that Jackson could ever be restored to competency.

Counsel for Jackson maintained that commitment under these circumstances amounted to a "life sentence" without his (Jackson's) ever having been convicted of a crime. The commitment therefore deprived Jackson of his Fourteenth Amendment rights to due process and equal protection and constituted cruel and unusual punishment under the Eighth Amendment to the Constitution of the United States. This now celebrated case set the precedent for limiting confinement of incompetents to a "reasonable period of time." If such defendants cannot be restored to competency in a foreseeable period of time with therapy, they must be treated like any other mentally ill person and either civilly committed or released.

The limitation on the term of commitment to a mental hospital was left to the discretion of the states. In New York, for example, a person accused of a misdemeanor and found incompetent may be committed for no longer than 90 days in a civil mental hospital, after which the charges are dropped.[10] A felony defendant in New York found incompetent may be committed for two-thirds of the maximum sentence he would have received if convicted of the crime of which he is accused. There is, however, periodic review of the patient's competency, and if competency is established, then the patient is returned to court to stand trial for the alleged crime.[11] Federal courts permit release of incompetent defendants after 18 months.[12]

THE INSANITY DEFENSE

While competency to stand trial addresses itself to a defendant's mental status at the time of the trial, the insanity defense proposes to assess mental status at the time of the commission of the crime itself. These issues are often confused by psychiatrists and lawyers and particularly by the public. Consequently, it is extremely important to recognize the difference between tests for incompetency and tests for insanity. Competency hearings characteristically take place without a jury and without public awareness. Insanity pleas, on the other hand, are much less frequent but are often reported in the media, giving the procedure "high visibility."[13] The insanity defense is usualy invoked only for serious crimes, whereas the competency issue can be raised, and often is, for the most trivial crimes as well as the most serious.

To return to our first example, Mr. Nathan was found to be suffering from a mental disease at the time his wife was killed, which exculpated him. He was therefore acquitted by reason of insanity. Why was he found not guilty? Again, criminal law has historically provided that a person who commits an offense is not legally responsible for his actions if at the time he commits the offense he is "insane." Insanity is an excusing condition. There are other excusing conditions in criminal law, for example, acting in self-defense, or offending because of an innocent mistake of fact. In each case, there is no intention to commit a crime. In criminal law, there cannot be a crime if the person did not have the requisite mental state, referred to historically as *mens rea* or "guilty mind." The reasoning for this is that illness may cause a mental impairment analogous to ignorance of the facts. Under the law, a person with such an impairment would not be considered blameworthy. It is unfair or unjust to convict such a person of a crime. A more appropriate dispositon, such as hospitalization for the illness, can be considered but not conviction for a crime. "Insanity" is a legal term that is not synonymous with mental illness. It does require, however, that a mental illness did exist and the person being accused suffered some kind of incapacity as a result of the illness. As Brooks points out, "It is the incapacity that is the critical excusing condition and not the mental illness."[14]

Tests of the Insanity Defense

There are several models of the insanity defense. Each model defines the excusing conditions based on one or more of following principles: The first is "I didn't know what I was doing" or "I didn't know that what I did was wrong." The second is "I couldn't help it." The third is "I was mentally ill when I did it."[14] The first is essentially the McNaughten Rule.

McNaughten

The McNaughten Rule was first used in England in 1843. To establish a defense of insanity under this test, there must be proof that at the time of committing the act, the defendant was "laboring under such a defect of reason from disease of the mind as not to know the nature and quality of the act he was doing; or, if he did know it, that he did not know that he was doing what was wrong."[15]

Mr. Nathan, who suffered from schizophrenia and was plagued by hallucinations, met the McNaughten criteria for insanity and was then acquitted.

Irresistible Impulse

The second test of insanity, "I couldn't help it," is never used by itself but in conjunction with the McNaughten Rule. Under the irresistible-impulse test, an individual might not be legally responsible even if he had the reason and the knowledge required in the McNaughten test if as a result of his mental illness he "so far lost the power to choose between right and wrong and avoid doing the act in question that his free agency was at the time destroyed."[16]

The Durham Decision

A third test of insanity, "I was mentally ill when I did it," was proposed in 1954 in federal court in the Durham case by Judge David Bazelon. Judge Bazelon felt that the existing legal tests, McNaughten and irresistible impulse, failed to take into account suffcient modern scientific knowledge about mental illness. He proposed that a defendant is not criminally responsible if the unlawful act is the "product of mental disease or defect."[17] The Durham decision did not define what constitutes mental disease or defect, nor was the meaning of the term *product* defined. The various aspects of the decision were challenged in a series of court cases resulting in the total elimination of this test in 1972.

American Law Institute

The American Law Institute develops model laws to be used by legal jurisdictions at their discretion. Under its model panel code, a defendant "is not responsible for criminal conduct if at the time of such conduct as a result of mental disease or defect he lacks substantial capacity either to appreciate the criminality of his conduct or to conform his conduct to the requirements of law." Furthermore, the terms *mental disease* or *defect* do not include "an abnormality manifested only by repeated criminal or otherwise antisocial conduct."[18] It should be noted that the American Law Institute's decision also did not define mental disease or defect.

Diminished Capacity

Another test, "diminished capacity," has been adopted by several states. Under this test, "evidence of abnormal mental condition would be admissible to affect the degree of crime for which an accused could be convicted. Specifically, those offenses requiring intent or knowledge could be reduced to lesser included offenses requiring only reckless or criminal negligence."[19]

All of these tests are based on the premise of the existence of mental disease and defect. Each suggest that a mental defect causes the defendant to commit acts over which he has no control. The Durham Rule was an attempt to use "science" to improve on McNaughten. The American Law Institute model was an attempt to improve on Durham. Yet despite these efforts to improve these tests, the jury ultimately makes the decision. After 8 years with the Durham decision, the court suggested a judicial definition of insanity. The court stated in *McDonald* v. *United States:*

> what psychiatrists may consider a "mental disease or defect" for clinical purposes, where their concern is treatment, may or may not be the same as mental disease or defect for the jury's purpose in determining the criminal responsibility. Consequently, for that purpose the jury should be told that a mental disease or defect includes any abnormal condition of the mind which substantially affects mental or emotional processes and substantially impairs behavior controls. Thus the jury would consider testimony concerning the development, adoption and functioning of these processes and controls. . . . The jury must determine for itself, from all the testimony, lay and expert, whether the nature and degree of the disability are sufficient to establish a mental disease or defect as we have now defined these terms. . . .[20]

What Happens to Those Found Not Guilty by Reason of Insanity?

A study cited in the *University of Pennyslvannia Law Review* indicates that the statutes in 15 states provide for the automatic, mandatory commitment of persons acquitted by reason of insanity, 30 states provide for such commitment at the discretion of the trial court or following a summary inquiry into the person's present mental condition, and only 5 states are required by statute to initiate and pursue a general civil commitment procedure in order to commit such persons.[21]

At the time Mr. Nathan was committed, New York State required automatic, mandatory commitment. (New York State no longer requires mandatory commitment.) From 1964 to 1972, Nathan was hospitalized because he was incompetent to stand trial; following his acquittal in 1972 he was rehospitalized for insanity, according to state mandatory commitment.

Recently, Mr. Nathan has filed for his release. In order to be released, he must establish that the mental condition for which he was committed has improved to the extent that he no longer is a danger to the safety of himself or others.

In New York, as in other states, the burden of establishing that he no longer needs hospitalization rests with the patient. The decision to release him can only be decided after a court hearing. The mechanisms for release are often difficult bureaucratic and legal procedures; expert opinions and testimony relating to the crucial matter of dangerousness are applied as the key criterion at each stage of the process.

DANGEROUSNESS

The concept of dangerousness has been a controversial issue at the intersection of psychiatry and the law. At the focal point of this controversy are the complexities inherent in the idea of dangerousness, involving (1) definitions of dangerousness, (2) predictability of dangerous behavior, (3) mental illness and dangerousness, (4) standard of proof required for deprivation of liberty, (5) *parens patriae* and police power functions, among others.[22]

The issue of dangerousness is critical not only in the psychiatric aspects of criminal law but also in civil law, particularly in certification status. These matters are briefly discussed in Chapter 26.

Since Mr. Nathan's liberty ultimately rests on the question of his future dangerous behavior, psychiatrists must also examine ways to assess it.

Mr. Nathan was subject to a series of three psychiatric examinations. When he was examined for competency to stand trial, his present mental status was the controlling issue. When he was examined for the insanity defense, his past mental status—that at the time of the commission of the crime—was the controlling issue. When he was examined for release, his future mental status—his future dangerousness—was the controlling issue.

Defining Dangerousness

Before dangerousness as a concept can be used, it must be defined. The term is at best ambiguous. Is it a trait that a person has, or is it a behavior that a person exhibits under certain conditions? Shah defines dangerousness as a behavior, as "acts that are characterized by an application of an overt threat of force and are likely to result in injury to other persons." To Shah, dangerous behavior is synonymous with violent behavior.[23] Schwitzgebel points out that legal definitions have focused on the individual: the origin of the dangerousness lies within him. He suggests that this "trait" approach fits well with psychoanalytic theories.[24] Both Schwitzgebel and Shah are proponents of an interactional approach to dangerousness. This view focuses on the interaction of a person and a social situation in producing a behavior. Some people may thus only be dangerous in particular situations and in particular social contexts.

According to the interactional approach, Mr. Nathan, for example, may not be dangerous *intrinsically* because of the dynamics of his mental disorder. He may *behave* dangerously, however, if placed in certain stressful situations, including certain interpersonal ones. If he were to remarry, for example, forget to take antipsychotic medication, and come home drunk, he might be more dangerous than if none of those conditions existed.

One attempt by the legal system to define dangerousness is found in *Lessard* v. *Schmidt* (1972). Here the U.S. Supreme Court defined dangerousness as a condition in which "there is an extreme likelihood that if the person is not confined, he will do immediate harm to himself or others." Elsewhere in the decision, the court used the term *imminent danger* to self or others and defined it as "based at minimum on a recent act, attempt, or threat to do substantial harm." The court declared that a "psychiatric opinion could not prevail absent a recent *act, attempt or threat*."[25]

Neither the law nor the social sciences have been able to come up with a definition of dangerousness on which all can agree. Brooks, in citing the vagaries of the legal criteria used to predict dangerousness, says that the determination involves consideration of (1) the magnitude of the harm to self, others, or property, (2) the likelihood or probability that the predicted behavior will occur, (3) the imminence of the behavior, and (4) the frequency with which such behavior is likely to occur.[26] Steadman and others have written extensively on the difficulty of predicting dangerousness.[27]

SPECIAL CATEGORIES OF OFFENDERS

Some legal jurisdictions provide statutes for special categories of offenders. These categories include "sexually dangerous person," "defective delinquents," "drug addicts," and "alcoholics." The aim of these special statutes is to provide treatment for so called psychopathic persons while protecting society from serious crimes.

According to Miller, these laws are really sentencing alternatives for persons involved in criminal conduct. If a continuum were constructed with the mental health system on one end and the criminal justice system on the other, programs for these special categories of offenders would fall somewhere in between.[21] Such statutes have been continually attacked on legal grounds, such as inadequate due process of law. Commitment of narcotics addicts and alcoholics, whose offenses have no victims, are criticized as being punitive without providing adequate treatment.[28]

Defective Delinquency

Defective delinquent laws are designed especially for those categories of offenders generally thought of as "psychopaths," that is, persons who are asocial, aggressive, or highly impulsive or who feel little or no guilt for their transgressions and generally are unable to empathize with others. Halleck tells us that since the psychopath is unconcerned with the feelings of others, his behavior is often antisocial. He is an activist who, in his efforts to mold the world to serve his own needs, often violates the law.[29]

The best-known "defective delinquent" statute was adopted in Maryland in 1951. This led to the opening of a now-famous (or notorious) treatment facility, Patuxant, designed as a model for the treatment of "psychopaths." Its therapeutic aim was to provide inmates with the internal controls needed to become useful citizens. Treatment focused on the rehabilitation of the entire individual, using a full range of psychotherapeutic techniques, including a therapeutic milieu and a structured system of rewards intended to develop desirable behavior.[30] The rationale for this program was that neither the penal system nor the state hospital was equipped to deal with the needs of the population. Since all its inmates were perceived to be dangerous to society, Patuxant was designed as a maximum security facility. The nature of this institution has been drastically altered by court challenges and by a reversal of the prevailing views toward the possibilities for psychiatric rehabilitation of the offender.

Sexual Offender Laws

Craig has reviewed legislation concerning sexual offenders in a report to the President's Commission on Law Enforcement and Administration of Justice. He found that approximately 30 states and the District of Columbia had enacted special legislation establishing commitment procedures for sex offenders, who, although they are not insane, are defined as being mentally abnormal.[31] (The Iowa and California Sexual Psychopath laws have been discussed in detail by Slovenko.[32]) Craig examined the background for these statutes, described how they operate, and offered critical evaluation of the statutes. Among other recommendations, he suggested that they be repealed.[31]

Sexual offender laws are frequently enacted following a particularly outrageous sex crime to protect society from such horrors.[33] Experts in the field, however, doubt that they serve the function for which they were designed, noting that offenders tend to be segregated as "sex offenders" based on their amenability to treatment rather than on their dangerousness to society.

Narcotics Addiction and Alcoholics

The U.S. Supreme Court has said little to the states about how to deal with drug addicts and alcoholics. Nonetheless, in *Robinson* v. *California* (1962), the supreme court made it clear that a person cannot be punished for being an addict.[34] Yet in *Powell* v. *Texas* (1968), the supreme court held that the alcoholic could be criminally prosecuted for public drunkenness.[35] In each case, the supreme court upheld the commitment law of these states.

The courts have not clarified procedure with regard to these special categories of offenders. In the future, Hicky expects the laws covering such offenders to be challenged based on the following criteria: (1) that due process in these proceedings is inadequate, (2) that treatment, which is the rationale of the proceedings, is not provided, (3) that the statutes are unconstitutionally vauge, and (4) that they permit action by the state exceeding its police powers.[36]

TRANSFER FROM CORRECTIONAL INSTITUTIONS

Another way an individual can enter the mental health system is by being transferred to a hospital from prison. The most frequent reason for such a transfer is that the prisoner becomes mentally ill while serving his sentence. Proper procedures for transfers are spelled out in *Schuster* v. *Herold* (1969)[37]

In 1941, while incarcerated in Clinton State Prison in New York, approaching the end of his sentence, Ray Schuster expressed his belief in the existence of "corruption" in the prison administration. Shortly thereafter, Schuster was found to be "paranoid" by a prison doctor. Solely on the strength of this finding, he was then transferred to Dannemora State Hospital for the Criminally Insane for an indefinite stay. In accordance with New York law at the time, Schuster was afforded no hearing on the issue of his sanity, was not permitted the assistance of counsel, was given no opportunity to call his own witnesses, and was given no advance notice of the transfer proceedings.

The Right to a Full Hearing

Schuster maintained that his transfer to Dannemora was in violation of his right to equal protection under the Fourteenth Amendment. His claim was grounded on the contention that he was not given the same procedural rights in contesting the transfer as are afforded civilians facing involuntary commitment. The court held for Schuster, stating that a substantial and unwarranted disparity existed between procedures available to civilians facing voluntary commitment and those available to Schuster, such that he was deprived of equal protection under the laws, within the meaning of the Fourteenth Amendment. The court cited *Baxtrom* v. *Herold* (1966) as the precedent that eliminated a dual system for criminal and noncriminal commitment procedures.[38] The Schuster court stated that "whether a man should be committed for mental illness has no relevance to the place where he happens to be at the time he becomes ill." They concluded that before a prisoner may be transferred to Dannemora, he is entitled to substantially the same procedures as are granted to civilians, including periodic review of the need for continued commitment in a mental institution and jury trial. Moreover, not only must Schuster be shown to suffer from a "mental disease," but also that mental disease must require care and treatment necessitating transfer.

Impact of Baxtrom

Following the Baxtrom decision, New York State officials rapidly released 967 patients confined at Dannemora and Matteawan hospitals for the criminally insane. After four years, a follow-up study by Steadman and Keveles showed that about half of the released patients were in civil mental hospitals, 27 percent were living in the community, and 14 percent were dead. Less than 3 percent had acted in a "dangerous way" and were in a correctional facility or a hospital for the "criminally insane."[39] A further follow-up study on those 27 persons who were returned to Dannemora and Matteawan established that they were different from those who did not return in that they had acted "in very violent ways."[40] In another article, Steadman concluded the Baxtrom patients as a group were not very dangerous.[41] The implications of the supreme court decision in Baxtrom and of the subsequent follow-up studies argue against both the rightfulness and the usefulness of special treatment for mentally ill criminal patients.

CONCLUSION

At this point, we can only speculate about the impact future court actions will have on mental patients committed under criminal law procedures. The inclination of the courts, however, is to lean in the direction of abolishing separate standards for involuntary commitments, relying on the equal protection clause of the U.S. Constitution. At the heart of the issue of involuntary commitment, which deprives persons of that liberty that is their constitutional right, lies the complex problem of the prediction of future dangerousness. Until science and the courts can come to some consensus on the nature and prediction of dangerous behavior, we will be forced to live with a degree of ambiguity regarding the treatment and release of committed patients.

REFERENCES

1. McGarry AL: Competency to stand trial and mental illness. DHEW Publication No. (ADM) 77-103, 1977
2. Howell TB (ed): State trials, London, 22:18009–26, p.307. Cited in group for the advancement of psychiatry: misuse of psychiatry in the criminal court: Competency to Stand Trial 8:89, 1974
3. Regina v. Dyson, Carrington and Payne 305:1 Lewin 64 (1931). Cited in group for the advancement of psychiatry: misuse of psychiatry in the criminal courts: Competency to Stand Trial 8:89, 1974
4. Walker W: Crime and Insanity in England. The Historical Perspective, vol. 1. The Edinburgh, Edinburgh University Press, 1968. Cited in group for the advancement of psychiatry: misuse of psychiatry in the criminal courts: Competency to Stand Trial 8:89, 1974
5. Dusky v. United States, 362, US 402 (1960)
6. Group for the advancement of psychiatry: misuse of psychiatry in the criminal courts: Competency to Stand Trial 8:89, 1974
7. Pate v. Robinson, 383, US 375 (1966)
8. Halpern AL: Use and misuse of psychiatry in competency examinations of criminal defendants. Psychiatr Ann 5:4, 1975
9. Jackson v. Indiana, 406 US 715 (1972)
10. New York Code criminal procedure: Article 730.50 (1) 1971
11. New York Code criminal procedure: Article 730.50 (3) 1971
12. Drendel v. United States, 403 F 2nd 55, 56 (5th Cir 1968)
13. Group for the advancement of psychiatry: misuse of psychiatry in the criminal courts: Competency to Stand Trial 8:862, 1974
14. Brooks A: Law Psychiatry and the Mental Health System. Boston, Little, Brown, 1974, p 112
15. The McNaughten Rule, 10 Cl & F 200, 8 Eng Rep 718 (HL 1843)
16. Fersch EA: Psychology and psychiatry in courts and corrections: New York, Wiley 1980, pp 94–133
17. Durham v. United States, 214 F 2nd 862 (DC 1954)
18. Fersch EA: Courts and Corrections, p 98
19. Fersch, Courts and Corrections, p 98
20. McDonald v. United States, 312 F 2nd 847 (DC Cir 1962)
21. Miller FW, Davidson RO, Dix GE, et al: The Mental Health Process: Mineola, NY Foundation Press, 1976, pp 161–162, 679–756
22. Frederick CJ: An overview of dangerousness: its complexities and consequences, in Dangerous Behavior: A problem in Law and Mental Health. DHEW No. (ADM) 78-563. 1978, pp 3–19
23. Shah SA: Dangerousness and mental illness: some conceptual, prediction and policy dilemas, in Dangerous Behavior: A Problem in Law and Mental Health. DHEW No. (ADM) 78-563. 1978, pp 153–191
24. Schwitzgebel RK: Legal and social aspects of the concept of dangerousness, in Dangerous Behavior: A Problem in Law and Mental Health. DHEW No. (ADM) 78-563. 1978, p 83–94
25. Lessard v. Schmidt, 349, F Supp 1978 (ED Wis., 1972)
26. Brooks A: Law Psychiatry and the Mental Health System. Boston, Little, Brown, 1974 p 680–682
27. Steadman H: Employing predictions of dangerous behavior: policy vs fact, in Dangerous Behavior: A Problem in Law and Mental Health. DHEW No. (ADM) 78-563. 1978 pp 133–136
28. Hicky L, Rubin S: Civil Commitment of Special Categories of Offenders. DHEW No (ADM) 74-15, 1973
29. Halleck S: Psychopathy, freedom and criminal behavior. Bull Menninger Clin 30 127–140, 1966
30. Director of Patuxant Institution v. Daniels, Circuit Ct. for Prince Georges. Maryland Co (1966)
31. Craig R: Sexual psychopath legislation. Report submitted to President's Commission on Law Enforcement and Administration of Justice, Washington DC, 1967, p 1
32. Slovenko R: Sexual Behavior and the Law. Springfield, Ill, Charles C. Thomas, 1965
33. Hicky L, Rubin S: Civil Commitment, p 11
34. Robinson v. California, 370 US 660, 82 Supt Ct 1415 (1962)
35. Powell v. Texas, 392, US 514, 88 Sup Ct 2145 (1968)
36. Hicky L, Rubin S: Civil Commitment, pp 11
37. United States ex rel. Schuster v. Harold, 410 F 2nd 1071 (2d Cir 1969)
38. Baxtrom v. Harold, 383, US 107 86, Sup Ct 760 15 L Ed 2d 620, (1966)
39. Steadman H, Keveles G: The community adjustment and criminal activity of the Baxtrom patients: 1966–1970. Am J Psychiatry 129:304–311, 1972
40. Steadman H: Follow-up on Baxtrom patients returned to hospitals for the criminally insane. Am J Psychiatry 130:317–319, 1973
41. Steadman H: Implications from the Baxtrom experience, Bull Am Acad Psychiatry and the Law. 189:191, 1973

Index

a
2 b
3 c
4 d
5 e
6 f
7 g
8 h
9 i
8 0 j